ANNUAL PROGRESS IN CHILD PSYCHIATRY AND CHILD DEVELOPMENT 1984

Edited by

STELLA CHESS, M.D.

Professor of Child Psychiatry
New York University Medical Center

and

ALEXANDER THOMAS, M.D.

Professor of Psychiatry
New York University Medical Center

BRUNNER/MAZEL, *Publishers* • New York

Library of Congress Card No. 68-23452

ISBN 0-87630-375-0

ISSN 0066-4030

MANUFACTURED IN THE UNITED STATES OF AMERICA

CONTENTS

ANNUAL PROGRESS IN CHILD PSYCHIATRY AND CHILD DEVELOPMENT 1984

Part I
INFANCY STUDIES

A major development in infancy studies in recent decades has been the dramatic demonstration of the competency of the young infant and even the neonate—in neuro-behavioral organization, in perceptual competence, in the ability to learn, in active social communication with caretakers, and in the selective responsiveness to environmental stimuli and demands. Thus, the first volume of this Annual Progress series in 1968 highlighted the report of the seminal work of Robert Fantz and his associates on the basic perceptual-cognitive development of young infants.

These complex competencies of the neonate and young infant indicate that the human infant is born with a "biological preprogramming" which provides the basis for the rapid development of all kinds of behavioral skills in the first year of life. However, as Stratton points out in his article "Biological Preprogramming of Infant Behavior," "it is not obvious that this recognition [of biological influences] has been of great practical value to those who care for young children." (We would make an exception in the value of the findings of temperamental individuality and their implications for child-care practices.) Stratton examines the various reasons for this lack of progress—the concentration on unproductive issues, the use of models which are unsuited for studies of human infants, the attempts to focus on simplistic explanations such as bonding and imprinting, and the insufficient attention paid to environmental influence. Stratton states this last issue clearly in his assertion that it is "a mistake to expect genetic influence to be revealed through behaviors which follow a strict program regardless of the environment . . . this may work for ants and embryos, but not for human infants."

Goldberg reviews the issue of "Parent-Infant Bonding: Another Look" by asking whether, in view of the large numbers of critical reviews and negative studies in the field, with a high degree of consensus among previous reviewers (see the 1982 and 1983 volumes of the Annual Progress), there is "any reason to examine this literature again." Her answer

3

is in the affirmative because of her judgment that the research work in this area, whether in support or in criticism of the bonding concept, has been flawed by a number of methodological details. She proceeds to document this thesis systematically and in detail. Considering the important theoretical and practical implications of the bonding concept, her review is valuable. Her conclusion actually is in line with those of most previous reviewers. The concept of bonding and the work it stimulated played an important role in bringing about needed changes in hospital practice surrounding birth. On the other hand, it created an expectation on the part of many parents that if they do not have this experience they have somehow failed and will never be fine parents. But as Goldberg and others emphasize, the parent-infant relationship is a complex system whose "success or failure does not hinge on a few brief moments in time. It would be irresponsible for us professionals to encourage this incorrect and extreme view."

In recent years, increasing attention has been paid in the developmental literature to "second-order" or indirect influence, that is, the influence that a third person may have on the interaction between the infant and caretaker, or for that matter on any dyadic interaction. Of special interest is the process of social referencing, in which an individual utilizes another's interpretation when appraising a person or situation. This phenomenon has been well identified in older children and adults, but Feinman and Lewis now report a study in which social referencing was manifest in the second half of the first year of life. Here, again, is further evidence of substantial social and cognitive skills in infancy, skills which are prerequisites for the development of social referencing. The relationship to the child's temperamental characteristics is also of interest.

PART I: INFANCY STUDIES

1

Biological Preprogramming of Infant Behavior

Peter Stratton

Department of Psychology, University of Leeds, England

OVERVIEW

ALTHOUGH there is at present a widespread acceptance of biological influence on infant behavior, this has rarely been translated into insights which could be of value to the practitioner. It is argued that this is because the models of genetic action used by developmental psychologists have been derived from situations which cannot represent the adaptability of the human infant or the variability of his/her environment. In the case of the newborn we can now achieve a realistic understanding of some of the ways that biological preprogramming facilitates adaptation, and the specific cases of feeding and the first stage of attachment are discussed. From these examples general principles are drawn to provide a basis for appreciating the ways that genetic influence is likely to be manifested during infancy.

LIMITATIONS OF THE BIOLOGY OF INFANCY

The extent to which biological influences are recognized within developmental psychology undergoes periodic oscillations, and at present we seem to be in a phase of acceptance in which genetic influences on behavior are widely perceived. However, it is not obvious that this rec-

---

Reprinted with permission from the *Journal of Child Psychology and Psychiatry*, 1983, Vol. 24, No. 2, 301-309. Copyright 1983 by the Association for Child Psychology and Psychiatry.

ognition has been of great practical value to those who care for young children. Part of the reason for this is that major efforts have been dissipated on unproductive questions. The chief example is, of course, the attempt to put a precise figure on the proportion of the variation in intelligence test scores which can be attributed to genetic variation within certain populations. It is difficult to imagine any practical utility of an answer to this question, whatever value is finally agreed (Levy, 1978), and I would suggest that the major ethical issue relates not so much to the possible social or political implications of particular answers as to the waste of resources which could have been directed to more fruitful issues.

Although the biometrical approach is relatively easy to apply to humans, it does have limitations (Fulker, 1981) which severely restrict its usefulness in explanations of individual behavior [see Fuller and Thompson (1978) for a discussion of compositionist vs. analytic approaches to individual differences]. Attempts to explain the mechanisms of genetic influence on human behavior have been made in a number of recent texts. Nash (1978) provides a review of development from a biological perspective in which all aspects of human functioning are found to have, at least potentially, biological determinants. Rather more restricted claims have been made particularly by students of social development. Bowlby (1980) continues to see attachment as an instinctive behavior, while Bower (1979) argues that "humans are born with specific social behaviors that have the characteristics of reaction-specific energy" (p. 309). Cairns (1979) also believes that the psychobiological orientation provides the basis for our present understanding of social development. However, he regards it as providing the foundation for a theory rather than a theory itself, and it is quite clear that the proponents of biological influence have had much greater success in showing the plausibility of genetic determination of human behavior than in identifying useful instances (Scarr-Salapatek, 1976). As an example, in his review of the highly specific and intricately organized connections between different parts of the nervous system, Nash (1978) concluded that "it is difficult to avoid the assumption that the precision with which the organism is wired up has strong influences on behavior" (p. 114). While agreeing, one must also note that it seems to be equally difficult to find specific instances of preprogrammed behavior. It may be for this reason that the major recent survey of infancy (Osofsky, 1979) has no serious discussion of genetic influences on normal behavior.

Sources of the Limitation

The lack of compelling examples of biological preprogramming in human infants is largely attributable to the use of models which have been derived from situations of relatively pure biological influence. The earlier biologically oriented theories of human development (Gesell, 1945; Werner, 1948) derived their principles by analogy with the physical growth of the embryo so that the only role of the environment was to allow or constrain genetic expression. More recent theorists such as those quoted above have drawn on the findings by ethologists of examples of genetically controlled behavior in other species, but are still arguing by analogy. True ethological observation depends on recording repeated instances of the same behavior in reliable association with other events, both intra and extra-organismic. Once the behavior has been identified and described, its significance is determined in terms of its contribution to evolutionary fitness. One of the few examples of a productive application of this method is Anderson's (1972) account of the attachment behaviors shown by 18-month-old infants out of doors. A number of consistent patterns were identified, particularly in terms of the ways in which the acceptable degree of separation from the mother varied according to circumstances. More typically, a large observational study of children in preschool (McGrew, 1972) found few instances of stereotyped behavior sequences, and was not able to interpret the significance of the recorded behaviors in evolutionary terms.

Ethological methods were taken up with enthusiasm in the 1960s and were widely believed to be particularly suitable for infants (Hutt and Hutt, 1970). With hindsight it is not too difficult to see why they have failed to live up to these expectations. The core phenomenon for the ethologist is the Fixed Action Pattern (FAP): a stereotyped sequence of behavior, independent from external control, spontaneous, and unmodifiable through learning (Moltz, 1965). FAPs will occur when an environmental demand operates consistently for long enough for a complex sequence of genetically determined behaviors to become established. The high degree of human adaptability ensures that the environment provided by parents will be variable, so we should not expect to find many instances in which FAPs would confer an advantage on the human infant.

Our dilemma, then, is that models of biological preprogramming which are taken from situations in which the genetic influence is identifiable are not very productive when applied to the human infant. Principles derived from the functioning of organisms of limited adaptability (e.g. ants or human embryos) in very stable environments are just as limited in accounting for the behavior of human infants as are principles of learning developed in contexts which have carefully excluded any possibility of provoking biologically adaptive modes of response. More sophisticated models of biological action have been available for a long time (e.g. Lehrman, 1953), but have not led to the discovery of examples of genetic determination of children's behavior. Our solution, I believe, lies in the advances which have been achieved recently in understanding the adaptive behavior of the human newborn. Although our understanding of the rest of infancy has suffered through the concentration of research during the last two decades on the neonatal period, the result has been a reasonably clear understanding of the complex interplay of biological and environmental factors at the beginning of infancy. Neonatal adaptation can now serve as a model through which the workings of biological influence in later infancy may be identified and understood.

PREPROGRAMMING OF NEWBORN BEHAVIOR

A genetic specification defines the phenotype which will result from interactions with particular kinds of environment, so the occurrence of more viable phenotypes can only be assured in the environment for which the genetic structure has evolved. In this sense, while the gene pool is an outcome of the evolutionary history of the species, it can also be viewed as a prediction that certain environmental features will be available for interaction with the genes to produce desirable outcomes in the phenotype. Genetic preprogramming of behavior will, therefore, become established through natural selection only when it allows more effective adaptation to an environmental feature which is important for fitness and which has remained stable over many generations. It will be revealed most clearly in the presence of such environmental features, whereas in interaction with novel environments, genes will produce effects which cannot be meaningfully related to the history of viability of the species. If we are to look for evidence of genetic preprogramming in the newborn, then breast feeding and contact with the mother appear to be significant functions which have been stable in something like their present form for a considerable time.

Feeding

The most important requirement for the newborn is to grow. Accordingly, Rovee-Collier and Lipsitt (1982) propose that any neonatal characteristic must be interpreted in terms of its implications for maximizing caloric intake and minimizing caloric expenditure. Many implications follow from this apparently simple principle. Because of physical constraints on the volume of milk that can be ingested at one time, the newborn must be able to elicit food regularly and must be able to respond appropriately when food is offered. Babies are, therefore, equipped with behaviors which range from very specific, such as the rooting reflex and precisely specified mechanisms of sucking (Crook, 1979), through those which provoke useful responses from the environment (crying, for example) to more general tendencies to control the timing and quantity of feeds (Wright and Crow, 1982).

The specificity of sucking mechanisms is possible because many characteristics of the lactating breast have remained constant between individuals and over a considerable period of time. Other aspects of feeding do not, however, allow such precise prediction. It seems that babies need to make anticipatory adaptations once feeding is imminent, but there is no reliable signal for this on which a genetic preprogramming could capitalize. However, the newborn does learn very quickly [usually within the first 6–10 feeds, according to Call (1964)] that being held in the particular posture that his/her mother characteristically uses signals that a feed is about to be offered. Such rapid learning could be "prepared" in the sense of a genetically determined readiness to acquire certain associations, as described by Seligman (1970), but rapid learning is so common at this age (Oppenheim, 1981) that Rovee-Collier and Lipsitt (1982) have argued for a more general tendency. The young infant must possess a limited repertoire of the responses most likely to have greatest adaptive value, and perceptual and other tendencies which maximize the probability that the response will come to be produced in the appropriate context.

Some of the most reliable consistency in the newborn's environment comes from adult behavior. Although costly in terms of energy, crying seems to be a highly efficient way of eliminating discomfort because it reliably elicits caretaker intervention. As Wolff (1969) has shown, adults are sensitive to different kinds of cry and find some patterns particularly difficult to ignore. The fact that this tendency is widespread across our species (there is no firm evidence on how widespread) should not lead us to posit a biologically preprogrammed tendency in the human adult. An intriguing possibility is that our sensitivity to the meaning of particular cries derives from repeated experiences in our own infancy in which producing (and therefore hearing) that crying pattern was reliably associated with particular somatic sensations. In this analysis the salience which certain newborn behaviors like crying, but possibly including others such as eye contact or smiling, have for adults derives from classical conditioning in infancy. Such cycles, in which an early preprogrammed behavior sets up long-term consequences which constrain the behavior of adult caretakers, may be a source of the environmental stability and predictability which is itself essential before genetic control can be of adaptive value.

This very restricted consideration of biological preprogramming of feeding in early infancy indicates that genetic prediction can be pointed towards many different forms of environmental stability. A consideration of mother-infant contact will help to make the principles more explicit.

Attachment

The ability of the human infant to develop strong emotional ties with adults within a few months of birth is an impressive performance which seems difficult to account for within our normal explanatory frameworks. Biologically oriented theorists have attempted to account for human attachment as a form of imprinting (e.g. Morris, 1967; Nash, 1978), but it is now apparent that this has added little to our understanding. The problem is not only, as Slukin (1974) discovered, that if the definition of imprinting is made broad enough to encompass the behavior of the human infant, it can no longer be assumed to carry the wider implications which make the term so powerful. Even more damaging is the fact that, since there is as yet no agreement on how imprinting occurs [Hess (1973) discusses several theories], labeling human socialization as an example of imprinting tells us nothing about its origins.

As Schaffer (1971) described, the first stage of attachment requires the infant to be attracted to other human beings. We now know that the young infant's perceptual and cognitive systems are specified at various levels in ways which maximize certain kinds of contact. At a very basic level, we know that a newborn's eyes have a relatively fixed focus at about 19 cm (Haynes *et al.*, 1965), which is approximately the distance to the mother's eyes when the baby is breast feeding, and eye contact is common in this situation. At a more general level, since Fantz (1961) showed that infants look longer at faces than at other stimuli, an enormous amount of research has been undertaken to discover what determines where a baby looks. From a very elegant analysis Haith (1980) rejects any notions of preference for particular stimuli and concludes that there is one basic rule: to maximize neural firing rate. But firing rate will be maximized when the image on the fovea is in focus, has multiple light-dark boundaries and is in motion. In other words, in the natural situation a baby is most likely to look at a face. The advance achieved by 20 years of careful research is in identifying the simple rule which combines with the structural characteristics of the newborn's visual system, and predictable features of the newborn's environment, to ensure the essential outcome.

A similar process can be seen at a rather higher level in the notion of contingency. Infants seem to be particularly sensitive to events which are contingent on their own behavior (Watson and Ramey, 1972). Given the motor incompetence of the human infant, most such contingencies will be associated with the responses of care-giving adults, so again we have a simple principle which exploits an inevitable characteristic of the normal caretaking environment to produce wide-ranging effects.

PRINCIPLES OF GENETIC INFLUENCE

The selective examples given above will serve to illustrate the ways genetic predisposition of behavior can be expected to operate.

1. Genetic preprogramming will capitalize on environmental consistency to achieve essential results with the simplest possible rules. For human infants much of the environmental consistency will be provided by adult caretakers.

2. To achieve a crucial effect in a variable environment, a number of independent mechanisms will converge. The discussion of attachment above provides just a few of the possible examples, and the generality and fail-safe nature of neonatal adaptation are discussed in more detail by Stratton (1982a). It is now clear that the search for a single mechanism of attachment, justified by a crude wielding of Occam's razor, is as misguided as the supposition that disruption of one mechanism of bonding necessarily causes permanent psychological damage. The more general principle, that an organism may have available a number of different developmental routes through which the same behavioral end-product may be achieved, is discussed by Bateson (1976).

3. Biologically preprogrammed behaviors are specified in such a way as to be elicited in appropriate environmental settings. It is apparent in recent accounts of early social behavior, both for newborns (Papoušek and Papoušek, 1982) and later (Dunn, 1981; Heard, 1981), that the consistency seen in the ontogenetic growth of attachment depends on the availability of the appropriate environmental support. It is, therefore, a mistake to expect genetic influence to be revealed through behaviors which follow a strict program regardless of the environment. This will only occur when the probability of the necessary environmental feature being present is so high that behaviors can be run off 'blind' with a high expectation of success. As already stated, this may work for ants and embryos, but not for human infants.

4. The obverse of the above principle is captured in Nash's (1978) principle of developmental efficiency. Individual development will proceed most efficiently if the environment fosters the inherent tendencies of the individual rather than demanding inappropriate adaptations. At the general level this means that biological tendencies are most likely to be useful (and interpretable) in the situation for which they have evolved. As a very concrete example, Prechtl (1965) describes how the Moro reflex seems pointless and incomprehensible in the usual test situation, but the adaptive utility becomes obvious if it is elicited while the baby is clinging to its mother. A child may, therefore, display biologically preprogrammed behavior while watching television or bottle feeding, but the nature and significance of the behavior may be difficult to identify.

5. A more general implication of Nash's principle concerns individual differences. We have evidence of genetic determination of temperamental characteristics of infants (Buss and Plomin, 1975; Torgersen and Kringlen, 1978), and the clinical findings of Thomas *et al.* (1968) support the proposal that development is stressful unless the environment is adapted to the needs of the individual child. From a comprehensive review of newborn individuality, Stratton (1982b) concluded that the longer-term significance of differences between babies at birth derived from their tendency to elicit differential treatment from the caregiver. This is an early example of the many instances in which the expression of genetic tendencies of the infant influences susceptible adults to provide an appropriate environment. In view of the complexity of these transactions, it would clearly be a mistake to demand linear relationships between characteristics of the individual at infancy and maturity.

6. Finally, once capacities have become established they may come to serve other purposes. The newborn's capacity for rapid learning may

have arisen entirely from the need to identify sources of food and to suppress wasteful responses to irrelevant environmental features, but the high level of cognitive competence which resulted is now intrinsic to the infant's social and information processing functions. An example which may have major significance for infancy is provided by contingencies. Response-contingent stimulation produces positive responses which parents find rewarding (Watson and Ramey, 1972), so infants may train their caregivers to increase the supply. This is important because the role of contingencies is no longer restricted to identifying conspecific adults. By 12 weeks, infants in more responsive environments have been found to be more efficient in the acquisition of new schemata (Lewis and Goldberg, 1969), while Finkelstein and Ramey (1977) found that exposure to response-contingent stimulation increased subsequent learning of 4½ to 9-month-olds.

CONCLUSION

The general implications which can be derived from this consideration of biological preprogramming in early infancy should dispel any expectations of discovering fixed action patterns later in life. However, the two-year-old is no less biological than the newborn: he/she merely has much greater variability in past history and present environment. Models derived from situations of simpler biological influence have not served us very well in understanding the infant, and in particular, the attempt to call human bonding "imprinting" neither carried useful implications nor helped our understanding of how it comes about. In fact, I would suggest that the situation could now be reversed. As our understanding of human bonding becomes more complete it provides a general explanatory framework within which imprinting can be seen as a special case arising when a single environmental feature is present with such predictability that a single, temporally constrained mechanism can guarantee success.

The most important lesson to be drawn from this review is that a realistic appreciation of the extent and nature of biological preprogramming in infancy enhances rather than diminishes our awareness of the significance of the environment. In demonstrating that it is the visual system which undergoes the most extensive maturational development in early infancy, Bronson (1982) concluded that for precisely this reason, appropriate visual stimulation is most important at this stage. More generally, Bowlby (1969) concluded that "heavily biased to develop in certain directions though behavioral equipment usually is, it does not develop so unless the infant animal is being cared for in the species' environment of evolutionary adaptedness" (p. 336).

Perhaps the days of "heredity versus environment" are at last over. We must now recognize that we can only properly evaluate the environments which we impose on our children when we take account of their biological predispositions, and that every increment in our awareness of biological influence sharpens our appreciation of the crucial role of the environment.

REFERENCES

Anderson, J. W. (1972). Attachment behaviour out of doors. In *Ethological Studies of Child Behaviour*. (Edited by Blurton Jones, N. G.), pp. 199–215. Cambridge University Press, Cambridge.

Bateson, P. P. G. (1976). Rules and reciprocity in behavioural development. In *Growing Pains in Ethology*. (Edited by Bateson, P. P. G. and Hinde, R. A.), pp. 401–421. Cambridge University Press, Cambridge.

Bower, T. G. R. (1979). *Human Development*. W. H. Freeman, San Francisco.

Bowlby, J. (1969). *Attachment and Loss*, Vol. I. *Attachment*. Hogarth, London.

Bowlby, J. (1980). *Attachment and Loss*. Vol. III. *Loss, Sadness and Depression*. Hogarth, London.

Bronson, G. W. (1982). Structure, status and characteristics of the nervous system at birth. In *Psychobiology of the Human Newborn* (Edited by Stratton, P. M.), pp. 99–118. Wiley, Chichester.

Buss, A. H. and Plomin, R. (1975). *A Temperament Theory of Personality Development*. Wiley, New York.

Cairns, R. B. (1979). *Social Development*. W. H. Freeman, San Francisco.

Call, J. D. (1964). Newborn approach behavior and early ego development. *Int. J. Psycho-Analysis* **45**, 286–294.

Crook, C. K. (1979). The organisation and control of infant sucking. In *Advances in Child Development and Behaviour* (Edited by Reese, H. W. and Lipsitt, L. P.), Vol. 14, pp. 209–252. Academic Press, London.

Dunn, J. (1981). Maturation and early social development. In *Maturation and Development: Biological and Psychological Perspectives* (Edited by Connolly, K. J. and Prechtl, H. F. R.), pp. 274–286. Heinemann, London.

Fantz, R. L. (1961). The origin of form perception. *Scient. Am.* **204**, 66–72.

Finkelstein, N. N. and Ramey, C. T. (1977). Learning to control the environment in infancy. *Child Dev.* **48**, 806–819.

Fulker, D. W. (1981). Genetics and behavioural development. In *Maturation and Development: Biological and Psychological Perspectives* (Edited by Connolly, K. J. and Prechtl, H. F. R.), pp. 32–49. Heinemann, London.

Fuller, J. L. and Thompson, W. R. (1978). *Foundations of Behaviour Genetics*. C. V. Mosby, St. Louis.

Gesell, A. (1945). *The Embryology of Behaviour*. Harper, New York.

Haith, M. M. (1980). *Rules that Babies Look By*. Lawrence Erlbaum, Hillsdale.

Haynes, H., White, B. L. and Held, R. (1965). Visual accommodation in human infants. *Science, N.Y.* **148**, 528–530.

Heard, D. H. (1981). The relevance of attachment theory to child psychiatric practice. *J. Child Psychol. Psychiat.* **22**, 89–96.

Hess, E. H. (1973). *Imprinting.* Van Nostrand Reinhold, New York.

Hutt, S. J. and Hutt, C. (1970). *Direct Observation and Measurement of Behavior.* C. C. Thomas, Springfield, Illinois.

Lehrman, D. S. (1953). A critique of Konrad Lorenz's theory of instinctive behavior. *Q. Rev. Biol.* **28**, 337–363.

Levy, P. (1978). The nature-nurture show. *Bull. Br. psychol. Soc.* **31**, 113–114.

Lewis, M. and Goldberg, S. (1969). Perceptual-cognitive development in infancy: a generalised expectancy model as a function of the mother-infant interaction. *Merrill-Palmer Q.* **15**, 81–100.

McGrew, W. C. (1972). *An Ethological Study of Children's Behaviour.* Academic Press, London.

Moltz, H. (1965). Contemporary instinct theory and the fixed action pattern. *Psychol. Rev.* **72**, 22–47.

Morris, D. (1967). *The Naked Ape.* Cape, London.

Nash, J. (1978). *Developmental Psychology* (2nd edition). Prentice-Hall, New Jersey.

Oppenheim, R. W. (1981). Ontogenetic adaptations and retrogressive processes in the development of the nervous system and behaviour: a neuroembryological perspective. In *Maturation and Development: Biological and Psychological Perspectives* (Edited by Connolly, K. J. and Prechtl, H. F. R.), pp. 73–109. Heinemann, London.

Osofsky, J. D. (1979). *Handbook of Infant Development.* Wiley, New York.

Papoušek, H. and Papoušek, M. (1982). Integration into the social world: survey of research. In *Psychobiology of the Human Newborn* (Edited by Stratton, P. M.), pp. 367–390. Wiley, Chichester.

Prechtl, H. F. R. (1965). Problems of behavioural studies in the newborn infant. In *Advances in the Study of Behaviour* (Edited by Lehrman, D. S., Hinde, R. A. and Shaw, E.), Vol. I, pp. 75–96. Academic Press, London.

Rovee-Collier, C. K. and Lipsitt, L. P. (1982). Learning, adaptation and memory in the newborn. In *Psychobiology of the Human Newborn* (Edited by Stratton, P. M.), pp. 147–190. Wiley, Chichester.

Scarr-Salapatek, S. (1976). Genetic determinants of infant development: an overstated case. In *Developmental Psychobiology* (Edited by Lipsitt, L. P.), pp. 55–79. Lawrence Erlbaum, Hillsdale.

Schaffer, H. R. (1971). *The Growth of Sociability.* Penguin Books, Middlesex.

Seligman, M. E. P. (1970). On the generality of the laws of learning. *Psychol. Rev.* **77**, 406–418.

Slukin, W. (1974). Imprinting reconsidered. *Bull. Br. psychol. Soc.* **27**, 447–451.

Stratton, P. M. (1982a). Emerging themes of neonatal psychobiology. In *Psychobiology of the Human Newborn* (Edited by Stratton, P. M.), pp. 391–414. Wiley, Chichester.

Stratton, P. M. (1982b). Newborn individuality. In *Psychobiology of the Human Newborn* (Edited by Stratton, P. M.), pp. 221–261. Wiley, Chichester.

Thomas, A., Chess, S. and Birch, H. (1968). *Temperament and Behavior Disorders in Children.* New York University Press, New York.

Torgersen, A. M. and Kringlen, E. (1978). Genetic aspects of temperamental differences in infants. *J. Am. Acad. Child Psychiat.* **17**, 433–444.

Watson, J. S. and Ramey, C. T. (1972). Reactions to response—contingent stimulation in early infancy. *Merrill-Palmer Q.* **18**, 220–227.

Werner, H. (1948). *Comparative Psychology of Mental Development.* Follett, Chicago.

Wolff, P. (1969). The natural history of crying and other vocalisations in early infancy. In *Determinants of Infant Behaviour* (Edited by Foss, B. M.), Vol. IV, pp. 81–109. Methuen, London.

Wright, P. and Crow, R. (1982). Nutrition and feeding. In *Psychobiology of the Human Newborn* (Edited by Stratton, P. M.), pp. 339–364. Wiley, Chichester.

PART I: INFANCY STUDIES

2

Parent-Infant Bonding: Another Look

Susan Goldberg

Hospital for Sick Children, Toronto

While previous reviewers of the literature on early parent-infant con-
tacts assume existing experiments are adequate tests of the sensitive
period hypothesis, this review asserts that the hypothesis has not been
tested on three counts: (1) there are no systematic studies of initial
mother-infant contacts, (2) the majority of the studies confound timing
and amount of contact, and (3) failure to consider underlying mech-
anisms resulted in the omission of designs and dependent measures
that could address the appropriate questions.

Parents' emotional ties to their children undergo many changes over
an extended period of time, beginning with the decision to have a child
and continuing through that part of their respective life spans that parents and children share. In recent years considerable emphasis has been
given to changes occurring shortly after birth, and the term "bonding"
as introduced by Klaus & Kennell (1976) has come to refer to unique
developmental changes thought to occur at this time and to have a lasting
effect on subsequent parent-child relationships and child development.
Many research studies have been devoted to demonstrating the presence
or absence of a special limited time period when these events occur and
the later effects of different experiences during this "sensitive" period.
Reviews and critiques of this literature have also proliferated (Campbell
& Taylor, 1980; Chess & Thomas, 1982; Harmon, 1981; Klaus & Kennell, 1982; Lamb & Hwang, 1982; Leiderman, 1982; Svejda, Pannabecker, & Emde, 1982; Vietze & O'Connor, 1981), and with the exception

Reprinted with permission from *Child Development*, 1983, Vol. 54, 1355–1382. Copyright
1983 by the Society for Research in Child Development, Inc.

of Klaus & Kennell (1982) most of the reviewers conclude that the evidence does not support the existence of a sensitive period for parent-infant bonding.

In the face of such a high degree of consensus among previous reviewers, is there any reason to examine this literature yet again? While previous reviews have generally taken the position that the existing research has indeed addressed the question of a sensitive period (though much of it is rightly criticized as methodologically flawed), I will take the position that, on at least three counts, the existence of a sensitive period is "not proven" (or disproven) because the relevant experiments have not been done: (1) there are few systematic studies on the actual initiation of maternal behavior, and none relate these experiences to subsequent maternal behavior; (2) the majority of studies confound the timing of early parent-infant contact with the amount of contact experience; and (3) the research has not considered mechanisms that could underlie the phenomenon being studied. While it might be argued that the failure to find long-term effects obviates the need to study explanatory mechanisms, hypotheses about mechanisms direct study designs and choice of outcome variables. The lack of hypothesis testing in existing studies means that important outcome variables have not been assessed and that study designs have often been inappropriate for the question they purport to ask.

Accordingly, the first part of this review considers observation of initial mother-infant contacts; the second part reviews in detail the few studies capable of providing evidence on the role that timing of initial contacts plays in establishing and/or maintaining the mother-infant relationship. A third section considers the remaining studies, those that investigated effects of contact irrespective of timing. Since they cannot inform us about sensitive periods and comprehensive reviews have been provided by others, these studies are not discussed in detail. The fourth section considers possibilities for future research that consider processes affecting the transition from pregnancy to parenthood. In the final section, practical implications of our current state of knowledge are discussed.

Since the bulk of the studies have been carried out with mothers, this paper will focus on maternal behavior, although studies of fathers will be considered in the fourth section. The discussion will be further restricted primarily to studies of parents with their full-term infants. Although some of the earliest studies were done with infants born prematurely, birth in this case occurs at a different point in mothers' physiological and psychological preparation for motherhood, and many other factors complicate their subsequent experience besides opportunities for contact. Studies of this group are therefore of limited value in understanding initiation of normal parental behavior. The primary question to be addressed in the next section is whether in the case of normal full-term births there is a sensitive period for mother-infant bonding.

INITIATION OF MATERNAL BEHAVIOR

Although Klaus & Kennell (1982) now use the term "bonding" to refer to the long-term process of the parents' developing emotional ties to the child in which the events of the sensitive period are but one ingredient, the more general usage has been to restrict the construct of bonding specifically to rapid irreversible changes in the parents' relationship to the infant that occur in a limited time period after birth (e.g., Campbell & Taylor, 1980; Svejda et al., 1982; Vietze & O'Connor, 1981). Phrased in this latter form, the construct suggests two separate testable propositions: (1) there are systematic changes in maternal responses to infants following birth such that mothers experience a period of peak responsiveness some time in the first few hours after birth, and (2) experiences during these first few hours have lasting effects on subsequent maternal behavior. This section focuses on the first of these propositions. The second will be taken up in the following section.

To ascertain whether maternal responsiveness to infants peaks within the first few hours after birth, the appropriate strategy is to observe initial mother-infant contacts in dyads meeting at different times after the delivery. Although there are numerous descriptions of initial mother-infant interactions (e.g., Carek & Capelli, 1981; Newton & Newton, 1962), few studies have employed the strategy of comparing these interactions in groups of mothers experiencing the first exposure to their infant at different times. Many investigators have manipulated the timing of first contacts, but these initial interactions have either not been observed or not been subjected to analysis.[1] One study that did make such comparisons (Klaus, Kennell, Plumb, & Zuelke, 1970) relied on a naturally occurring experiment—preterm versus full-term birth. However, because these groups differ in so many other respects, the comparisons cannot shed much light on possible changes in maternal responsiveness to infants after delivery under normal conditions.

One of the more striking descriptions of delivery room behavior comes from a preliminary report of a larger British study (Packer & Rosenblatt,

---

[1] In many studies this was deliberately not done because the investigators felt that privacy was essential for the most rewarding and beneficial initial contacts.

1979). In these primarily descriptive data, the actual amount of mother-infant interaction in the delivery room was quite low. As many as 50% of the mothers did not touch or stroke their babies in the first 20 min., and 18% did not look at their infants, while 50% of the mothers looked at the baby for less than 5 min. However, the conditions under which these early contacts occurred were less than supportive. The authors report their impression that the infant was offered to the mother at times that were convenient for the delivery room staff (e.g., during episiotomy repair to distract her from discomfort) rather than at a time that would be convenient or comfortable for the mother. The modal pattern in this group was for the mother to hold the baby while conversing with the father, looking occasionally at the infant as she made reference to him or her.

A U.S. study by Taylor, Taylor, Campbell, Maloni, and Dickey (Note 1), which meticulously recorded what mothers did when offered their babies in the delivery room, also showed considerable individual variation in mothers' enthusiasm for interacting with their infants. For example, only 35 of 65 mothers touched the infant, and only 13 of the 65 actually held the baby. Additionally, Craig, Tyson, Sampson, and Lasky (1982) and de Chateau and his colleagues (see de Chateau, 1980) found that a small number of mothers refused contacts offered in the delivery room. These reports go a long way toward dispelling the notion that delivery room mother-infant contacts are necessarily characterized by intimacy or euphoria, an idea implicit in much of the popular literature on the subject. They also indicate large individual differences in experiences of mothers and babies during delivery room contacts. This raises the question of what it means to say a group of mothers experienced "early contact" when only half of them touched the baby when given the opportunity and less than one-quarter held their infants (as in Taylor et al., Note 1). If the hours after birth have a special impact on later mother-child relationships, these individual differences should have measurable consequences.

Gaulin-Kremer, Shaw, and Thoman (Note 2) observed the first feeding for 28 mother-infant pairs. In this study, mothers had been able to see and touch their swaddled baby in the delivery room and had had a brief (2–3 min) contact when mother and baby were moved to the maternity floor (about 6 hours after delivery), but the first prolonged contact, depending on the nursery feeding schedule, occurred 10–25 hours after delivery. Correlations between the duration of the separation interval and maternal behavior variables (ranging in magnitude from .39 to .50) revealed that the sooner after birth the first prolonged contact occurred, the more the mother caressed, talked to, and held her baby before beginning the actual feeding. There were no systematic changes in infant behavior that accounted for this finding. Although these data do not emanate from the very first contact, they suggest that maternal social or affectionate behavior is more easily elicited closer to the delivery, while latency to feed decreases as the separation lengthens. This study indicates that there may be systematic changes in maternal responsiveness during delays in mother-infant contact following delivery.

The above data, as indicated earlier, are extremely meager. The only evidence of changes in maternal responsiveness (Gaulin-Kremer et al., Note 2) is not from initial contacts. The studies with data on initial contacts did not vary timing of contacts. Thus, there is no evidence from which we can make inferences about a sensitive period for initiating maternal behavior.

TIMING OF INITIAL CONTACTS: EFFECTS ON SUBSEQUENT BEHAVIOR

The second proposition introduced above concerns the effects of experiences during the first few hours after birth on subsequent maternal behavior. Is there any evidence that these early experiences have persisting effects? One appropriate test would be comparison of behavior occurring at initial contacts in the delivery or recovery room with interactions observed at a later time. Although the meager information reviewed in the previous section indicates wide variation in maternal behavior at first contacts, no studies have sought to relate these early individual differences to subsequent differences in mother-infant interaction. In the studies that have made observations of later mother-infant interactions, data on behavior during initial contacts have not usually been recorded or analyzed. Thus, the majority of studies compare the effects of differences in opportunity for contact without examining how or whether such opportunities were utilized.

A second strategy is to compare the effects of a given amount and type of opportunity for contact within the supposed sensitive period with the effects of the same opportunity at a later time by observing subsequent mother-infant interactions. Only one study (Hales, Lozoff, Sosa, & Kennell, 1977) has actually done this. Three other studies (Grossmann, Thane, & Grossmann, 1981; Kontos, 1978; Hopkins & Vietze, Note 3) compared two different types of contact that also differed in timing. Table 1 summarizes these four studies that attempted to assess *timing* of contacts apart from the *amount* of contact available. In all of the remaining studies the control groups had experienced less contact than

TABLE 1

STUDIES OF THE TIMING OF EARLY CONTACT INDEPENDENT OF AMOUNT

References	Population	Contact Condition (N)	Comparison Condition (N)	Time of Outcome	Outcome Measures	Findings	Comments
Hales et al., 1977	Low-SES, Guatemalan, breastfeeding	Early—45-min contact immediately after birth, daytime rooming in (20); delayed—45-min contact at 12 hours, daytime rooming in (20)	(20) Glimpse at birth 12 hours separation, daytime rooming in (20)	36 hours	Ratings of caregiving plus observation of mother-infant interaction	Early-contact group—more kiss, smile, talk, en face, no differences in proximity or caregiving, though in expected direction, little difference between early and delayed, though in expected direction	First study to look at timing of extra contact
Hopkins & Vietze, 1977	Lower-class, primiparous, U.S.	Early—10–45 min within 3 hours of delivery (26); extended—daytime rooming in 8 hours per day (26); early and extended—both of above (26); routine contact-neither of above (26)	Fourth or fifth feeding 4 months	Feeding observation, Brazelton scales, Carey Temperament survey	Early-contact infants obtain better Brazelton scores, more attentive to mother physically less active, described by mother as less distractible, mother spends more time in optimal feeding position, less simultaneous responding, more mother act alone, less infant act alone	Most findings favor early-contact groups, interactive data less clear

TABLE 1—(*Continued*)

References	Population	Contact Condition (N)	Comparison Condition (N)	Time of Outcome	Outcome Measures	Findings	Comments
Kontos, 1977	Canadian (English & Italian descent), primiparous	Early—1 hour beginning within 45 min of birth (12); extended—rooming in from Day 1 (12); early + extended—both of the above (12)	Routine care—not described	1 month 3 months	Play observations, summary attachment score	Both early- and extended-contact conditions lead to higher attachment scores; for individual behaviors, early contact led to increased smiling, no effect of extended contact, similar effects for en face and play	Rooming in could not be assigned at random, one experimenter (of two) knew group assignments
Grossmann, Thane, & Grossmann, 1981	Middle-class, mixed-parity, German	Early—30 min on delivery table (12); extended—partial rooming in 4 hours, in AM & 1 hour in PM (13); early & extended—both of above (13)	Brief view or touch after birth, infant next to mother's bed 2 hours, then 30-min feeding five times daily	2–3 days 4–5 days 7–9 days	Feeding Feeding Feeding	No group differences in caregiving; for affectionate touch: early > early + extended > control > extended; controls initially lowest, show dramatic increase in last days; effects significant only for those with planned pregnancy	Overall effect did not last through 10-day hospital stay effect of planned pregnancy suggests importance of psychological mechanisms in early contact effects

the experimental group(s) when the outcomes were assessed. This may not be important several weeks or months after the birth, but 15–60 min extra represents a large proportion of the interactive experience of mothers and infants in the first days when four to six 30-min periods is the typical daily ration. Thus, this larger group of studies provides information on the effects of *extra* contact but is not relevant to the question of how timing of contact affects later interactions.

In reviewing the studies in Table 1 and those in subsequent sections, two types of manipulated opportunities for mother-infant contact in hospitals will be distinguished. "Early contact" will refer to opportunities for contact provided in the delivery or recovery room—that is, within the first few hours of birth, hypothesized to be the sensitive period for mother-infant bonding. "Extended contact" will refer to opportunities for additional contact during the remainder of the period in the hospital. This includes rooming in, partial rooming in (e.g., days only, mornings only), and extra time together during routine feedings.

The first study to look at the timing of early contact was carried out in Guatemala with 60 lower-class mothers randomly assigned to three groups (Hales et al., 1977). One group of 20 mothers was given 45 min of skin-to-skin contact beginning in the delivery room followed by daytime rooming in. A second group of 20 was given 45 min of similar contact at 12 hours postpartum plus daytime rooming in. The third group was separated for the first 12 hours and then had only daytime rooming in. Mothers were observed with their infants 36 hours after delivery by a naive observer. Summary frequency scores for three classes of behavior were analyzed. There were no differences in proximity or caregiving behavior among the three groups, but there were significant differences in affectionate behavior. The early-contact group obtained the highest score, followed by the delayed-contact and then the routine-care group. Only the difference between the early and routine groups was significant. Further tests on the six individual behaviors making up the affection score (en face, look, talk, fondle, kiss, smile) revealed that only en face differed significantly among the three groups.

Most critiques of this study point out that only one of 19 behaviors recorded showed a significant group difference (e.g., Lamb & Hwang, 1982; Vietze & O'Connor, 1981), and they suggest that this could well be a chance finding. However, the presentation by Hales et al. (1977) indicates that they followed an appropriate strategy of reducing the 19 initial measures to three composite scores. Having found a significant group difference for one of the composite scores, affection, they then proceeded to ask which were the primary individual measures contributing to the effect. Unfortunately, the means for all of the items in the affection cluster were not presented, as the interpretation of the significance of the en face difference depends on whether the other measures showed the same pattern, albeit of weaker extent, or were distributed differently. In this study, rooming in, sometimes used as the contact condition in studies of extra contact, was the routine condition available for all groups. Therefore, it demonstrates an effect of early contact above a baseline of extended contact. This is the only study that can be considered a "pure" test of the timing of contact, as the same type and amount of contact were available at different times for two different groups. In the remaining three studies, type and timing of contact are confounded.

In the second study, Hopkins & Vietze (Note 3) assigned 104 lower-class primiparous mothers to four different conditions: (1) early contact, which consisted of 10–45 min of extra contact within the first 3 hours following birth; (2) extended contact, which consisted of daytime rooming in of about 8 hours per day; (3) early and extended contact, which included both of the above conditions; and (4) a routine contact condition, which provided 30 min every 4 hours for feeding. Observations were made of both mother and infant behavior at the fourth or fifth hospital feeding. Infant behavior was independently evaluated on the Brazelton (1973) Neonatal Behavioral Assessment Scales, and the mothers later completed the Carey (1973) Infant Temperament Survey. (It is not clear when the Carey survey, designed for 4–8-month-olds, was used.)

Although some differences were attributable to extended contact (extended-contact mothers completed more of the items on the temperament survey), most of the differences that were found differentiated the two groups that had early contact from those that did not. However, only the means for the early-contact comparisons are provided. In the early-contact groups, infants obtained more optimal scores in response to physiological stress on the Brazelton scales, were more visually attentive to their mothers while physically less active, and were perceived by their mothers as less distractible. Mothers in the early-contact conditions spent more of the feeding time in what was considered the optimal feeding position ("mother's eyes on a plane with the infant's, bottle perpendicular, and nipple full") than those in the remaining groups. Analysis of interactive patterns indicated that the early-contact dyads were characterized by less simultaneous responding, more mother acting alone, and less infant acting alone than the remaining dyads. Although some of these data suggest more harmonious interactions in the early-contact groups (e.g., greater infant visual alertness and more optimal feeding position for the mothers), this last analysis cannot clearly be interpreted in this fashion. For example, the pattern in the early-contact groups is similar to what Brown and Bakeman (1979) described as characteristic of preterm dyads (considered to experience much early stress) in contrast with full-term dyads. However, in these data there are differences in both mother and infant behavior that are related to the timing of first contacts apart from the amount of contact experienced.

The inclusion of data on baby behavior is one of the unique features of this study. Since early contact opportunities may affect the baby, who in turn elicits particular patterns of maternal behavior, such data are essential to any explanation of sensitive-period effects. Because Hopkins and Vietze (Note 3) was a presented paper rather than a published one, some important details have been omitted that limit the conclusions to be drawn. First, it is not clear whether the observer(s) knew the group assignments of mothers and/or the purpose of the study. Second, data are provided only for the early- versus no-early-contact comparisons, and although the comparisons for the effects of extended contact are described as insignificant, there are no data to substantiate this point. Third, because only a selected portion of the data is reported and details of analyses are glossed over, it is not clear how many statistical tests were done and what proportion were significant in this complex body of data. Evaluation of these data must therefore await a published and more detailed account of the study.

A similar design was used by Kontos (1977) in a study of primiparous Canadian mothers.[2] The early contact in this study was 1 hour in duration, beginning within 45 min of the delivery. One of the experimenters was usually present during this time. Mother-infant play was observed in the home at 1 and 3 months, and the main outcome measure was the total amount of "attachment behavior" on the mother's part. This measure included en face, touching, smiling, vocalizing, and so forth. Both early and extended contact were found to have independent additive effects of increasing the total amount of maternal attachment behavior observed. When individual behaviors were examined, early but not extended contact was associated with increased smiling, en face, and play behavior. Two methodological problems qualify the findings of this study. The first is that rooming in was not assigned randomly but by mothers' choice. Thus, the extended-contact groups may include moth-

---

[2] Although this study has been published (Kontos, 1978), I had access to the dissertation itself and found the details included there more useful than the published report.

ers who were initially more enthusiastic about interacting with their babies. Second, one of the two experimenters who coded outcome data had been with mothers following delivery and was therefore aware of the group assignments. However, interobserver reliability determined as percentage agreement on occurrence of individual behaviors was consistently high, suggesting that this knowledge did not bias the data coding.

The last and most recent (also most methodologically careful) study was carried out in Germany by Grossmann et al. (1981). Like the previous two, it assigned mothers to four groups: (1) early contact of 30 min on the delivery table; (2) extended contact of partial rooming in (4 hours in the morning plus 1 hour in the afternoon); (3) early and extended contact, which included both of the foregoing; and (4) the routine treatment of a brief view of the baby after the birth, the infant in the crib next to the mother for the 2 hours after the birth, and then 30-min feedings five times daily. This middle-class mixed-parity group of 54 mothers was followed intensively through the first 10 days of life as that is the normal hospital stay in Germany. Feedings were observed by coders naive to group membership at 2–3 days, 4–5 days, and 7–9 days. There were no group differences in caregiving behavior, but for all observations combined affectionate touching behavior in the early-contact group ranked highest, followed by the early-and-extended-, the routine-, and then the extended-contact groups. These differences were largest at the first feeding and then declined, so that by the end of the hospital stay, there were no group differences. The routine-care group, which was initially lowest in affectionate contact, showed a dramatic increase over time, ranking highest by the end of the study. A further finding of this study was that, when mothers were divided into those who had versus those who had not planned the pregnancy, early contact was shown to affect only the planned pregnancy group. Again, there is an effect of early contact on affectionate behavior, but it is qualified as being short in duration and restricted only to those who had planned their pregnancies.

Among these four studies that made some effort to separate amount of opportunity for contact from the timing of such opportunities, two (Hales et al., 1977; Hopkins & Vietze, Note 3) have little to say about persisting effects since they only observed mothers and infants in the first 2 days of life. While both sets of authors interpret their data as evidence for effects of early contact, both presentations are characterized by omission of details essential to support this interpretation. Furthermore, in the data of Hales et al. (1977), the early-contact group did not differ significantly from the delayed-contact group in composite affectional behavior score or in the one individual measure (en face) for which there were group differences, though the differences were in the predicted direction. Thus, on the basis of these data alone an effect of timing of contact cannot be inferred even for the short term. However, the most careful and methodologically sophisticated study (Grossmann et al., 1981) did show a similar effect of early contact within the first 3 days, corroborating the findings of Hales et al. (1977) and Hopkins & Vietze (Note 3).

Careful review of the dependent variables reveals little similarity in these three studies in the behaviors affected by early contact. Grossmann and her colleagues (1981) examined only touch (caregiving and affectionate), arguing that the effects of contact should be seen in the domain of affectionate touch. Hopkins and Vietze (Note 3) note effects on maternal feeding position and infant alertness, while Hales et al. (1977) report an effect on total affectionate behavior of which the primary component seems to be en face. Thus, though there is some agreement on a short-term effect of early contact, there is little consensus on the behaviors that are affected.

Grossmann et al. (1981) provide further follow-ups of their dyads in the next week, indicating that the effect of early contact was short-lived; it is no longer present by days 7–9. Even this brief effect was restricted only to mothers who planned their pregnancies. The fourth study considered above (Kontos, 1977) did collect data beyond the hospital stay and seems to suggest that timing of contact was unimportant: both early and extended contact had the effect of increasing total amount of attachment behavior. However, the generalizability of these findings is limited because mothers were not assigned randomly to groups. In short, there is little data in these studies from which one could confidently make inferences about persisting effects of early contact.

STUDIES OF EXTRA CONTACT DURING THE HOSPITAL STAY

The majority of existing studies are best characterized as studies of extra contact during the hospital stay. In all of these studies, one group was provided with extra opportunities for mother-infant interaction during the hospital stay and was subsequently compared with controls lacking these opportunities. Thus, not only did the contact group experience earlier mother-infant interaction than the controls; they also experienced more interaction. Hence, the effects of amount cannot be separated from effects of the timing of contact. In most cases, these extra opportunities occurred in the delivery or recovery room. In some cases, these contacts were supplemented by some form of rooming in or lengthened feeding periods (extended contact). In one series of studies (O'Connor, Vietze, Sandler, Sherrod, & Altemeier, 1980a, Note 4; O'Connor, Vietze, Sherrod, Sandler, & Altemeier, 1980b) only extended contact was provided in the form of rooming in, which began 6–12 hours after the delivery. For the most part, these studies have used two major classes of outcome variables. The first is frequency of maternal affectionate behavior (including body contact, en face positioning, gaze, vocalizing, and touching). The second is some measure of success at breast feeding, such as length of time breast feeding was continued or extent of supplementary feeding.

While breast feeding is physically beneficial for the infant and can be emotionally rewarding for mother and infant, its value as an index of mother-infant bonding has been questioned. Leiderman (1982) points out that a mother's decision to breast feed and how long she does so are subject to multiple influences (e.g., cultural expectations, maternal physical health, availability of alternative foods, the need for mother to earn income). Thus, while there may be persistent effects of extra contact opportunities on feeding practices, these may not be relevant to the construct of bonding.

Indeed, one of the problems in this body of research is that there is little agreement on how maternal bonding or attachment can be operationally defined. Because an emotional bond or attachment is not directly observable, a variety of discrete behaviors thought to reflect maternal feelings and attitudes have been recorded, and it is not always made clear how these behaviors are interrelated or relate to the construct of bonding or attachment. There have been no efforts to show that any of the objectively observable behaviors are systematically related to reported maternal feelings or attitudes.

Since these studies contain little direct information on the effects of timing of initial mother-infant contact and have also been carefully reviewed by others (the most detailed reviews are Vietze & O'Connor, 1981, and Lamb & Hwang, 1982), they will be discussed more briefly than the previous group. They are divided into three groups on the basis of the experimental conditions utilized: those studies investigating presence or absence of early contact alone (Table 2); those combining early and extended contact (Table 3); and those that used other designs (Table 4).

The studies reviewed below cannot be adequately evaluated or integrated without considering the methodological problems noted by previous reviewers. Both the tables and the summary therefore note information addressing presence or absence of the following problems: (a) failure to assign mothers randomly to treatments and/or to test similarity of treatment groups with respect to influential factors (e.g., sex and weight of infant, labor and delivery experience, maternal age, education), (b) failure to ensure and/or assess similarity of treatment for mothers in all groups for aspects of care not relevant to the experimental treatment per se, (c) failure to ensure that those assessing outcome are unaware of mother's treatment group, (d) incomplete reporting confined to the few statistically significant tests when a large number of additional tests have been done, and (e) inconsistent choice of experimental manipulations and control groups. Since "contact" could mean as little as 15 min offered at various times, in various places, with different people present and the infant clothed or unclothed and "routine care" could include 12-hour separations (e.g., Sosa, Kennell, Klaus, & Urutia, 1976), 10 min contact at the delivery (Craig et al., 1982), and 2 hours of the infant's cot next to the mother (Grossmann et al., 1981), the routine-care groups in some studies were similar to the experimental groups in others.

Early contact alone.—Table 2 summarizes all of those studies in which the primary comparison was between presence and absence of opportunities for contact in the delivery or recovery room. Two of these studies have been reported in formats with limited description of methodology (Taylor et al., Note 1; Anisfeld & Lipper, Note 5); therefore, they cannot be adequately evaluated. However, Taylor et al. (Note 1) is of great value in detailing the actual amount of contact that occurred in both contact and control groups in the delivery room and on subsequent days.

Unless otherwise noted in the "Comments" column, all of these studies assigned mothers randomly to experimental groups, and later data were collected by individuals unaware of these initial assignments. Most authors have also documented the similarity of experimental and control groups on important factors (e.g., maternal age, education, labor and delivery experience, infant sex, weight), and in two cases (Sosa et al., 1976; Thomson, Hartsock, & Larson, 1979) these comparisons reveal group differences that lead the authors themselves to question the inferences that can be made about the effects of the experimental manipulations. Because the experimental manipulation in these studies is introduced at a time when mothers are generally cared for individually, there is little opportunity for them to be aware of different group treat-

TABLE 2
STUDIES OF EXTRA CONTACT IN DELIVERY OR RECOVERY ROOM

References	Population	Contact Condition (N)	Comparison Condition (N)	Time of Outcome	Outcome Situation or Measures	Findings	Comments
Taylor et al., 1979	Primiparous, white middle-class U.S.	50-min private contact after transfer to recovery room (35)	Mother and infant separated after arrival in recovery room (30)	2 days 1 month	Klaus & Kennell's interview, Broussard neonatal perception inventory, feeding	No differences except for males; contact group has "better" feeding scores	First detailed account of actual contact—both groups alike until recovery, controls actually had more contact on Day 1 (from figures in tables), feeding scores seem judgmental, no description of group assignments or observation conditions
Campbell & Taylor, 1980		(50)	(50)	1 year	"Strange situation" (Ainsworth)	No differences between groups on any measure of infant behavior	
Anisfeld & Lipper, Note 4	U.S.	1 hour on mother's abdomen after birth (30)	Glimpse in delivery room (30)	2 days 3 months	Feed Physical exam	Contact group showed more affectionate behaviors but other variables (e.g., medical complications, sex of infant, social support) determined how strong effect of contact was fewer contact mothers schedule baby's day, contact mothers report more frequent pickups to cry	Methodological details not available

TABLE 2—(Continued)

References	Population	Contact Condition (N)	Comparison Condition (N)	Time of Outcome	Outcome Situation or Measures	Findings	Comments
Sosa et al., 1976	Poor, urban, Guatemalan primiparous	Mother given baby after episiotomy repair for 45 min alone in private room	First contact 6–12 hours after birth	Follow-ups at 35 days and 3, 6, 9, 12 m.	Weight gain, infections, breast feeding	In Social Security hospital contact infants had gained more weight at 6 and 12 months, contact infants had fewer infections in Roosevelt I and Social Security (marginally in Roosevelt II) contact infants were breast fed longer	Chapter also include Hales et al. (1977) study described in Table 1; authors find SES differences between contact and controls observer reliability?
	Roosevelt I Roosevelt II Social Security	(30) (34) (20)	(30) (34) (20)				
Thomson et al., 1979	Primiparous, mixed ethnicity, Canadian, breast-feeding	15–30 min holding in delivery room, feed if mother wishes (15)	Held briefly in delivery room, seen at 12–20 hours, modified rooming in from Day 2 (15)	After delivery 2 months	Mother reaction to baby Home interview, breast feeding	13 contact us, nine control showed "happier" reaction to infant—not significant but lack of happy reaction related to cessation of breast feeding by 2 months more contact mothers were breast feeding without supplement	Sex distribution differs in the two groups, group differences hold up within sex groups
de Chateau & Wiberg, 1977a	"Healthy" mothers and infants, Swedish, married, breast-feeding	15-min skin-to-skin contact and nursing immediately after delivery, mother, father, and infant together 2 hours in delivery with infant in crib next to mother (22)	Routine care contact once every 4 hours first 2 days then daytime rooming in for 1 week (20, primiparous) (20, multiparous)	36 hours	Feeding	Contact primiparous infants behaved like multiparous infants sat up more, cradled more, infants cried less effects stronger for male babies contact group more en face, kiss, baby smile (males only) for males & females combined, contact mothers did more en face kiss, less cleaning, more infant smile, less cry	Contact effects attributable mainly to effects for males

TABLE 2—(Continued)

References	Population	Contact Condition (N)	Comparison Condition (N)	Time of Outcome	Outcome Measures	Findings	Comments
de Chateau & Wiberg, 1977b........				3 months	Feeding, interview	Contact group report more breast feeding, longer continuation in night feeds, fewer feeding problems	
de Chateau et al., 1977 ...				1 year	Interview	Contact group breast fed for 175 days vs. 108 for controls, variability too high to be significant	Changes in hospital procedure—e.g., not weighing baby after feeds, father participation in information sessions about breast feeding *are* significantly related to length of breast feeding
Ali & Lowry, 1981	Lower-SES, Jamaican	45-min immediately after birth (37)	Glimpse at delivery, mean separation of 9 hours then "regular" care giving (37)	6 weeks	Interview, exam, dress, and feed observation	More of contact mothers breast feeding, no other differences	Observer reliability?
		(35)	(37)	12 weeks		More contact mothers breast feeding, contact group stays closer during exam, more gaze & vocalizing during feed	
Craig et al., 1982..........	Indigent, U.S.	1 hour skin to skin after delivery (26)	≤10-min contact, baby wrapped (28)	1 month	Neonatal Perception Inventory Interview (after Klaus & Kennell and de Chateau) mothers' recording of infant behavior	No differences between groups on any measures	Controls have more early contact than most controls in other studies

ments. In most hospitals, those caring for the mother or baby on the maternity floor would be unlikely to know whether mothers had participated in an experimental treatment in the delivery room. However, few investigators have actually taken steps to ascertain or ensure that this was indeed the case.

Although none of these studies can be considered entirely free of some methodological limitations, the majority have been carefully done. With the exception of Craig et al. (1982), to be discussed below, all have reported some effects of presence versus absence of early contact opportunities. While two studies report effects mainly for male infants (de Chateau & Wiberg, 1977a, 1977b; Taylor et al., Note 1), one reports effects primarily for female infants (Anisfeld & Lipper, Note 5). Four sets of authors (Ali & Lowry, 1981; de Chateau, Holmberg, Jacobsson, & Winberg, 1977; de Chateau & Wiberg, 1977b; Sosa et al., 1976; Thomson et al., 1979) report more "success" at breast feeding in the experimental groups, while three (Ali & Lowry, 1981; de Chateau & Wiberg, 1977a, 1977b; Anisfeld & Lipper, Note 5) report increased maternal affectionate behavior in the experimental group. However, there is little consistency in the time of assessment or specific measures for which differences are found. These inconsistencies would be of less concern if there were a universally accepted operational definition of maternal attachment or a clearly documented developmental pattern of maternal behavior that could lend a coherent interpretation to the pattern of findings. In the absence of clear consensus on these issues, it appears that even among studies that report positive effects, there is little replication of findings for specific measures.

The one study which differs from the others in finding no effects of early contact (Craig et al., 1982) is unusual in several respects. First, the control group had a relatively long period of early contact (up to 10 min), albeit clothed rather than skin to skin. However, more importantly, the authors posited a mechanism for previously reported effects of early contact and sought to test it. They hypothesized that maternal perceptions of the infant would be changed in the positive direction by early contact. At 1 month postpartum, however, they found no differences between groups on responses to the Neonatal Perception Inventory, interview questions patterned after those of Klaus and Kennell, or mothers' recording of infant behavior.

The overall evaluation of this group of studies is that the effects of early contact opportunities have not been consistently or clearly demonstrated. However, with the exception of the most recent study by Craig et al. (1982) the absence of such effects has also not been convincingly demonstrated.

Early plus extended contact.—The initial studies by Klaus and his colleagues, which stimulated most of the research discussed here, provided mothers not only with skin-to-skin contact within the first 3 hours after birth but 5 hours extra of contact over each of the next 3 days. These studies have been described and evaluated in most of the previous reviews and will not be detailed here, although they are summarized in Table 3.

Table 3 includes studies in which the major comparison was between an experimental group receiving both early and extended contact and a control group with neither. In these designs, the experimental and control groups differ maximally in amount of contact opportunity. Thus, these studies are most likely to be informative about the effects that *amount* of contact during the hospital stay has on later maternal behavior. However, the role that timing of such opportunities plays is totally obscured, as these opportunities are presented at numerous times during the hospital stay. Unless otherwise noted, all of the studies in the table assigned mothers to groups randomly and used observers naive to these assignments. In these designs hospital staff could not be naive as to group assignments since whether the infant roomed in or not or remained in the room for extended feedings would be obvious. Thus, differential treatment by hospital staff may confound apparent effects of experimental treatment. Unless otherwise noted, mothers roomed with others receiving the same treatment so that awareness of special treatment was minimized.

In addition to the original studies by Klaus and Kennell, the studies in this group include one that found no effects of extra contact opportunities (Svejda et al., 1980), one that found small effects on maternal and infant behavior at 4 and 12 months (Siegel, Bauman, Schaefer, Saunders, & Ingram, 1980), and one that reported effects on maternal behavior in the first week that had dissipated by 6 weeks (Carlsson, Fagerberg, Horneman, Hwang, Larsson, Rödholm, Schaller, Daniellson, & Gundewal, 1978, 1979; Schaller, Carlsson, & Larsson, 1979;. One additional study that reported effects on breast feeding (Sousa, Barros, Gazalle, Begères, Pinbeiro, Menzes, & Arruda, 1974) confounded the contact manipulation with other procedures designed to encourage breast feeding and cannot be clearly interpreted. Thus, the studies in this group show little concordance of findings.

Other studies.—There is some evidence that extended contact alone can

TABLE 3

STUDIES OF EXTRA CONTACT: EARLY PLUS EXTENDED

References	Population	Contact Condition (N)	Comparison Condition (N)	Time of Outcome	Outcome Situation or Measures	Findings	Comments
Klaus et al., 1972	Low-SES, black, predominantly single, bottle-feeding, U.S.	1 hour in first, 3 & 5 hour/day for 3 days (14)	Routine care, brief contact at 6–12 hours, 30 min every 4 hours for feed (14)	1 month	Interview	Extra-contact mothers report greater response to cries, more concern about baby when away; contact mothers stay clear more en face and contact for contact group	Interview questions a weak measure; possible effects of mother-staff relationship may explain some findings
					Pediatric exam feeding		
Kennell et al., 1974	...	...	...	1 year	Interview	More contact mothers return to work but report missing baby more than routine care group	Exact data analyses not always clear as to single vs. pooled behavior measures; one finding (number of mothers working) could be considered to be in opposite direction
					Pediatric exam	contact mothers stay closer spent more time soothing baby, more kissing	
					Free play, Bayley exam, feeding	No differences	
Ringler et al., 1975	...	(5)	(5)	1 and 2 years	Maternal speech during interview and free play	At 1 year contact group used fewer statements, no other difference; 2-year contact group used more adjectives, asked more questions, gave fewer commands, used more words per proposition (contact mothers increase in these domains from 1 to 2, routine care group does not)	Extremely small number; not clear how these behaviors relate to parent bonding construct

TABLE 3—(Continued)

References	Population	Contact Condition (N)	Comparison Condition (N)	Time of Outcome	Outcome Situation or Measures	Findings	Comments
Svejda, Campos & Emde, 1980	Lower middle-class, married, primiparous, breast-feeding, fathers at delivery, U.S.	15–25 min after birth in own room, extra hour at each feed (10 extra hours in first 36) (15)	Saw baby at delivery held 5 min during transfer, then 30 min every 4 hours (15)	36 hours	Feeding	No differences in any discrete behaviors or in categories of behavior	Only study with no early effects at all
Siegel et al., 1980	Low-SES, 1/4 white, 1/3 married, U.S.	45 min in first 3 hours + 5 hours/day home visitor (47); Same as above with no home visits (50)	"Brief" contact at delivery the 2½ hours/day routine contact, home visitor (53); Same as above with no home visits (52)	Pregnancy, 4 months; 12 months	Interview, home observation; Home observation	Contact condition accounted for 2.5% variance in maternal acceptance and consoling behavior at 4 months and 3.2% of variance in infant behavior at 12 months; background variables contributed larger portion of variance, no differences in rates of abuse or neglect	Gives some sense of how contact compares with other contributing variables in size of effect; reliability of observers?
Carlsson et al., 1978	Middle-class Swedish, married, planned pregnancy, breast-feeding	A. Mother keeps baby 1–2 hours after delivery fed on demand every 2–4 hours, help with breast-feeding (20) B. same as A in delivery room, no extended contact or help with feeds (22)	C. 5 min after birth in crib next to mother for 4 hours, fed every 4 hours (20)	First 4 days (days 2 & 4)	Feeding	Contact group made more physical contact, more affectionate behaviors, no difference between A and B	

TABLE 3—(Continued)

References	Population	Contact Condition (N)	Comparison Condition (N)	Time of Outcome	Outcome Situation or Measures	Findings	Comments
Carlsson et al., 1979	. . .	A. 17 B. 17	C. 16	6 weeks	Home feeding	No differences in any behaviors	
Schaller et al., 1979	. . .				Reanalysis of pooled feeding measures from above sessions	Confirms above findings contact group engages in more proximal behavior in 1st week no differences by 6 weeks	
Sousa et al., 1974	Brazil, breast-feeding	Continous contact beginning right after birth, crib next to mother support with breast-feeding (100)	Glimpse at birth; 12–24-hour separation 30 min/3 hours (100)	2 months	Breast-feeding	77% of contact mothers breast-feed vs. 27% comparison group	Cannot attribute differences to early contact alone; other treatment differences

have long-term positive effects on parental behavior. O'Connor et al. (1980b) followed 301 low-SES primiparous U.S. mothers through the first 2 years. Of this group, 143 had been randomly assigned to rooming in beginning 6–12 hours postpartum, while 158 had been assigned to half-hour feeding contacts only. Within the first 2 years, reports from hospitals, protective services, and other agency records indicated that 10 control infants versus two rooming-in infants were mistreated by parents, $p < .05$. Furthermore, five of the control infants versus none of the rooming-in infants had a nonparent as primary caregiver, $p < .05$. A follow-up study with similar treatment conditions (O'Connor et al., 1980a, Note 4) and more detailed measures of infant development and parent-infant interaction has reported preliminary findings of differences between the groups on many measures. The majority of these favor the rooming-in group (see Table 4), but this is not always the case, and some differences are difficult to interpret. Additionally, differences do not remain consistent from one assessment to the next. Unlike the previous studies, the initial study in this series relied on an extremely large sample to examine differences in extreme and low-frequency events. A similar attempt in the study by Siegel et al. (1980) with a somewhat smaller sample did not find contact-control differences in child mistreatment.

Two additional studies best described as separation studies should also be considered here. Both were preliminary reports and cannot yet be adequately evaluated. In each of these, the early-contact group received routine hospital treatment similar to the controls in the previous studies. The late-contact mothers were those for whom the first contact was delayed 1–14 days because of minor medical problems. In the first study, Whiten (1977) followed a British sample of mixed-SES primiparous mothers making home observations at 3 weeks and 1, 2, and 3 months postpartum. Except for the 3-month visits, when there were no reported differences, the early-contact group had more mutual looking and smiling and more contingent responsiveness of both mother and baby to each other than was the case in the separated group.

In the second study, Sostek & Scanlon (Note 6) studied a primiparous group of mixed-SES mothers in the United States observing mother-infant interaction and assessing maternal feelings and attitudes over the first 6 months. The separated group of mothers was found to have lower self confidence in their maternal roles at 4–6 weeks and 6 months than their counterparts who had experienced routine hospital contacts beginning on Day 1. This study was the first attempt to assess maternal attitudes and feelings that might be mediators of effects observed in other studies.

TABLE 4

OTHER STUDIES

References	Population	Contact Condition (N)	Comparison Condition (N)	Time of Outcome	Outcome Situation or Measures	Findings	Comments
O'Connor et al., 1980b	Low-SES, primiparous, mixed-race, married, & single	Glimpse in delivery room, 7–12-hour separation then room in 8 hour/day, mean of 11.44 hours contact in first 2 days (143)	Same except for no rooming in; mean of 2.15-hour contact in first 2 days (158)	12–21 months	Reports of abuse and neglect, hospital records, Protective Service Reports, etc.	Evidence of parent inadequacy for 10 control vs. two rooming-in babies ($p < .05$); five controls vs. zero rooming-in babies, have non-parent as primary caregiver ($p < 05$)	Extended contact rather than early contact largest sample followed more extreme outcome measures
O'Connor et al., 1980a	Same as above but new sample	(62)	(90)	48 hours	Brazelton scale, mother-infant interaction	Rooming-in babies more alert, slept more, mothers in rooming-in speak more softly to infant, do more nonfeed care	Methodological details not available from report
				1 month	Home observation	Control babies cry more, control mothers do more nonfeed care	
				3 months	Home observation	Rooming-in mothers show more negative emotion	
				6 months	Home observation	Rooming-in mothers look at baby more, respond more rapidly to distress, their babies are more alert	Mixed findings; sometimes rooming-in, sometimes controls have "advantage"; not always clear what "advantage" is
				9 months	Bayley scales	Rooming-in babies have higher motor scores	
				12 months	Home observation	Rooming-in mothers smile more, look and talk to baby more, infants are more drowsy but interact more with mother	

TABLE 4—*(Continued)*

References	Population	Contact Condition (N)	Comparison Condition (N)	Time of Outcome	Outcome Situation or Measures	Findings	Comments
O'Connor et al., Note 4....	Dyadic state	Analysis of data from same sample		1, 3, 6, 12, & 18 months	Based on home observations	Rooming-in groups had more coaction, controls had more acting alone and more frequent occurrence of partner dropping out of interaction	
Whiten, 1977	Mixed-SES, primiparous, married, British	Routine care, touched and fed baby on day 1 (11)	Separated for minor medical reasons, 2–14 days	3 weeks 1 month 2 months	Home observations at all points	Contact group had more mutual look and smile, reply to infant vocalization, more interaction; contact group had more interaction, more mother respond to baby smile or vocalization and more baby smile to mother's touch or smile	Looking at different part of early experience, longer separations than other studies
				3 months		No significant differences	
Sostek & Scanlon, 1980	Mixed-SES and race primiparous, U.S.	Routine care, mother keeps baby all day if desired (34) > 22 hours contact in first 2-1/2 days (17)	18% separated 24 hours or more because of mother's fever < 22 hours contact in first 2½ days (17)	2–3 days 4–6 weeks 6 months	Mother-infant play, Brazelton scales Same as above Maternal confidence questionnaire and anxiety measure Maternal confidence	Separated group had lower self-confidence at 4–6 weeks and 6 months, though not significant Low contact mothers had more overt anxiety, less covert anxiety	Suggests maternal self-confidence or attitude as possible mediator of early contact effects

Although there is also a literature on parent separation based on studies of parents with prematurely born infants, these families are confronted with numerous other assaults to the early parent-infant relationship and cannot be considered an appropriate comparison group for parents of normal full-term infants. The studies above do indicate that amount of contact available to mothers and their infants may affect subsequent parent-child interactions when the initial contacts are much delayed after the delivery or recovery room experience.

Social class as a mediating variable.—Although not explicit in most of the above reports, several previous reviewers of the literature on parent-infant bonding (e.g., Goldberg, 1982; Leiderman, 1982; Klaus, Kennell, & Sosa, Note 7) have suggested that sample characteristics that differ between studies, particularly social class, account for differences in findings. Studies of lower-class mothers are considered to show stronger or longer lasting effects of early contact than those of middle-class mothers. It has been argued that middle-class mothers, having fewer stresses, engage in nurturing behavior that is close to the maximum possible, whether afforded opportunities for early contact or not. Among lower-class mothers, a higher level of stress and fewer social supports can depress maternal affectionate behavior, allowing the effects of in-hospital contact to be more readily demonstrable.

Although this is a plausible and reasonable argument, Tables 1–4 indicate no clear-cut pattern of social class effects in the existent literature. First, a number of studies do not provide enough information about sample characteristics to make a determination of social class (de Chateau & Wiberg, 1977a, 1977b; Kontos, 1977; Sousa et al., 1974; Thomson et al., 1979; Anisfeld & Lipper, Note 5). Second, because there is variation in procedures, design, and age of infants at assessments, there are few examples of studies that are similar enough in all but social class to make useful direct comparisons. Finally, none of the existing studies utilized social class as an independent variable. The impression that early contact has more powerful or longer lasting effects among lower-class mothers may reflect that mothers from lower-income groups have been studied more extensively than middle-class mothers. There are, in all, eight studies of lower-class mothers (Ali & Lowry, 1981; Craig et al., 1982; Hales et al., 1977; Klaus, Jerauld, Kreger, McAlpine, Steffa, & Kennell, 1972; O'Connor et al., 1980a; Siegel et al., 1980; Sosa et al., 1976; Hopkins & Vietze, Note 3), four studies of middle-class mothers (Carlsson et al., 1978; Grossmann et al., 1981; Svejda, Campos, & Emde, 1980; Taylor et al., Note 1), and two studies of mixed-SES groups (Whiten, 1977; Sostek & Scanlon, Note 6). Furthermore, two studies with no effects of early contact (Svejda et al., 1980; Taylor et al., Note 1) are of middle-class samples. One (Craig et al., 1982) is of lower-class mothers. These studies also share the feature of having provided both contact and comparison groups a 5–10 min contact in the delivery room and en route to the recovery room before the experimental manipulation proper was introduced. Thus, failure to find positive effects of early contact could be explained by this limitation of the experimental manipulation rather than social-class status of the sample. In addition, the more recent of the studies of middle-class mothers (Svejda et al., 1980) only reported data for Day 2 observations, a point in development where only two of the studies of lower-class mothers collected data (Hales et al., 1977; Hopkins & Vietze, Note 3). Although both of these studies did find positive effects of early contact, they can readily be matched by two studies of middle-class mothers (Carlsson et al., 1978; Grossmann et al., 1981) that found comparable effects in the same time period.

In the same way, the most dramatic long-term finding, that of a relationship between child maltreatment and in-hospital contact, by O'Connor and her colleagues (1980a), must be weighed against the failure of Siegel and his colleagues (1980) to find such a relationship in a similar lower-class sample. In the latter study, an extensive, carefully carried out investigation with a relatively large sample, in-hospital contact was associated with aspects of maternal behavior at 4 months and infant behavior at 12 months, but this manipulation accounted for an extremely small proportion of the variance (2%–3.5%) in contrast with background variables such as maternal age, race, and education, which accounted for most of the explained variance. Although this is one of two studies of lower-class mothers in which in-hospital contact did not have clear effects on maternal behavior, the finding that background variables that contribute to stress did predict maternal behavior indirectly supports the arguments of those who have seen social-class differences as an explanation for variations in study findings. However, this brief overview indicates that the data on social-class effects are equivocal. Although it seems likely that social class is a factor that can mediate the impact of early contact, the literature does not provide adequate information for evaluating this proposition.

Summary.—The main points that emerge thus far are as follows:

1. There has been no systematic study of a possible sensitive period for the initiation of maternal behavior. Data on initial interactions have been primarily descriptive. Studies with data on initial interactions have generally not related these data to later maternal behavior.

2. Only four studies investigated subsequent effects of early contact

in a fashion that allows inferences about the *timing* of contact opportunities apart from the *amount* of opportunity. Among these, there is consistent report of effects within the first 3 days but no consensus on the precise nature of these effects. The possibility of effects persisting beyond the first three days has not been adequately studied.

3. Consistent effects of extra contact opportunity in the delivery or recovery room have not been convincingly demonstrated. However, with the exception of Craig et al. (1982), the absence of such effects has not been convincingly demonstrated either. Inability to reject the null hypothesis because a study is methodologically flawed does not have the same logical status as inability to reject the null hypothesis in a well-designed, well-executed study.

4. The studies in the best position to provide evidence on subsequent effects of *amount* of in-hospital contact opportunity are those in which mothers in the experimental group received both early and extended contact. There is no consensus of findings within this group of studies.

5. While several previous reviewers have felt that social-class effects explained the inconsistent findings, the evidence necessary to determine whether social class mediates effects of in-hospital contact opportunity is not available.

DIRECTIONS FOR FUTURE RESEARCH

The above summary indicates that we do not know much more about initial parent-infant contacts and effects on later behavior than we knew in the early 1970s, when the first of these studies was published. Since then public awareness of the bonding ideas and changes in hospital practice in response to this awareness have combined to create a climate in which it is impossible to do the experiments that can properly answer the questions we should have been asking in the last 10 years. As an alternative to accepting perpetual ignorance, we can exploit another limitation in the existent literature, the failure to consider processes that link initial contact to later parent-infant relationships. Whether we consider these initial experiences as particularly influential or simply one step in an ongoing process that is no more or less influential than other steps (and the available data supply little help in making this choice), an understanding of the role that initial contacts play for parents and infants is of interest.

One of the striking features of the reviewed literature is that, although much effort has been directed toward establishing that early contact affects subsequent maternal behavior, there has been little conceptualization of causal mechanisms underlying such effects and little hypothesis testing of alternative explanations. Studies by Curry (1979), who showed that skin contact was no more effective than interacting with the clothed infant, Gewirtz (Note 8), who showed that clothing or lack of it and duration of contact did not have differential effects, and Craig et al. (1982), who did not find a postulated effect of early contact on maternal perceptions as measured on the Neonatal Perception Inventory, are exceptions to this general phenomenon. Of course, these studies do not exhaust possible routes to understanding the process underlying the transition from pregnancy to parenthood. While there are many ethical and practical barriers to carrying out some of the ideal studies, it would be useful to speculate on possible processes that might occur in initial contacts, to evaluate the existing evidence with respect to such mechanisms, and to consider what kinds of additional evidence would be useful to support, rule out, or illuminate multiple causal factors.

Physiological changes in the mother.—Many of the studies discussed above are introduced with a few references to animal studies with the implicit suggestion that the proposed study will determine whether similar mechanisms (e.g., hormonal changes) underlie the initiation and maintenance of human maternal behavior (for a comprehensive review of the animal research, see Lamb & Hwang, 1982). However, the discussions, conclusions, and suggestions for further research rarely return to this theme. There has been no work on the role that hormonal changes may play in maternal responsiveness to human infants. Hormonal assays following delivery might bracket points in the course of the reproductive cycle when changes in maternal responsiveness would be expected and observations of first interactions that occur within different time brackets could be compared. Of course, the ideal strategy would be to relate individual differences in patterns of hormonal change to individual differences in maternal behavior, though this would pose methodological and ethical problems.

However, there has been a tradition of research relating events and conditions of labor and delivery to infant status following delivery and to subsequent infant development. Many of these variables, such as length of labor, medications received, and number of risk factors, can be considered indicators of the physiological state of the mother during and following delivery. As the preliminary report of Anisfeld and Lipper (Note 5) suggests, relationships between these measures and early maternal behavior is one route through which physiological influences on initial maternal behavior could be established. Additional data on this point come from two studies of the effect of a supportive companion on labor and delivery experience (Sosa, Kennell, Klaus, Robertson, & Urutia, 1980; Klaus, Kennell, & Sosa, Note 7). Women who had a supportive companion during labor and delivery did more talking, stroking, and smiling in first contacts with their infants than those who labored alone. However, the presence of a supportive companion was also associated with a shorter labor, fewer delivery complications, and more time awake for the mothers during the subsequent interaction period with their infants. While the experimental design does not allow for separation of physiological and psychological influences, the authors suggest the following plausible mechanisms.

Presence of a supportive companion reduces anxiety and tension. This in turn reduces catecholamine levels, which lead to increase in uterine contractile activity and uterine blood flow. The result is a shorter and easier labor for both mother and baby so that both are in more optimal states at their first encounter. Given these data and the research showing influences of labor and delivery conditions on infant behavior and development, it is surprising that few of the early contact studies mention the conditions of labor and delivery and that individual differences in this domain have generally not been related to initial maternal responsiveness.

Interview studies of the transition to parenthood (e.g., Leifer, 1980; Shereshefsky & Yarrow, 1973) indicate that many women are unprepared for the physical limitations they encounter immediately following delivery (e.g., exhaustion, discomfort of stitches, afterpains). Although such symptoms are familiar to everyone who has had a baby and those who care for new mothers, there has been little attention to how the physiological changes accompanying recovery from the effort and the process of delivery affect maternal behavior and may play a role in effects of early contact. It is possible, for example, that the occasionally apparent tendency for extended contact to depress the effects of early contact (Grossmann et al., 1981) may reflect that for some mothers extended contact demands more energy than they have available at the time. It would be informative to examine individual differences in the recovery process as possible mediators of maternal behavior in relation to time from delivery.

Physiological and behavioral changes in the infant.—There is some evidence that in the unmedicated delivery there is a period of newborn alertness following delivery during which the infant can be expected to be more responsive to adult social interactions than in subsequent hours and days (Desmond, Rudolph, & Phitakophraiwan, 1966; Emde, Swedberg, & Suzuki, 1975). It is possible that interacting with the infant during this period is more rewarding for the mother and makes a more lasting positive impression than attempts to rouse a drowsy baby later. Indeed, it seems likely that the optimal situation is for both baby and mother to be in an appropriate physiological state for social interaction at the first meeting. That catching both participants in such a state is difficult and that there are probably large individual differences in the time course of responsiveness may account for the inconsistency in research findings. Once again, it is striking that few of the presented or published reports have attended to baby behavior during the initial interactions. The one study in which this was done (Gaulin-Kremer et al., Note 2) did not find effects of baby behavior explaining differences in maternal behavior over time.

It is also possible that the primary effects of early or extended contact are on the infant, who in turn elicits different feelings or behaviors from the parents. De Chateau and his colleagues (de Chateau et al., 1977; de Chateau & Wiberg, 1977b) and Hopkins & Vietze (Note 3) provide some data suggestive of contact effects on infant behavior. In tracing such mechanisms, it is important to document both initial infant behavior and its effect on parents. That is, the existence of differences in infant behavior alone cannot be used to infer effects on parental behavior as these may not in fact follow. An example of this is found in the work of Butterfield and her colleagues (Butterfield & Emde, 1978; Butterfield, Emde, & Svejda, 1981; Butterfield, Emde, Svejda, & Naiman, 1982) concerning the administration of silver nitrate to the eyes of the newborn. While application of silver nitrate depressed visual alertness and pursuit in neonates, there were few measurable differences in maternal behavior toward the infant or maternal descriptions and feelings concerning the infant that could be attributed to amount of eye opening by infants during initial contacts. This was surprising, as Grossmann (1978) reported that, in typical mother-neonate interactions, the infants' eye openings were reliably used by mothers as cues to initiate interactions. However, fathers were more likely to look closely, touch affectionately, pick up, and talk to the more visually alert newborns.

In considering possible physiological and behavioral changes in mother and baby following delivery as explanatory mechanisms for the effects of early contact (and indeed for all of the following alternative mechanisms), to establish that such changes contribute to differences in the quality of initial interactions does not at all explain why such differences might persist. It seems necessary to postulate a "law of behavioral inertia": patterns of interaction, once established, tend to persist more often than they change, or the affective quality (positive or negative) of interactions tends to persist. Such a principle predicts that there should be a relationship between the quality of the first interactions and those observed at subsequent times. Some mothers who have had early delivery room contact have certainly had more positive experiences than others (e.g., recall the descriptions of Packer & Rosenblatt [1979] of mothers given their infants during episiotomy repair), and some mothers participate more extensively than others during opportunities for early contact (Taylor et al., Note 1). Are the positive effects of early contact stronger for those who have had more positive experiences? By the same token, does a negative or disappointing initial contact lead to less positive interactions at later times?

Psychological changes in the mother.—A literature exists on psychological changes during pregnancy and the postpartum period (e.g., Benedek, 1970; Bibring, 1961; Leifer, 1980; Robson & Moss, 1970; Shereshefsky & Yarrow, 1973), largely based on interviews with mothers and, in some cases, fathers. Although much of the early-contact research has invoked the concept of parental attachment or bonding, only one study (Sostek & Scanlon, Note 6) attempted to assess maternal feelings or attitudes as a consequence of early contact. However, the two literatures taken together suggest (1) that some of the documented psychological changes create a state of readiness to respond to the infant following delivery, and (2) that whatever lasting effects early contact has depends on influencing attitudes or feelings of the mother. Some of the variables found to mediate early-contact effects, such as the planned versus unplanned status of the pregnancy (Grossmann et al., 1981), are consonant with psychological rather than physiological mechanisms.

It is particularly interesting in this respect to consider the slowly growing data on early father contact. While many of the psychological experiences and expectations of fathers and mothers necessarily differ (since the mother has an internal physiological connection to the baby and an active traditional social role, while the father has neither), many features are also similar. Indeed, to the extent that fathers and mothers are similarly affected by early contact with the infant, psychological rather than physiological mechanisms would seem to be implicated.

The one published study of early father contact (Rodholm, 1981) compared play behavior of two groups of Swedish fathers whose infants had been delivered by Caesarean section. In one group ($N = 29$) the father was allowed to handle the infant for a 10-min period 15 min after the delivery. In the second ($N = 15$), the father had only a brief glimpse of the baby after the delivery. When the infants were 3 months old, the fathers in the contact group were found to engage in more face-to-face play and affectionate touching than those in the control group.

The preliminary report of a recent U.S. study (Keller, Hildebrandt, & Richards, Note 9) compared three groups of fathers who had different delivery experiences. In two groups fathers had been present at the delivery, and in one of these groups fathers were also given 4½ hours of private extended contact with their babies during the hospital stay. In the third group of unplanned Caesarean section deliveries, fathers were neither present at the delivery nor offered extended contact. Play and feeding observations at 3 months indicated few differences in infant behavior among the three groups. However, the extended-contact fathers engaged in significantly more face-to-face activity and vocalization during the feeding. There were no differences during the play observations in the three groups. Additionally, the extended-contact fathers responded more positively to a variety of questionnaire items concerning feelings about the birth experience, child care, and their infants. There was some evidence that extended-contact fathers of first-borns experienced an increase in self-esteem (Keller & Hildebrandt, Note 10).

A third study (Pannabecker, Emde, & Austin, 1982) compared three groups of middle-class fathers of first-borns. All had been present at the delivery and held the baby at that time. In one group, fathers and babies spent two 30-min periods with one of the investigators, who demonstrated items from the Brazelton scales with the infant. In a second, the fathers received the same information by viewing a prepared videotape with the investigator. In the third group, fathers had neither of these opportunities. At the 4-week pediatric visit, father and infant behaviors were coded as well as videotaped for further coding. All coding was done by observers unfamiliar with the group assignments. A large number of different individual and composite behaviors were analyzed, revealing few significant group differences. Although this study did not use a traditional contact manipulation (all fathers had held their babies at delivery), it explores the effects of a different type of father-infant-professional interaction.

The role that psychological factors can play in overriding early-contact effects for fathers is illustrated by a Canadian study that compared 12 fathers of preterm infants (of whom three had been present at the delivery) with 12 fathers of full-term infants (eight of whom had been present at the delivery). While one might predict that the full-term fathers should be more actively engaged with their infants as a result of more extensive early contact, the reverse was the case (Marton, Minde, &

Perrotta, Note 11). The fathers of preterm babies held them longer during the feeding and were more involved in their overall care than were fathers of full-term infants. Similar anecdotal evidence is reported by Goldberg (1979), in which fathers of preterm infants were more likely to participate in home and laboratory visits than those of full-term infants. Thus, particular concern for the well-being of the infant or awareness of special needs of the infant seemingly overcomes lack of early contact for fathers with preterm infants.

These studies suggest that data on effects of early or extended contact on fathers are not yet clear enough to demonstrate similarities and differences between father and mother experiences. Nevertheless, this appears to be a fruitful area of investigation.

Several reasons for the potential psychological importance of the hours shortly after birth can be offered. First, parenthood represents a major transition in adult development, during which parents may be especially vulnerable to events signifying their new status. First interactions with the infant may therefore be influential in setting the pattern for future interactions or in developing expectations about future interactions. Richards (1979) has suggested that, when professionals whisk the baby away in the delivery room, they convey to the parents that they (professionals) are competent to care for the baby whereas parents are not. Indeed, much of the traditional hospital system for newborn care carries this message. Allowing and encouraging parents to handle and care for their baby at this time signifies to the parents that they are being recognized as competent and responsible for their infants. If this is the case, effects of early contact should be more powerful in primiparous than multiparous parents (a comparison that has not yet been made). In addition, parental self-confidence and expectations should be affected by amount and type of early contact. Only Sostek and Scanlon (Note 6) and Keller and Hildebrandt (Note 10) have reported self-confidence data and did indeed find some relationships between self-confidence or self-esteem and contact experiences. Data on the presence of a supportive companion during labor (Sosa et al., 1980; Klaus et al., Note 7) can also be interpreted to indicate that an intervention that enhances mothers' feelings of being important and supported enhance her ability to engage in affectionate behavior toward the infant after delivery.

Second, it is well documented that parents, especially mothers, develop an idealized image of their baby during pregnancy (e.g., Leifer, 1980). When the actual baby arrives, this idealized image must be reconciled with reality. One function of early or extended contact may be to allow the mother to complete this reconciliation process sooner and therefore to leave the hospital with more realistic expectations of what is to follow. If this is the case, we should find cognitive differences between contact and control groups in perceptions of their infants and in expectations of infant behavior. Although the one study that collected data in this domain (Craig et al., 1982) did not find differences attributable to early contact at 1 month, only one possible area of cognitive effects—the mother's perception of her baby as average, "better," or "worse" than average—was investigated. This by no means exhausts the questions that can be asked in this domain.

And third, as in any dyadic relationship, a certain amount of "getting acquainted" may be necessary before a parent can feel "attached" to the baby. Parents who have had more interaction with their infants via early or extended contact may be further along in the process of getting acquainted than those who have not had this experience. If this were the case, we would expect to find larger effects of extra contact early in development (where a short period of time can represent a large percentage of the actual experience) and smaller or dissipating effects later on. Three of the reviewed studies (Carlsson et al., 1978, 1979; Grossmann et al., 1981; Whiten, 1977) do report this pattern of findings. In general, the short-term effects of extra contact are better documented than long-term effects, but the number of studies with long-term follow-ups is still relatively small. Very little is known as to whether positive effects of early contact exist and whether they eventually disappear. In addition, the provision of early plus extended contact or extended contact alone should have greater effects than early contact alone. This does not appear to be the case (Grossmann et al., 1981).

The above discussion is by no means exhaustive, and the proposed processes are not necessarily mutually exclusive. However, even this brief excursion into possible explanations has indicated some important directions for future research.

1. The study of individual differences can be profitably used in future research to determine how conditions surrounding labor, delivery, and recovery affect maternal responsiveness, how factors such as parity, sex of infant, planned versus unplanned delivery enhance or depress effects of early contact, and whether the affective quality of the first experience is continued in later interactions.

2. Interview and questionnaire data, as well as experimental procedures to assess parental feelings and attitudes and cognitive expectations and perceptions of the infant, are needed to supplement dependent variables in current studies.

3. The study of effects of early contact on adults other than mothers,

particularly fathers, can be helpful in separating physiological and psychological processes underlying effects of contact.

4. Documentation of the actual procedures involved in offering early contact and of the behaviors during the first interactions for both infants and parents is necessary for the adequate interpretation of both existing and future studies.

PRACTICAL IMPLICATIONS

The notion of bonding and the work stimulated by Klaus and Kennell (1976) played an important role in bringing about needed changes in hospital practices surrounding birth. Instead of being regarded as the culmination of a 9-month illness, birth is increasingly recognized and treated as a normal, healthy, and potentially rewarding human experience. However, the popularization of the ideas and work behind these changes has often led to the distorted view that the first hours after birth are critical for the establishment of parent-infant bonding, that parents who miss such opportunities will be impaired in their ability to care for their infants, or that the relatively low-cost "intervention" of 15–60 min of contact in the delivery room can substitute for continuing and more expensive forms of support for disadvantaged parents. The foregoing review suggests that there is no scientific evidence to support these more extreme views and only minimal support for more modest claims concerning the effects of early contact. Most of the important questions have not been asked experimentally, let alone been answered. What does this state of affairs imply for hospital policies?

First, there is minimal evidence that extra contact has negative effects and some evidence of positive effects. Even among these who feel that early contact has been overrated, there are few who would argue that it is unimportant. Initial contacts are one phase in an ongoing process, and parents should be supported in this phase as well as others. Therefore, when not medically contraindicated, the opportunity for early interaction in the delivery or recovery room should be offered in order to make the experience of birth more humane, more positive, and more rewarding for parents.

Second, individual differences in enthusiasm for immediate or even extended contact are normal. Insofar as possible, it is desirable to offer or allow contacts to occur when comfortable and convenient for the parents. The mother who wants or needs time to rest before holding her baby should not be made to feel that she is abnormal for not wanting to do so immediately. The mother who does not prefer rooming in or who does not keep the baby in her room as much as possible should also be made to feel comfortable with her decision.

Finally, the notion of early contact as critical rather than potentially beneficial needs to be dispelled. The emphasis on "early bonding" has already created an expectation on the part of many parents that if they do not have this experience they have somehow failed and will never be fine parents. For all of those who cannot have these experiences because of medical interventions during delivery (e.g., Caesarean section) or problems with the infant's health (e.g., premature birth), it is important to emphasize that the parent-infant relationship is a complex system with many fail-safe or alternative routes to the same outcome. Its success or failure does not hinge on a few brief moments in time. It would be irresponsible of us as professionals to encourage this incorrect and extreme view.

REFERENCE NOTES

1. Taylor, P. M., Taylor, F. H., Campbell, S. B., Maloni, J., & Dickey, D. (1979, March). *Effects of extra contact on early maternal attitudes, perceptions, and behaviors.* Paper presented at the biennial meeting of the Society for Research in Child Development, San Francisco.
2. Gaulin-Kremer, E., Shaw, J. L. & Thoman, E. B. (1977, March). *Mother-infant interaction at first prolonged encounter: Effects of variation in delay after delivery.* Paper presented at the biennial meeting of the Society for Research in Child Development, New Orleans.
3. Hopkins, J. B. & Vietze, P. (1977, March). *Postpartum early and extended contact: Quality, quantity, or both?* Paper presented at the biennial meeting of the Society for Research in Child Development, New Orleans.
4. O'Connor, S., Vietze, P., Sandler, H., Sherrod, K., & Altemeier, W. (1981, April). *Response transitions during mother-infant interaction after extended postpartum contact.* Paper presented at the biennial meeting of the Society for Research in Child Development, Boston.
5. Anisfeld, E., & Lipper, E. (1981, April). *Effects of perinatal events on mother-infant bonding.* Paper presented at the biennial meeting of the Society for Research in Child Development, Boston. (Available from first author at Columbia School of Public Health, New York, New York 10027.)
6. Sostek, A. M., & Scanlon, J. W. (1980). *Effects of postpartum contact on maternal attitude.* Paper presented at the International Conference on Infant Studies, New Haven, Conn.
7. Klaus, M., Kennell, J., & Sosa, R. (1981). *Child health and breast feeding: The effect of a supportive woman (doula) during labor and the effect of early suckling.* Unpublished paper, Pediatrics Department, Case Western Reserve University.
8. Gewirtz, J. L. (1979, March). *Maternal "attachment" outcomes.* Paper presented at the biennial meeting of the Society for Research in Child Development, San Francisco.
9. Keller, W. D., Hildebrandt, K. A., & Richards, M. (1981, April). *Effects of extended father-infant contact during the newborn period.* Paper presented at the biennial meeting of the Society for Research in Child Development, Boston.

10. Keller, W. D., & Hildebrandt, K. A. (1982). *Changes in father's self-concepts as a function of presence at birth and extended postpartum contact.* Manuscript submitted for publication.
11. Marton, P., Minde, K., & Perrotta, M. (1981). *The interaction of fathers with infants at risk.* Manuscript submitted for publication.

REFERENCES

Ali, Z. & Lowry, M. (1981). Early maternal-child contact: Effects on later behavior. *Developmental Medicine and Child Neurology*, **23**, 337–345.

Benedek, T. (1970). The psychobiology of pregnancy. In E. J. Anthony & T. Benedek (Eds.) *Parenthood: Its psychology and psychopathology.* Boston: Little, Brown.

Bibring, G. L. (1961). A study of the psychological processes in pregnancy and the earliest mother-child relationship. *Psychoanalytic Study of the Child*, **16**, 9–44.

Brazelton, T. B. (1973). *Neonatal Behavioral Assessment Scales.* London: Heinemann.

Brown, J., & Bakeman, R. (1979). Relationships of human mothers with their infants during the first year of life. In R. W. Bell & W. P. Smotherman (Eds.), *Maternal influences and early behavior.* Jamaica, N.Y.: Spectrum.

Butterfield, P. M., & Emde, R. N. (1978). Effects of silver nitrate on initial visual behavior. *American Journal of Diseases of Childhood*, **132**, 426.

Butterfield, P. M., Emde, R. N., & Svejda, M. J. (1981). Does the early application of silver nitrate impair maternal attachment? *Pediatrics*, **67**, 737–738.

Butterfield, P. M., Emde, R. N., Svejda, M. J. & Naiman, S. (1982). Silver nitrate and the eyes of the newborn. In R. N. Emde & R. J. Harmon (Eds.), *Attachment and affiliative systems.* New York: Plenum.

Campbell, S., & Taylor, P. M. (1980). Bonding and attachment: Theoretical issues. *Seminars in Perinatology*, **3**, 3–14.

Carek, D. J., & Capelli, A. J. (1981). Mothers' reactions to their newborn infants. *Journal of the American Academy of Child Psychiatry*, **20**, 16–31.

Carey, W. B. (1973). Measuring infant temperament in pediatric practice. In J. C. Westman (Ed.), *Individual differences in children.* New York: Wiley.

Carlsson, S. G., Fagerberg, H., Horneman, G., Hwang, P., Larsson, K., Rödholm, M., Schaller, J., Danielsson, B., & Gundewal, C. (1978). Effects of amount of contact between mother and child on the mother's nursing behavior. *Developmental Psychobiology*, **11**, 143–150.

Carlsson, S. G., Fagerberg, H., Horneman, G., Hwang, P., Larsson, K., Rödholm, M., Schaller, J., Daniellson, B., & Gundewal, C. (1979). Effects of various amounts of contact between mother and child on the mother's nursing behavior: A follow-up study. *Infant Behavior and Development*, **2**, 209–214.

Chess, S., & Thomas, A. (1982). Infant-parent bonding: Myth or reality. *American Journal of Orthopsychiatry*, **52**, 213–222.

Craig, S., Tyson, J. E., Samson, J., & Lasky, R. E. (1982). The effect of early contact on maternal perception of infant behavior. *Early Human Development*, **6**, 197–204.

Curry, M.A. (1979). Contact during the first hour with the wrapped or naked newborn: Effect on maternal attachment behaviors at 36 hours and 3 months. *Birth and the Family Journal*, **6**, 227–236.

de Chateau, P. (1980). Effects of hospital practices on synchrony in the development of the infant-parent relationship. In P. M. Taylor (Ed.), *Parent-infant relationships.* New York: Grune & Stratton.

de Chateau, P., Holmberg, H., Jacobsson, K., & Winberg, J. (1977). A study of factors promoting lactation. *Developmental Medicine and Child Neurology*, **19**, 575–584.

de Chateau, P., & Wiberg, B. (1977). Long-term effect on mother-infant behavior of extra contact during the first hour post-partum, I: First observations at 36 hours. *Acta Paediatrica Scandinavica*, **66**, 137–143. (a)

de Chateau, P., & Wiberg, B. (1977). Long-term effect on mother-infant behavior of extra contact during the first hour post-partum, II: A follow-up at three months. *Acta Paediatrica Scandinavica*, **66**, 145–151. (b)

Desmond, N. M., Rudolph, A. J., & Phitakophraiwan, P. (1966). The transitional care nursery: A mechanism for preventive medicine in the newborn. *Pediatric Clinics of North America*, **13**, 651–668.

Emde, R., Swedberg, J., & Suzuki, B. (1975). Human wakefulness and biological rhythms after birth. *Archives of General Psychiatry*, **32**, 780.

Goldberg, S. (1979). Pragmatics and problems of longitudinal research with high risk infants. In T. Field, A. Sostek, S. Goldberg, & H. H. Shuman (Eds.), *Infants born at risk*. Holliswood, N.Y.: Spectrum.

Goldberg, S. (1982). Some biological aspects of early parent-infant interaction. In S. G. Moore & C. R. Cooper (Eds.), *The young child: Reviews of research*. Washington, D.C.: National Association for the Education of Young Children.

Grossmann, K. (1978). Die wirkung des augenöffnens von neugebornen auf das verhatten ihrer mütter. *Geburtschifte und Frauenheilkunde*, **38**, 629–635.

Grossmann, K., Thane, K., & Grossmann, K. E. (1981). Maternal tactual contact of the newborn after various conditions of mother-infant contact. *Developmental Psychology*, **17**, 158–169.

Hales, D. J., Lozoff, B., Sosa, R., & Kennell, J. H. (1977). Defining the limits of the maternal sensitive period. *Developmental Medicine and Child Neurology*, **19**, 454–461.

Harmon, R. J. (1981). The perinatal period: Infants and parents. In E. Brody (Ed.), *Clinical medicine*. (Vol. **12**): *Psychiatry*. Hagerstown, Md.: Harper & Row.

Kennell, J. H., Jerauld, R., Wolfe, H., Chesler, D., Kreger, N. C., McAlpine, W., Steffa, M., & Klaus, M. H. (1974). Maternal behavior one year after early and extended postpartum contact. *Developmental Medicine and Child Neurology*, **16**, 172–179.

Kennell, J. H., Trause, M., & Klaus, M. H. (1975). Evidence for a sensitive period in the human mother. In *Parent-infant interaction*, CIBA Foundation Symposium No. 33. Amsterdam: Elsevier.

Klaus, M. H., Jerauld, R., Kreger, N., McAlpine, W. Steffa, M., & Kennell, J. H. (1972). Maternal attachment: Importance of the first postpartum days. *New England Journal of Medicine*, **286**, 460–463.

Klaus, M. H., & Kennell, J. H. (1976). *Maternal-infant bonding*. St. Louis: Mosby.

Klaus, M. H., & Kennell, J. H. (1982). *Parent-infant bonding*. St. Louis: Mosby.

Klaus, M. H., Kennell, J. H., Plumb, N., & Zuelke, S. (1970). Human maternal behavior at first contact with her young. *Pediatrics*, **46**, 187–192.

Kontos, D. K. (1977). *The effects of mother-infant separation in the early postpartum hours and days on later maternal attachment behavior.* Unpublished doctoral dissertation, Ontario Institute for Studies in Education.

Kontos, D. (1978). A study of the effects of extended mother-infant contact on maternal behavior at one and three months. *Birth and Family Journal*, **5**, 133–140.

Lamb, M. E., & Hwang, C. P. (1982). Maternal attachment and mother-neonate bonding: A critical review. In M. E. Lamb & A. L. Brown (Eds.), *Advances in developmental psychology* (Vol. **2**). Hillsdale, N.J.: Erlbaum.

Leiderman, P. H. (1982). The critical period hypothesis revisited: Mother to infant social bonding in the neonatal period. In K. Immelman, G. Barlow, M. Main, & L. Petrinovich (Eds.), *Issues in behavioral development: The Bielefeld Interdisciplinary Conference.* Cambridge: Cambridge University Press.

Leifer, M. (1980). *Psychological effects of motherhood: A study of first pregnancy.* New York: Praeger Science.

Newton, N., & Newton, M. (1962). Mothers' reactions to their newborn babies. *Journal of the American Medical Association,* **181**, 206–211.

O'Connor, S., Vietze, P., Sandler, H., Sherrod, K., & Altemeier, W. (1980). Quality of parenting and the mother-infant relationship following rooming in. In P. Taylor (Ed.), *Parent-infant relationships.* New York: Grune & Stratton. (a)

O'Connor, S., Vietze, P. M., Sherrod, K. B., Sandler, H. M., & Altemeier, W. A. (1980). Reduced incidence of parenting inadequacy following rooming-in. *Pediatrics,* **66**, 176–182. (b)

Packer, M., & Rosenblatt, D. (1979). Issues in the study of social behavior in the first week of life. In D. Shaffer & J. Dunn (Eds.), *The first year of life.* New York: Wiley.

Pannabecker, B. J., Emde, R. N., & Austin, B. C. (1982). The effect of early extended contact on father-newborn interaction. *Journal of Genetic Psychology,* **141**, 7–17.

Richards, M. P. M. (1979). Effects on development of medical interventions and the separation of newborns from their parents. In D. Shaffer & J. Dunn (Eds.), *The first year of life.* New York: Wiley.

Ringler, N. M., Kennell, J. H., Jarvella, R., Navojosky, B. J., & Klaus, M. H. (1975). Mother-to-child speech at 2 years: Effects of early post-natal contact. *Journal of Pediatrics,* **86**, 141–144.

Robson, K. S., & Moss, H. A. (1970). Patterns and determinants of maternal attachment. *Journal of Pediatrics,* **77**, 976–985.

Rodholm, M. (1981). Effects of father-infant post-partum contact on their interaction 3 months after birth. *Early Human Development,* **5**, 79–86.

Schaller, J., Carlsson, S. G., & Larsson, K. (1979). Effects of extended post-partum mother-child contact on the mother's behavior during nursing. *Infant Behavior and Development,* **2**, 319–324.

Shereshefsky, P., & Yarrow, L. (1973). *Psychological aspects of a first pregnancy and early postnatal adaptation.* New York: Raven.

Siegel, E., Bauman, K. E., Schaefer, E. S., Saunders, M. M., & Ingram, D. D. (1980). Hospital and home support during infancy: Impact on maternal attachment, child abuse and neglect, and health care utilization. *Pediatrics,* **66**, 183–190.

Sosa, R., Kennell, J., Klaus, M., Robertson, S., & Urutia, J. (1980). The effect of a supportive companion on perinatal problems, length of labor, and mother-infant interaction. *New England Journal of Medicine,* **303**, 597–600.

Sosa, R., Kennell, J., Klaus, M., & Urutia, J. (1976). The effects of early mother-infant contact on breast-feeding, infection, and growth. In *Breast-feeding and the mother,* CIBA Foundation Symposium No. 45. Amsterdam: Associated Scientific.

Sousa, P. L. R., Barros, F. C., Gazalle, R. V., Begères, R. M., Pinbeiro, G. N., Menzes, S. T., & Arruda, L. A. (1974). Attachment and lactation. In *Proceedings of the Fourteenth International Congress of Pediatrics, Buenos Aires.* Paris: International Pediatric Association.

Svejda, M. J., Campos, J. J., & Emde, R. N. (1980). Mother-infant bonding: Failure to generalize. *Child Development,* **51**, 775–779.

Svejda, M. J., Pannabecker, B. J., & Emde, R. N. (1982). Parent-to-infant attachment: A critique of the early "bonding" model. In R. N. Emde & R. J. Harmon (Eds.), *Attachment and affiliative systems*. New York: Plenum.

Thomson, M. E., Hartsock, G., & Larson, C. (1979). The importance of immediate post-natal contact: Its effect on breast-feeding. *Canadian Family Physician, 25,* 1374–1378.

Vietze, P. M., & O'Connor, S. (1981). Mother-to-infant bonding: A review. In N. Kretchmer & J. Brasel (Eds.), *Biomedical and social bases of pediatrics*. New York, Masson.

Whiten, A. (1977). Assessing the effects of perinatal events on the success of the mother-infant relationship. In H. R. Shaffer (Ed.) *Studies of mother-infant interaction*. New York: Academic Press.

3

Social Referencing at Ten Months: A Second-Order Effect on Infants' Responses to Strangers

Saul Feinman
University of Wyoming

Michael Lewis
Rutgers Medical School

One pathway through which second-order effects may proceed is social referencing, a process in which the individual utilizes another's interpretation when appraising a situation. This phenomenon is well identified in adults and older children. There are indications that the necessary cognitive and social skills for social referencing may emerge in the second half of the first year. 87 10-month-old boys and girls received positive or neutral nonverbal messages, or no message, about a stranger either directly from the mother when she spoke to the infant, or indirectly when the infant observed her speaking to the stranger.

Reprinted with permission from *Child Development*, 1983, Vol. 54, 878–887. Copyright 1983 by the Society for Research in Child Development, Inc.

During the course of this project, the first author was supported by NIMH National Research Service award 1F32MH07625–01 while at Educational Testing Service, and by NIMH grant 1R03MH35384–01A1 at the University of Wyoming. Additional support was provided by an Arts and Sciences Basic Research Grant from the University of Wyoming. The second author was supported by BEH grant 300–77–0307. Research assistance was provided by Judith Hayes, Sung-Young Hong, Susan Jones, Robin Adelstein, Vickie Martin, Edie Plancher, and especially by Pam Ritter. Thanks are extended to Steve Bieber, Gary Hampe, Ceva Katz, Marsha Weinraub, and the anonymous reviewers for their helpful comments and suggestions. The present paper is based, in part, on a paper prepared for the symposium on "Conceptualizing Second Order Effects in Infancy" at the biennial meeting of the Society for Research in Child Development, Boston, Massachusetts, April 1981.

Infants were friendlier to the stranger when the mothers had spoken positively rather than neutrally, but only when the message had been provided directly to the infants. This effect was especially strong for infants of easy temperament classification. These results are discussed with regard to the process of social referencing and alternative explanations as well.

The location of dyads within broader social contexts renders them susceptible to "second-order" or "indirect" effects (Bronfenbrenner, 1974; Lewis & Weinraub, 1976; Parke, 1979), that is, the influence that a third person has on dyadic interaction. Indeed, the presence, stimulation, and support of a third person often influences the infant's interaction within a dyad (Clarke-Stewart, 1978a; Lamb, 1978; Lewis & Feiring, 1981; Parke, 1979; Pedersen, Anderson, & Cain, 1980). For example, infant response to strangers can be affected by the caregiver's presence and proximity (Campos, Emde, Gaensbauer, & Henderson, 1975; Feinman, 1980).

A primary caregiver is often viewed as the infant's "secure base," providing emotional comfort (Ainsworth, Blehar, Waters, & Wall, 1978). In addition to being a *base of security*, a caregiver may also serve as a *base of information*, influencing the infant's appraisal of ambiguous and new events, for example, meeting a stranger. This social influence process, long recognized in older humans, has been called *social referencing* (Feinman, 1982; Klinnert, Campos, Sorce, & Emde, 1982). The present study considers whether social referencing occurs when 10-month-olds and their mothers meet an unfamiliar adult.

Social referencing is characterized by the use of one's perception of other persons' interpretations of the situation to form one's own understanding of that situation. Such interpretations may be requested by the individual, or they may be received and used although not actually solicited. Social referencing information can be conveyed directly, when others inform the individual of their interpretations, or it can be acquired indirectly, when the individual infers others' interpretations from their behavioral responses. Indeed, social referencing is the hallmark of a multitude of social psychological theories such as those of social comparison (Festinger, 1954), affiliation (Schachter, 1959), conformity (Sherif, 1958), and the looking-glass self (Cooley, 1902).

There is evidence that social referencing may emerge in the second half year. First, during this period, infants begin to evaluate events as if judging their likely consequences, and then basing action upon appraisal (Piaget, 1952; Schaffer, Greenwood, & Parry, 1972). Second, infants often look toward caregivers when encountering a new toy or person (e.g., Carr, Dabbs, & Carr, 1975; Rheingold & Eckerman, 1973), which may reflect the infant's use of the caregiver as a base of information. Similarly, while infants' distress when mothers are present but do not interact with their infants (Fein, 1975; Sorce & Emde, 1981) may be due to the caregiver's emotional unavailability (Sorce & Emde, 1981), such responses might occur because the caregiver is informationally unavailable.

Third, infants 6 months or older imitate unfamiliar behaviors (e.g., Eckerman, Whatley, & McGhee, 1979), which may indicate that others' responses are being used by the infant as a guide for interpretation of the situation. Fourth, by 6 months, infants distinguish among and react appropriately to emotional expression (Charlesworth & Kreutzer, 1973). Since verbal comprehension during the second semester appears to be minimal (e.g., Bates, Benigni, Bretherton, Camaioni, & Volterra, 1979), the emergence of sensitivity to emotion is a significant development inasmuch as early social referencing probably relies heavily on nonverbal affective cues.

Other studies provide more specific indications of infant social referencing. Clarke-Stewart (1978b) found no significant differences in the behavior of 30-month-olds to a stranger after viewing either a friendly or a hostile stranger-mother interaction. In contrast, Lewis and Feiring (1981) noted that 15-month-olds were more receptive to a stranger who was seen interacting positively with their mothers than to one who had done so with another stranger or not at all. The relative influence of mother's and stranger's behavior in this situation could not be determined. In data reported by Feinman (1980), 7–15-month-olds were especially likely to move either toward or away from an approaching stranger after looking toward or touching their mothers. But the data did not allow for the examination of whether such patterns were due to affective variations provided in mothers' facial and tactile cues.

In the present study, infants received nonverbally positive or neutral messages about a stranger from their mothers. The message was conveyed either directly when mothers spoke to their infants about the stranger, or indirectly when their infants saw them greet the stranger. Mothers also completed an infant temperament questionnaire.

The central prediction was that the infant would be friendlier to the stranger when the mother provided a positive rather than a neutral message. But infants may have difficulty understanding indirect messages, as suggested by the finding that when mothers interact pleasantly with a stranger, 18-month-olds avoid the stranger (Fein, 1975). Infants may not perceive the caregiver's interaction with a new person as an opportunity to learn about that person but, rather, may use such interaction to judge the mother's availability. This study also evaluated the relative efficacy of direct compared to indirect messages about the stranger.

Since it was also important to consider whether there were infant characteristics that could account for individual differences in social referencing, the effect of temperament was investigated. While there is some evidence that older children's learning and school performance are affected by temperament (Carey, Fox, & McDevitt, 1977; Thomas & Chess, 1977), there is a dearth of research concerning the effect of temperament on infant learning and receptivity. It seems reasonable, though, to suspect that features ascribed to easier-temperament infants, for example, adaptability and calmness, might incline them to greater receptivity to their mothers' communication about the stranger.

METHOD

Participants.—Eighty-seven 10-month-old infants—46 girls and 41 boys—participated in the study. Two boys participated with their fathers, both of whom were significant caregivers. One father insisted that he, rather than his wife, accompany their child. Since 98% of the infants participated with their mothers, the term "mother" is used in place of the term "caregiver."

Setting and procedure.—At the onset of the experimental session, the infant was in a high chair, and the mother sat to the infant's right. The chair in which the stranger would sit was to the infant's left. The door through which the stranger entered faced the infant. Four tape marks were placed on the floor to indicate to the stranger where to stop during the approach.

Two components of the study were of interest in the analysis presented below: the stranger approach and the nonintrusive phase. In the approach, the stranger—a 23-year-old female—entered the room, and in sequence, walked and stopped for 5 sec at each mark. The mother provided a message each time the stranger paused. In the control condition, the mother did not speak during the approach. After standing at the fourth mark—which was located in front of the empty chair—the stranger sat down, initiating the nonintrusive phase, and looked through a magazine for the next minute. The mother gave her infant a toy when the stranger sat down but did not interact with infant or stranger. The experimental session was videotaped by two cameras in the corner of the room to the left of the door. One camera focused on the infant's face and the other included infant, mother, and stranger.

The direct-influence conditions called for mothers to speak to their infants in either a positive or a neutral tone about the stranger. In the indirect-influence conditions, they spoke to the stranger in either a positive or neutral voice tone. Thus, nonverbal affect—positive or neutral—and direction of communication—to the infant or to the stranger—were varied in the experimental design.

Temperament questionnaire.—Mothers' responses to Carey and McDevitt's (1978) Revised Infant Temperament Questionnaire (RITQ) were used to classify infants as easy or difficult. The former category consisted of Carey and McDevitt's easy and intermediate-low groups, and the latter consisted of the intermediate-high, difficult, and slow-to-warm-up groups. Slightly less than half of the 87 infants (49%) were in the easy temperament category.

Coding of infant behavior.—For coding purposes, the 1-min nonintrusive period was divided into four 15-sec segments. In each period, coding was performed for the presence of the following behaviors: (1) smiling to the stranger, (2) smiling to the mother, (3) proximity to the stranger (moved toward or stayed near the stranger), (4) proximity to the mother (moved toward or stayed near the mother), (5) toy offer to the stranger, and (6) toy offer to the mother. Proximity was measured by the infant's movement within the range permitted by the high chair restraints, that is, leaning over the side of the chair toward stranger or mother.

Intercoder agreement, based on the judgments of one coder who considered all cases, and a second coder who viewed half of the cases, was 90% or better for all behaviors. Dependent measures that indicated the number of 15-sec periods in which the infant had performed each behavior to the stranger were created from these codes. Three additional variables were created: (1) smiles to the stranger minus smiles to the mother, (2) proximity to the stranger minus proximity to the mother, and (3) toy offers to the stranger minus toy offers to the mother. Two summed measures were also constructed: (1) the sum of smiles, proximity, and toy offers to the stranger, and (2) the sum of behaviors to the stranger minus the sum of behaviors to the mother. Crying was coded but was not included in data analysis because of its extremely low frequency (less than 1% of coded responses).

RESULTS AND DISCUSSION

Independent variable manipulation checks.—Nonverbal affective quality and length of mother's message were coded in order to evaluate the manipulation of the affect conditions and to determine whether affect and length were correlated. Since the 17 mothers in the control condition did not speak, these procedures could not be performed for them. Length of message was measured by two ways—by the number of words and by the number of syllables. Intercoder agreement, indicated by the correlation between one coder who listened to all 70 cases and another who listened to 35 cases, was .99 for both measures of length. Syllables and words were highly correlated ($r = .99$); the number-of-words measure was used in analysis since it possessed clearer natural meaning. Affect was coded on a scale from -8 (extremely negative) to $+8$ (extremely positive) with an intercoder correlation of .95 for the 35 cases considered by both coders.

For two mothers, the rated affects were found to be inappropriate for the assigned affect condition, and these two participants were excluded from further analysis. Mothers spoke more words in the positive than in the neutral condition, $F(1,60) = 5.74$, $p < .02$, and were marginally more talkative to their infants than to the stranger, $F(1,60) = 3.45$, $p < .07$. Length of message was negatively correlated with several measures of infant behavior, either significantly or at a level approaching significance. Consequently, length of message was used as a covariate in further analyses. Rated affect was higher in the positive than in the neutral condition, $F(1,59) = 311.63$, $p < .001$, indicating that affect of mother's message had been effectively manipulated.

Analysis of variance.—The key consideration of the social referencing hypothesis logically focuses on whether infant behavior to the stranger is influenced by affect of the mother's message. Therefore, the major thrust of data analysis was directed to the 68 infants whose mothers spoke during the stranger's approach and did not include the 17 control-condition infants. The primary data analysis consisted of analyses of variance that included: the measures of infant behavior as the dependent criteria; affect (positive or neutral) and direction (to the infant or to the stranger) of the mother's message, and infant temperament (easy or difficult) as the independent factors; and length of message as a covariate. Means presented in Table 1 were derived from these analyses and adjusted to remove the effect of message length (see Dixon, Brown, Engelman, Frane, Hill, Jennrich, & Toporek, 1981, pp. 675–677, for the computational procedure used in the computer generation of the adjusted means). Several of the dependent measures had positively skewed distributions, and therefore ANOVAs were also calculated using a $\log_{10} (x + 1)$ transformation (Winer, 1971, p. 400). Since these results did not differ from those for the raw data, only the results for the nontransformed data are presented here. For comparison purposes, results involving the control condition are presented in Table 2.

TABLE 1

MEAN FREQUENCIES OF INFANT SMILING, PROXIMITY, AND TOY OFFERS BY
AFFECT AND DIRECTION OF MOTHER'S MESSAGE AND INFANT
TEMPERAMENT ADJUSTED TO REMOVE THE EFFECT
OF LENGTH OF MESSAGE

Mother's Message to: Temperament Category:	Infant Easy (8/8)[a]	Infant Difficult (8/9)[a]	Stranger Easy (9/9)[a]	Stranger Difficult (9/8)[a]
Smiles to stranger:				
Positive affect	1.81	1.17	.44	1.04
Neutral affect	.12	.46	1.15	.92
Positive − neutral	1.69	.71	− .71	.12
Smiles to stranger − smiles to mother:				
Positive affect	.28	.36	− .45	.44
Neutral affect	− .88	− .41	− .08	− .58
Positive − neutral	1.16	.77	− .37	1.02
Proximity to stranger:				
Positive affect	1.77	.97	.45	.55
Neutral affect	.37	1.03	.04	.57
Positive − neutral	1.40	− .06	.41	− .02
Proximity to stranger − proximity to mother:				
Positive affect	− .18	−1.37	− .44	− .53
Neutral affect′..............	−1.01	.04	−1.46	− .62
Positive − neutral	.83	−1.41	1.02	.09
Toy offers to stranger:				
Positive affect	.39	.01	.11	.23
Neutral affect	.00	.11	.10	.11
Positive − neutral	.39	− .10	.01	.12
Toy offers to stranger − toy offers to mother:				
Positive affect	.44	− .08	− .22	.26
Neutral affect	− .38	− .33	− .52	− .20
Positive − neutral	.82	.25	.30	.46
Behavior[b] to stranger:				
Positive affect	3.96	2.15	1.00	1.82
Neutral affect	.50	1.60	1.29	1.60
Positive − neutral	3.46	.55	− .29	.22
Behavior[b] to stranger − behavior[b] to mother:				
Positive affect	.53	−1.09	−1.11	.18
Neutral affect	−2.25	− .70	−2.07	−1.40
Positive − neutral	2.78	− .39	.96	1.58

[a] In each pair, the first N refers to the positive-affect condition and the second N refers to
the neutral-affect condition.
[b] The sum of smiles, proximity, and toy offers.

Effects of affect, direction, and temperament on infant behavior to the stranger: noncontrol conditions.—The overall effect of mother's affect on infant smiling to the stranger was not significant, but there was an affect × direction interaction, $F(1,59) = 6.07$, $p < .01$. Infants whose mothers spoke directly to them smiled more often in the positive ($M = 1.49$) than the neutral condition ($M = 0.30;F[1,59] = 7.63$, $p < .01$; Table 1). But when mothers spoke to the stranger, affect did not influence smiling. Proximity to the stranger was influenced by mother's affect at a level approaching conventional significance, $F(1,59) = 3.76$, $p < .06$, and by the interaction of affect and temperament, $F(1,59) = 4.86$, $p < .04$. While affect did not influence difficult infants' proximity to the stranger, easy infants were near the stranger more often after positive ($M = 1.07$) than after neutral communication ($M = 0.19$; $F[1,59] = 8.66$, $p < .01$; Table 1).

The ANOVA for toy offers to the stranger detected a three-way interaction of affect, direction, and temperament that approached significance, $F(1,59) = 3.19$, $p < .08$. It was only when mothers spoke directly to easy infants that there were more toy offers after positive than after neutral messages, $F(1,59) = 5.17$, $p < .03$ (Table 1). For the summed measure of behavior to the stranger (smiles, proximity, and toy offers), infants displayed friendly behavior more often in the positive ($M = 2.18$) than in the neutral condition ($M = 1.26$; $F[1,59] = 5.00$, $p < .03$). Affect and direction interacted, $F(1,59) = 5.82$, $p < .02$; affect had no influence in the indirect condition, but infants whose mothers spoke directly to them displayed more friendly behavior to the stranger in the positive condition ($M = 3.06$) than in the neutral condition ($M = 1.08$; $F[1,59] = 10.75$, $p < .005$; Table 1). There was also a significant inter-

TABLE 2

MEAN FREQUENCIES OF THE SUM OF INFANT BEHAVIOR BY AFFECT AND DIRECTION
OF MOTHER'S MESSAGE AND INFANT TEMPERAMENT

Mother's Message to: Temperament Category:	Infant Easy (8/8)[a]	Infant Difficult (8/9)[a]	Control Easy (8)[a]	Control Difficult (9)[a]	Stranger Easy (9/9)[a]	Stranger Difficult (9/8)[a]
Behavior[b] to stranger:						
Positive affect	3.75	2.00	...	...	1.00	1.67
Control	...	...	1.75	1.22	...	...
Neutral affect	.50	1.56	...	...	1.56	1.88
Behavior[b] to stranger − behavior[b] to mother:						
Positive affect	.13	−1.38	...	...	−1.11	− .11
Control	...	...	− .25	−1.11	...	...
Neutral affect	−2.25	− .78	...	...	−1.56	− .88

[a] In each pair, the first N refers to the positive-affect condition and the second N refers to the neutral-affect condition.

[b] The sum of smiles, proximity, and toy offers.

action of affect with direction and temperament, $F(1,59) = 4.08, p < .05$. Of the four direction × temperament conditions, a significant impact of affect was found only when mothers spoke directly to infants of easy temperament, $F(1,59) = 15.92, p < .001$ (Table 1).

Social referencing and alternative explanations.—Rather than understand the mother's message as information about the stranger, the infant might take the mother's nonverbal affect as an indication of her interest in interacting with the infant, particularly when the mother speaks to the infant. An invitation-to-interact hypothesis predicts that infants will be friendlier to the mother but not to the stranger in the positive than in the neutral condition. But the positive influence of mother's affect on infant behavior to the stranger indicates that this alternative explanation does not account for the results.

A more compelling alternative is that the mother's message modifies the infant's mood, which in turn shapes behavior to the stranger. There still would be a second-order effect, but not due to an alteration of the infant's appraisal of the stranger. In the mood-modification hypothesis, the positive message elicits a more favorable mood leading to higher frequencies of friendly behavior to mother as well as to the stranger than does the neutral message. In social referencing, mother's affect is used by the infant as information about the stranger specifically. There is a positive impact of mother's affect on infant behavior to the stranger but no such effect, or a much smaller one, for behavior to the mother.

In order to compare the social referencing and the mood-modification hypotheses, analyses of variance were calculated for the measures of behavior to the stranger minus behavior to the mother. In mood modification, mother's affect will not have a significant effect on measures of infant's behavior to the stranger minus behavior to the mother. But if social referencing occurs, the frequency of friendly behavior to the stranger minus that to the mother will still be higher in the positive condition than in the neutral condition.

For the measure of smiling to the stranger minus smiling to the mother, there was no affect × direction interaction. But when mothers spoke directly to their infants, this measure was still greater in the positive $(M = 0.32)$ than the neutral condition $(M = -0.63; F[1,59] = 4.28, p < .05$; Table 1). There was no such effect when mothers spoke to the stranger. For easy infants, the measure of proximity to the stranger minus proximity to the mother was marginally greater after positive communication $(M = -0.32)$ than after neutral communication $(M = -1.25; F[1,59] = 2.81, p < .10)$. The affect × temperament interaction was also maintained, $F(1,59) = 4.02, p < .05$ (Table 1). The measure of toy offers to the stranger minus those to the mother did not display the three-way interaction found for toy offers to the stranger. But it was only when mothers spoke directly to easy infants that a significant impact of mother's affect was detected for this measure, $F(1,59) = 7.97$, $p < .01$ (Table 1). This result was similar to that found for toy offers to the stranger.

For the summary measure, the overall influence of affect on behavior to the stranger was maintained when behavior to the mother was subtracted, $F(1,59) = 4.06$, $p < .05$. The affect × direction interaction was not significant for the measure of summed behaviors to the stranger minus those to the mother, and the previously noted tendency for infants in the direct condition to be friendlier to the stranger when mother spoke positively was no longer significant. Although the three-way interaction was not significant for the measure of behaviors to the stranger minus behaviors to the mother, a significant impact of mother's affect was still found only when she spoke directly to easy infants, $F(1,59) = 5.05$, $p < .03$ (Table 1), as had been noted for the summed behaviors to the stranger.

The influence of affect on the sum of behaviors to the stranger was, in general, maintained even after behavior to the mother was subtracted. The only exception was the absence of an overall affect of affect when the mother spoke directly to the infant. But even for behaviors to the stranger, this result was the statistical combination of a sizable significant effect for easy infants and a small nonsignificant effect for difficult infants. Overall, the influence of mother's affect on infant behavior seemed to be more accurately predicted by the social referencing hypothesis.

Methodological considerations.—Could the greater impact of mother's affect on infant's behavior to the stranger than to the mother derive from a restricted range or very low frequency of behavior to the mother in a situation where the stranger is the infant's primary focus? Inspection of the data suggested that behavior was not any less frequent to the mother than to the stranger. Indeed, for the summary measures there was actually more friendly behavior to the mother than to the stranger, $F(1,62) = 9.84$, $p < .01$. Similarly, the ranges and variances were not larger for behaviors to the stranger than to the mother.

Another question is raised by the finding that mothers' rated affect was more positive when they spoke to their infants than to the stranger, $F(1,59) = 26.00$, $p < .001$. Could this difference account for the greater social referencing effect in the direct than in the indirect condition? This explanation seems unlikely given that the distance between rated affect for the positive and neutral conditions did not vary as a function of communication direction.

One further possibility is that the relationship of mother's affect and infant behavior is curvilinear, in that influence emerges only at highly positive affect. If so, then the rated affect differences between mother's communication to the infant and to the stranger might account for the absence of an effect of affect in the indirect condition. To consider this explanation, all ANOVAs were repeated, but with infants whose mothers had spoken very positively excluded from the sample. The results were consistent with those reported above, with no indication that the impact of mother's affect was found only at the highest levels of that variable.

Since receptive word comprehension appears to be very limited at 10 months (Bates et al., 1979; Benedict, 1979; Thomas, Campos, Shucard, Ramsay, & Shucard, 1981), it seems unlikely that the semantic content of the message could explain the impact of the mother's message. Inasmuch as mothers' speech to their infants has been found to be more semantically repetitious and less syntactically complex (Messer, 1980; Phillips, 1973; Snow, 1972), could the absence of an effect of the mother's communication in the indirect condition have been due to such variations? To consider this possibility, the mother's message was coded for three measures of repetition and complexity: (1) the number of syllables divided by the number of words; (2) the type token ratio, that is, the number of different words divided by the total number of words; and (3) the number of words per utterance.

The use of polysyllabic words did not vary as a function of affect or direction of message, or of infant temperament. Although mothers used shorter utterances when speaking to their infants, $F(1,60) = 5.26$, $p < .03$, and when speaking positively, $F(1,60) = 5.21$, $p < .03$, the words-per-utterance measure was not correlated with any of the infant behavior measures. Mothers' speech also displayed a greater variety of words (type token ratio) to the stranger, $F(1,60) = 11.77$, $p < .002$, and there were borderline positive correlations between the type token ratio and three infant behaviors. But repetition of the ANOVAs for all infant behavior measures, with the three complexity indicators included as additional covariates, did not yield results that differed from those reported above, suggesting that complexity and repetition could not explain the impact of the mother's message on infant behavior.

Since temperament classifications were based on mothers' perceptions of infant behavior, could the effects ascribed to temperament be due not to temperament per se but, rather, to differences in the way mothers spoke to easy and difficult infants? Temperament classification did not have an overall effect on rated affect. Furthermore, the significant interaction of affect, direction, and temperament, $F(1,59) = 6.37$, $p < .02$, was due primarily to the larger magnitude of the positive-neutral difference in rated affect when mothers of difficult infants spoke to the stranger as compared to the other three direction $\times$ temperament conditions, $F(1,59) = 5.96$, $p < .02$. When mothers spoke to their infants, scored temperament did not significantly influence rated affect. While some investigators have suggested that parents' reports of infant behavior may not yield accurate ratings of infant temperament (Bates, Bennett Freeland, & Lounsbury, 1979; Vaughn, Taraldson, Crichton, & Egeland, 1981), the impact of direction and temperament on rated affect in the present study did not account for the influence of these factors on the relationship between affect of mother's message and infant behavior.

Control condition infants.—When the control condition is considered, length of mother's message cannot be utilized as a covariate. The unadjusted means for the two summary measures of infant behavior are presented in Table 2 for all infants, including the 17 control infants. Comparison of control infants to the direct condition, in which the mother spoke to the infant about the stranger, indicated a significant overall effect of mother's affect (positive, control, neutral; $F[2,44] = 5.90$, $p < .01$), and a significant interaction of affect with temperament, $F(2,44) = 3.29$, $p < .05$, for infant behavior to the stranger. For easy temperament infants, there was significantly less friendly behavior to the stranger in the control condition than in the positive condition, $F(1,44) = 6.24$, $p < .01$. In addition, the neutral message to the infant elicited a lower frequency of friendly behavior to the stranger than did the control condition, although this difference was not significant. This pattern was maintained for the measure of behavior to the stranger minus behavior to the mother, although the control condition did not differ significantly from either affect condition.

When mothers spoke directly to difficult-temperament infants, the differences between the positive and control conditions and between the neutral and control conditions were not significant for the summary measure of behavior to the stranger or the measure of behavior to the stranger minus behavior to the mother. Similarly, comparison of control infants to the indirect condition, in which the mother let the infant observe her speak to the stranger, did not yield any significant differences for either measure of behavior. Thus, behavior of the control infants was intermediate to the neutral and positive conditions for those circumstances under which a significant influence of mother's affect had been noted previously in the major analysis, that is, when mothers spoke about the stranger directly to infants of easy temperament.

Social referencing and response to strangers.—In general, the results indicated that affect of the mother's message influenced infant response to the stranger when the mother spoke directly to the infant, and especially when infants were of easy temperament. The greater consistency of the results with the social referencing hypothesis than with alternative explanations increases the likelihood that this process is at work in 10-month-old infants.

Infant behavior to the stranger was not influenced by mother's affect when the infant saw her speak to the stranger. Perhaps second-semester infants do not realize that observation of mother's behavior to the stranger can provide information about the stranger. But infants were friendlier to mothers who spoke neutrally to the stranger than to those who spoke positively, $F(1,59) = 4.09$, $p < .05$, suggesting that the mother's greeting to the stranger may be interpreted as information about the mother's emotional unavailability (Sorce & Emde, 1981). It might be that the mother's positive greeting to the stranger was threatening to the infant or elicited feelings of annoyance or jealousy. Perhaps the importance of attachment at 10 months (Ainsworth et al., 1978) biases the infant to understand social interaction of primary caregivers with other people in terms of the implications for the caregiver-infant relationship.

The influence of temperament classification on infant behavior was nested within the direction of communication effect. When mothers spoke to the stranger, temperament did not influence infant response. But when mothers spoke to the infant, the social referencing effect was stronger for easy infants. Although other studies have failed to find correlations of temperament scores with caregiver-infant interaction (Vaughn et al., 1981) or have found modest relationships (Taraldson, reported in Vaughn et al., 1981), those investigations did not focus on situations in which the mother attempted to influence her infant's response to a new situation. The current results suggest that temperament classifications are of value in detecting individual differences in infants' utilization of mothers' communications about an unfamiliar person.

CONCLUSIONS

While earlier studies had found that infants look to their caregivers when they meet an unfamiliar person, the common practice of asking the caregiver not to converse with infant or stranger prevented the caregiver from influencing the infant's response. When caregivers are asked to provide information about the stranger, a second-order effect occurs in that 10-month-olds are influenced by the message when it is provided directly to infants classified as being of easy temperament. The failure of the mood-modification hypothesis to offer an adequate alternative explanation heightens the possibility that social referencing does indeed occur in 10-month-old infants. In addition to the secure-base effect of the caregiver's presence when the infant meets a stranger, the caregiver may also influence the infant's appraisal of the stranger by serving as a base of information.

REFERENCES

Ainsworth, M. D., Blehar, M. C., Waters, E. & Wall, S. (1978). *Patterns of attachment.* Hillsdale, N.J.: Erlbaum.

Bates, E., Benigni, L., Bretherton, I., Camaioni, L., & Volterra, V. (1979). *The emergence of symbols: Cognition and communication in infancy.* New York: Academic Press.

Bates, J., Bennett Freeland, C., & Lounsbury, M. (1979). Measurement of infant difficultness. *Child Development, 50,* 794–803.

Benedict, H. (1979). Early lexical development: Comprehension and production. *Journal of Child Language, 6,* 183–200.

Bronfenbrenner, U. (1974). Developmental research, public policy, and the ecology of childhood. *Child Development, 45,* 1–5.

Campos, J. J., Emde, R. N., Gaensbauer, T., & Henderson, C. (1975). Cardiac and behavioral interrelationships in the reactions of infants to strangers. *Developmental Psychology, 11,* 589–601.

Carey, W. B., Fox, M., & McDevitt, S. C. (1977). Temperament as a factor in early school adjustment. *Pediatrics, 60,* 621–624.

Carey, W. B., & McDevitt, S. C. (1978). Revision of the Infant Temperament Questionnaire. *Pediatrics, 61,* 735–739.

Carr, S., Dabbs, J., & Carr, T. (1975). Mother-infant attachment: The importance of the mother's visual field. *Child Development, 46,* 331–338.

Charlesworth, W. R., & Kreutzer, M. A. (1973). Facial expressions of infants and children. In P. Ekman (Ed.), *Darwin and facial expression.* New York: Academic Press.

Clarke-Stewart, K. A. (1978). And daddy makes three: The father's impact on mother and young child. *Child Development, 49,* 466–478. (a)

Clarke-Stewart, K. A. (1978). Recasting the lone stranger. In J. Glick & K. A. Clarke-Stewart (Eds.), *The development of social understanding.* New York: Gardner. (b)

Cooley, C. H. (1964). *Human nature and the social order.* New York: Schocken. (Originally published, 1902.)

Dixon, W. J., Brown, M. B., Engelman, L., Frane, J. W., Hill, M. A., Jennrich, R. I., & Toporek, J. D. (1981). *BMDP statistical software 1981.* Berkeley: University of California Press.

Eckerman, C. O., Whatley, J. L., & McGhee, L. J. (1979). Approaching and contacting the object another manipulates: A social skill of the 1-year-old. *Developmental Psychology, 15,* 585–593.

Fein, G. G. (1975). Children's sensitivity to social contexts at 18 months of age. *Developmental Psychology*, **11**, 853–854.

Feinman, S. (1980). Infant response to race, size, proximity, and movement of strangers. *Infant Behavior and Development*, **3**, 187–204.

Feinman, S. (1982). Social referencing in infancy. *Merrill Palmer Quarterly*, **28**, 445–470.

Festinger, L. (1954). A theory of social comparison processes. *Human Relations*, **7**, 17–40.

Klinnert, M., Campos, J. J., Sorce, J., & Emde, R. N. (1982). Social referencing: An important appraisal process in human infancy. In R. Plutchik & H. Kellerman (Eds.), *The emotions* (Vol. **2**). New York: Academic Press.

Lamb, M. E. (1978). Infant social cognition and "second order" effects. *Infant Behavior and Development*, **1**, 1–10.

Lewis, M., & Feiring, C. (1981). Direct and indirect interactions in social relationships. In L. Lipsitt (Ed.), *Advances in infancy research*. New York: Ablex.

Lewis, M., & Weinraub, M. (1976). The father's role in the infant's social network. In M. E. Lamb (Ed.), *The role of the father in child development*. New York: Wiley.

Messer, J. (1980). The episodic structure of maternal speech to young children. *Journal of Child Language*, **7**, 29–40.

Parke, R. D. (1979). Perspectives on father-infant interaction. In J. D. Osofsky (Ed.), *Handbook of infant development*. New York: Wiley.

Pedersen, F. A., Anderson, B. J., & Cain, R. L., Jr. (1980). Parent-infant and husband-wife interactions observed at age 5 months. In F. A. Pedersen (Ed.), *The father-infant relationship: Observational studies in the family setting*. New York: Praeger.

Phillips, J. R. (1973). Syntax and vocabulary of mothers' speech to young children: Age and sex comparisons. *Child Development*, **44**, 182–185.

Piaget, J. (1952). *The origins of intelligence in children*. New York: International Universities Press.

Rheingold, H. L., & Eckerman, C. O. (1973). Fear of the stranger: A critical review. In H. W. Reese (Ed.), *Advances in child development and behavior* (Vol. **8**). New York: Academic Press.

Schachter, S. (1959). *The psychology of affiliation*. Stanford, Calif.: Stanford University Press.

Schaffer, H. R., Greenwood, A., & Parry, M. H. (1972). The onset of wariness. *Child Development*, **43**, 165–175.

Sherif, M. (1958). Group influences upon the formation of norms and attitudes. In E. Maccoby, T. Newcomb, & E. Hartley (Eds.), *Readings in social psychology*. New York: Holt, Rinehart & Winston.

Snow, C. E. (1972). Mothers' speech to children learning language. *Child Development*, **43**, 549–565.

Sorce, J. F., & Emde, R. N. (1981). Mother's presence is not enough: Effect of emotional availability on infant exploration. *Developmental Psychology*, **17**, 737–745.

Thomas, A., & Chess, S. (1977). *Temperament and development*. New York: Brunner/Mazel.

Thomas, D. G., & Campos, J. J., Shucard, D. W., Ramsay, D. S., & Shucard, J. (1981). Semantic comprehension in infancy: A signal detection analysis. *Child Development*, **52**, 798–803.

Vaughn, B. E., Taraldson, B. J., Crichton, L., & Egeland, B. (1981). The assessment of infant temperament: A critique of the Carey Infant Temperament Questionnaire. *Infant Behavior and Development*, **4**, 1–17.

Winer, B. J. (1971). *Statistical principles in experimental design* (2d ed.). New York: McGraw-Hill.

Part II

HEREDITY-ENVIRONMENT INTERACTION

Concepts regarding the relationship between heredity and environment in shaping human behavior have themselves gone through a number of developmental stages. For many centuries the debate raged on an all-or-nothing basis. Either the newborn infant was considered a *homunculus*, an adult in miniature who already possessed by inheritance all that would characterize him as an adult or, in the other view, the neonate was a *tabula rasa*, a clean slate on which the environment would inscribe its influence until the adult personality was etched to completion. When these unidimensional views proved inadequate, a simple additive view took over. It was agreed that both heredity and environment were important, that each contributed a certain percentage in shaping behavior, and that the goal of research was the determination of the precise percentages of each in various types of normal or pathological behavior. In recent decades this simplistic mechanical model has been rejected by biologists, developmental psychologists, and psychiatrists as inadequate in explaining the complexities of the dynamic interplay between heredity and environment and between biology and culture at all stages of the individual's life. As one leading psychiatrist has put it, "Attempts at quantitative partition of phenotypic variance into genetic and environmental components require the assumption of linear models, single causes and additive effects, assumptions which ignore the ubiquity of interactions and correlations between genotype and environment" (L. Eisenberg, *British Journal of Psychiatry*, 131: 226, 1977).

The agreement on an interactional/transactional model of the continuously evolving dynamic interplay of heredity and environment provides a new perspective for the examination of specific genetic and environmental features in human behavioral development. This approach, and the fruits of the research activities stemming from it, are exemplified in the various papers in this section. Wilson reviews a number of recent

73

concepts from the fields of evolutionary theory and developmental genetics to illuminate the contradictory aspects of human behavior—the similarity of the distinctive behavioral programs that characterize all human beings, combined with the variations that mark each individual person as unique. He emphasizes the distinctive episodes of spurt and lag which characterize sequences of child development, and reminds us of Waddington's cogent remark that a developmental process is one that involves progressive change as time passes, not one that simply persists—formulations which have highly significant implications for developmental theory and research strategies.

Scarr and McCartney define three types of genotype-environment correlations and discuss their implications for individual differences in developmental course. They indicate how their formulations may account for certain seemingly anomalous findings from research on twins and families, suggest some of the research strategies that can flow from their concepts, and at the very least encourage more developmentalists to study more than one child per family, genetically unrelated families, and individual differences in experience.

McCall provides another of his challenging and stimulating discussions in his examination of the influence that environmental variation within families not shared by siblings has on a child's mental performance—an influence largely ignored in most studies. He concludes with the proposition that major contributors to the field of mental development are idiosyncratic, and then poses and answers the question of whether such idiosyncratic influences are outside the realm of science, which seeks general laws. This discussion is highly pertinent for all of us who have struggled with the challenge of a systematic approach to the idiosyncratic influences which are so evident in long-term longitudinal studies.

Finally, the paper by Robinson and his associates provides additional substantial data on the developmental patterns of a sample of children with sex chromosomal abnormalities. The practical implications of the findings, which include such issues as anticipatory guidance and support for the families, are discussed clearly, with specific recommendations from the research findings.

4

Human Behavioral Development and Genetics

Ronald S. Wilson

University of Louisville School of Medicine, Louisville, Kentucky

*Behavioral development during childhood is examined in relation to
recent concepts and data from evolutionary theory and developmental
genetics. The epigenetic framework of Waddington is proposed as a
powerful tool for analyzing the progressions in behavior, particularly
for recognizing that development involves coordinated pathways of
change over time. Many of these pathways appear to depend upon
the activity of timed gene-action systems that switch off and on according to a predetermined plan. Behavioral development thus gives
expression to the dynamics of preprogrammed change; and in this
perspective, behavioral discontinuities may be as strongly rooted in
the epigenetic ground plan as the continuities are. The present paper
aims to pull together some common themes from different areas that
bear on the central issues of behavioral development—the neural
foundations, the time course followed, the interplay of maturation and
experience, the extent of preorganization furnished by the genetic
program, and the adaptive significance of such behaviors in an evolutionary perspective. The final section touches on some hypotheses
drawn from developmental neurobiology and developmental genetics
that may enrich the analyses of human behavioral development.*

Reprinted with permission from *Acta Geneticaa Medicae et Gemellologiae*, 1983, Vol. 32,
1–16. Copyright 1983 by Alan R. Liss, Inc.

INTRODUCTION

The topic of this paper is at once an inquiry into the distinctive behavioral programs that characterize all members of Homo sapiens, and at the same time an inquiry into the variations that mark each specimen as unique. If there is a basic species prototype on which each member is modeled, it is also true that variations on the main theme are equally important attributes. Each specimen thus represents a rough casting from the species mold, as shaped by the long course of evolution, but with substantial sculpting added by the genetic diversity among species members. Both aspects are ultimately rooted in the genetic core of the population—the species main effect and the dispersion of individual differences—and it is to these principal factors that the present paper is addressed.

Recent advances in evolutionary theory and developmental genetics have revitalized a fresh interest in the intrinsic determinants of behavior. The distinctive behavioral attributes of Homo sapiens must have been shaped by natural selection as surely as the physical characters were and must be as strongly rooted in the evolutionary history of the species [25]. Indeed, Waddington [48] has argued that behavior is the driving force in evolution, and in this sense the behavioral repertoire of man is at least as distinctive and as genetically rooted as the physical morphology.

Mayr [51,52] remarks on the genetic basis of certain characteristic behaviors in each species, and how these distinguishing behaviors may help identify which species or subgroup a particular animal belongs to. He concludes that in their genetic basis as well as in their phylogenetic history, such behavioral characters are completely equivalent to morphological characters that are distinctive to each subgroup. Mayr further notes the striking and persistent individual differences in behavior which often seem to be genetic in origin.

Evolutionary theory has made several fundamental contributions to the analysis of human behavior. First, it has brought to bear questions of adaptive significance in infant behavior, and the extent to which such behaviors are intrinsic in the sense of being preprimed and readily evoked under most conditions. Second, it has focused on certain of these behaviors as facilitating the bond with the caretaker, upon whom the infant is massively dependent for survival.

Third, it has brought to bear the techniques of ethology, with its emphasis on detailed observation of emergent behaviors in the natural habitat, as a means of assaying the patterning and adaptive significance of early behavior [53–55]. Finally, it has highlighted the central issue of development as an ongoing, dynamic process by which a single zygote ultimately becomes transformed into a multibillion-cell organism of extraordinary differentiation and detail. Insofar as these manifold growth processes are initiated and regulated by programs in the genetic code, the resultant behaviors must be guided by the same processes.

From this perspective, the powerful concepts from embryology and developmental genetics may furnish a stimulating framework for the analysis of human behavioral development. In particular, this framework keeps attention focused on development as a continuous dynamic process, with episodes of differentiation and growth being switched on and off in accordance with the detailed instructions in the genetic program.

We might suggest that the principles of developmental regulation applicable to biological structures also apply equally to emergent behaviors. Caspari, after surveying the wealth of evidence for gene-controlled regulatory processes that guide cell differentiation, then concluded: "If the general properties of developmental systems are applied to the development of behavioral characters, it does not appear as if any additional principles have to be involved" [7:p 9].

<h2 style="text-align:center">WADDINGTON ON DEVELOPMENT</h2>

Few workers have contributed as much to the understanding of developmental processes as the distinguished embryologist C.H. Waddington [45–48]. His concepts have been profitably employed by several investigators in the area of behavior genetics and child development, notably Gottesman [17], McClearn [27], Scarr-Salapatek [37], Bateson [1], and particularly, Fishbein [12].

Waddington himself describes the ideas from embryology as potentially useful analogies for model building in developmental psychology, and he remarks on two important features:

> Note first that any concept applicable to development must be one which involves progressive change as time passes; thus we are thinking not of a constellation of processes which just persists, but of a pathway of development.
> The characteristic of the pathways of development . . . is that the course they pursue is resistant to modification. If we act . . . to divert it from its normal course, we find that it tends, after the initial fluctuation, to get back to the trajectory along which it had begun to travel [47:pp 19–20].

These general concepts led Waddington to more detailed ones such as chreods or stabilized pathways of development, of canalization and buffering to protect against disruptive influences, of sensitive periods in which development is most readily accomplished, and of time-linked gene-action systems that are switched on and off in sequential order. Developmental processes thus give expression to the dynamics of pre-programmed change, constantly incorporating new episodes of growth into the preexisting phenotype, and being selectively attuned to certain dimensions of environmental input.

This paper presents a highly selective review of several topic areas which seem to offer fruitful concepts and analogies for analyzing human behavioral development. No attempt is made to itemize all relevant studies from behavior genetics which display concordance among twins or family members for various categories of behavior. Excellent reviews may be found in McClearn [27,56], Lindzey et al [57], Broadhurst, Fulker, and Wilcock [58], Scarr-Salapatek [37,59], DeFries and Plomin [60], Willerman [61] and Henderson [62].

Rather, the aim is to pull together some common themes from different areas which seem to bear on the central issues of behavioral development—the neural foundations, the time course followed, the interplay of maturation and experience, the extent of preorganization furnished by the genetic program, and the adaptive significance of such behaviors in an evolutionary perspective. We shall consider first several integrative papers that touch on these themes, then turn to more specific analyses within each topic area.

FISHBEIN ON EVOLUTION AND CHILD DEVELOPMENT

Fishbein [12] has written a stimulating book in which he traces the progressive increments of brain structure that have evolved for Homo sapiens, and how these newly evolved structures of the neocortex only gradually become functional during childhood. One recurrent theme concerns the different rates of maturation for these structures and their effect upon the specific behavioral capabilities supported by these structures.

Fishbein provides an illustration by showing that, while language and other motor skills are correlated on a species-wide basis, there may be considerable asynchrony for a given child—that is, language development may be delayed while other motor skills are not, or vice versa. Bateson [1] has remarked on the same phenomenon and also noted that early or late development is rarely significant for the ultimate level attained. These data suggest different gradients of maturation for particular capabilities which may be partially out of phase, but which have no necessary influence on the level attained at maturity. It is a theme that will reappear in several contexts.

Fishbein [12] has also provided a comprehensive translation of Waddington's concepts [46] into the area of developmental psychology, and he proposes that behavioral development is guided by epigenetic processes that have been mapped out by evolution in the genetic blueprint. Development proceeds towards certain targets or end-states—guided by an intrinsic template, so to speak—and it maintains this directional focus by means of canalization. Fishbein defines canalization as follows:

> Canalization involves a set of genetic processes which insure that development will proceed in normal ways, that the phenotypic targets will be attained despite the presence of minor abnormal genetic or environmental conditions. Canalization processes operate at each point in development to correct minor deflections from the sought-for phenotypic targets [12:p 7].

Canalization means that certain patterns of behavior are easily, almost inevitably, acquired by all species members under the normal circumstances of life. Such behaviors come with a high degree of preorganization and priming laid down in the brain structure by evolution, and they are actuated in straightforward fashion except in the most extreme circumstances. In this sense, canalization underwrites the species-specific behavioral programs that push each member along a common developmental pathway. However, canalization also preserves the dispersion of individual differences by buffering the zygote against early insult and reorienting each infant along its unique developmental pathway if once deflected.

BATESON ON SELF-STABILIZING DEVELOPMENTAL PATHWAYS

Bateson [1] gives a thoughtful interpretation of Waddington's epigenetic model as it pertains to the capacity of a developing system to correct itself after some disruption. He illustrates with a model for weight regulation and recovery after early deficit, and he relates this self-correcting process to a similar concept from systems analysis, whereby the same final state may be reached by convergence via different routes.

Bateson then considers whether there may be two or more alternative systems controlling the development of a particular behavior pattern. Clearly, redundant developmental systems would be highly adaptive, with the added systems helping to protect against failure or to cope with a changed environment. Such redundant systems would provide a degree of plasticity in the face of different environmental conditions, and the actual behavior patterns would be guided by control systems that match actual input values with some intrinsic end-state values. This is also the essence of the canalization concept, whereby development is impelled along a particular pathway with constant self-correcting adjustments until some targeted end-state is reached.

It might be noted that these concepts touch on some fundamental questions related to gene activity—for example, what furnishes the signal that a particular developmental mission is accomplished and that the differentiating processes can stop rather than running on unchecked? The whole concept of targeted end-states, or intrinsic templates to be matched, implies that developmental processes are self-limiting and are constantly involved in a match-to-model process with the inherent growth equation.

Further, these targeted end-states are not "known" in any teleological sense. They must reflect evolved mechanisms that terminate the ongoing process via the same material agents that also initiated the process. An adequate explanation must encompass all three features—the dynamics of growth itself, with its extraordinary differentiation of form and function; the capability to preserve the prescribed developmental pathways in the face of deflecting agents; and the precise termination of developmental episodes as each subroutine of the developmental program is accomplished. Some speculative hypotheses from developmental genetics and neurobiology will be briefly considered at a later point.

GOTTESMAN ON DEVELOPMENTAL GENETICS AND CHILD DEVELOPMENT

Gottesman [17] provided a stimulating paper which, in his words: " . . . has as one of its main objectives the communication of my conviction that we must start now to build a bridge between developmental genetics and ontogenetic psychology" (p 55). Gottesman reviews the recent work in developmental genetics concerning the switching on and off of gene-action systems, and he then illustrates how these concepts can enrich the interpretation of individual growth curves. The differences in timing of rapid growth spurts brings to the forefront questions about the differential switching on and off of maturational processes and stages.

Gottesman also notes that only a small portion of the genotype is active at any given time, a feature that in itself contributes to time-linked phases of development and thus may generate different developmental trajectories even for closely related zygotes. The dispersion of individual differences is further emphasized by Gottesman for the concepts of canalization and buffering against deviant conditions: some behavior patterns are canalized species-wide, but with significant individual variations in the strength of canalization and resistance to deflection.

MANNING ON GENES AND BEHAVIORAL DEVELOPMENT

Manning [26] moves a step further in relating individual differences in development to the effects of genes. He states the central question as follows: "How is behavioural potential encoded in genetic terms and expressed in the course of development?" (p 327). He adds that there must be a strategy to behavioral development, and different sets of genes may be operating at different times.

Manning (p 338) then makes a trenchant observation: " . . . we must also look for genetic discontinuities in the course of development. Such discontinuities could indicate the existence of distinct sets of genes becoming activated that would in turn have a bearing on the units problem" [i.e., the changes in behavior measured over successive ages]. This particular observation has direct bearing on several current theories that emphasize discontinuities in behavioral development [eg, 63–65], and it suggests that some discontinuities may be plausibly related to the time-ordering of developmental processes in the genetic program.

The point may be illustrated by mental development data obtained for a large sample of monozygotic and dizygotic twins. The twins were tested from 3 months to 6 years of age, and several representative curves are shown in the Figure (from Wilson [49]).

The curves show that many individual twins made substantial changes in their test scores from age to age—a graphic illustration of behavioral discontinuities, and a reflection of age-linked spurts and lags in mental development for each twin. But in the case of monozygotic twins, these spurts and lags were synchronized over age, and to a significantly greater degree than for dizygotic twins [49]. These synchronies in the course of mental development suggested that the underlying processes were guided by timed gene-action systems, which became activated in sequential fashion and which followed a parallel course for two zygotes

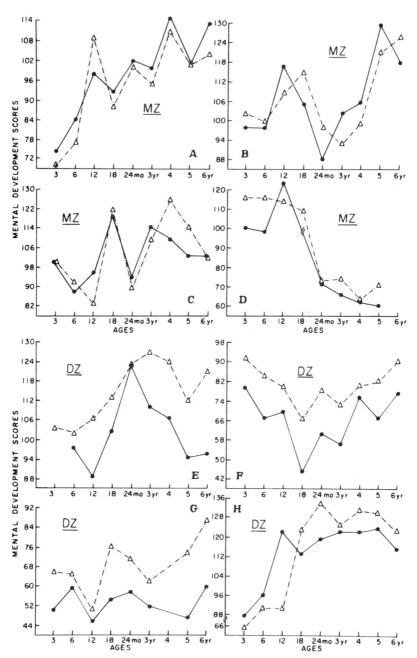

Figure. Illustrative mental development curves for monozygotic (MZ) and dizygotic (DZ) twins. From Wilson [49].

sharing the same genotype. The behavioral discontinuity, therefore, had its roots in time-ordered developmental processes originating in the genotype.

FREEDMAN ON HUMAN INFANCY

We turn now to studies that focus upon the adaptive significance and survival value of infant behavior. Freedman [13] builds upon the same background of evolution and natural selection as the previous studies, but he gives special emphasis to the characteristic behaviors of the human infant and what adaptive function these behaviors serve. In fact, adaptive significance is the principal theme in Freedman's analysis, and it is at the core of his interpretation of infant smiling and attachment. Freedman concludes [13:p 45]: "Some of the capabilities of the newborn . . . are clearly adaptive from the infant's viewpoint in the sense that they strengthen the social bonds and elicit caretaking on the part of the parent."

The newborn's capabilities extend beyond these socially facilitative behaviors, however. After reviewing the data on perceptual constancies as demonstrated in infants, Freedman remarks:

> Given the basic adaptive value of the perceptual constancies, is it possible that they have to be relearned in each lifetime? Evolutionary logic yields a negative answer and it seems that learning proceeds easiest in directions determined by phylogenetic evolution; that is, evolution has dug the major channels through which the river of experience runs. Said another way, natural selection frequently yields differential thresholds for learning rather than full-blown species-specific behaviors [13:p 28].

Freedman furnishes several notable illustrations of canalization in infant development and the powerful self-directing tendencies of these developmental pathways. He further notes the striking individual differences among infants in strength of attachment and response to separation, a point that is also confirmed by Sroufe and Waters [66] and by Mineka and Suomi [67].

SUPER ON CROSS-CULTURAL DEVELOPMENT

If the various features of infant behavior are an end-product of evolutionary adaptations, and if these are uniformly represented among all populations of infants, then it is of interest to see how strongly the communalities are represented across cultures. Super [40] has just completed such a survey, which in the number of titles cited (over 500) gives an indication of how prolific such studies have become.

He remarks that each cultural niche does seem to have some bearing on the rate at which certain capabilities develop, but perhaps the strongest theme is the species-wide regularity in the way stations of development. While there is no aspect of human development unaffected by culture, the hallmark of cognitive abilities is perhaps the least malleable by our cultural variety. As with motor skills, there is a fine patterning in the timing of universal developments [40:p 160].

PIAGET ON COGNITIVE DEVELOPMENT

Super's reference to the species-wide regularities in cognitive development may be coordinated with the Piagetian conception of successive stages unfolding in invariant order and building upon the experiences of the preceding stages. Piaget's theory [32] touches on the fundamental operations and transformations accomplished by all human infants, and indeed his detailed microanalysis of cognitive functioning may be regarded as the basic itinerary for the species.

Since some of Piaget's interpreters in this country, notably J. McV. Hunt [20,21], have given very heavy emphasis to the role of cumulative experience in initiating the progressions in cognitive development, it is instructive to consider Piaget's own statements about the foundations of cognitive processes. The issue is addressed principally in *Biology and Knowledge* [33]. Piaget opens by remarking that knowledge does not imply making a mere copy of reality, but rather of transforming the input in accordance with the basic programming of the brain, and in accordance with prior experiences and actions. He adds:

> It goes without saying that these regulatory mechanisms, in knowledge at all levels, raise the problem of their relationship with organic regulations. The central problem with which this book will have to deal is, therefore, that of the relationships between cognitive and organic regulations at all levels [33:p 12].

Piaget then draws specifically from Waddington for developmental concepts applicable to growth of intelligence. He employs the term chreods (or necessary routes) to describe how an embryo becomes progressively differentiated into a complex organism, then concludes:

It is impossible to take note of such a picture without immediately thinking of the far-reaching analogies it has with
the development of schemata or ideas in the intelligence. . . .
Briefly, intellectual growth contains its own rhythm and its
"chreods" just as physical growth does. The epigenetic process
which is the basis of intellectual operations is rather closely
comparable to embryological epigenesis. . . . [33:pp 21–23].

Piaget's further application of epigenetic concepts to the growth of
intelligence is detailed and extensive, and he draws at length on many
recent works in developmental biology, population genetics, and evolutionary theory. It is perhaps time to acknowledge this fundamental
framework within which Piaget's theory has been formulated, and to
recognize that the premise of genetic regulation of cognitive development is not the anathema for Piaget that it is for some who cite him
frequently.*

A balanced discussion of Piaget's theory from a psychobiological perspective may be found in Kohen-Raz [68], and this volume also provides
coverage of other topics and theorists that attend to the biological foundations of cognitive development. The conclusion seems inescapable that
the integrative power of the brain is the end product of developmental
processes that have been endlessly sharpened and refined by evolution,
and that are played out according to a unique chronogenetic schedule
for each specimen.

THOMAS AND CHESS ON TEMPERAMENT

Perhaps no aspect of infant behavior is more obvious to parent or
professional than the earliest patterns of irritability and reactivity in the
neonate. They seem to reflect intrinsic response characteristics, and they
exert a marked influence on the developing infant-caretaker relationship
[3,24].

A detailed and provocative body of research on temperament has been
conducted by Thomas and Chess and their colleagues at the New York

---

*A recent paper by Kitchener [23] also examines the concept of epigenesis and whether
it might be applicable to behavioral development. After an extended discussion of organic
epigenesis as being relatively impervious to environmental fluctuations, Kitchener then
argues that the concept cannot apply to behavioral development, since everyone agrees
that environmental factors play a powerful role in human behavior. This conclusion,
however, seems to rely mainly upon implied consensus and personal conviction, and it
does not furnish a persuasive reason for excluding the concept of epigenesis from developmental psychology.

Longitudinal Study [42,43]. The focus of the program was upon behavioral differences found among infants in the early months of life, and how these differences influenced later development. For many infants, individualized patterns of reactivity were evident at this early stage, and certain behavioral clusters were observed that seemed to reflect different styles of temperament—easy, difficult, and slow to warm up.

In considering the origins of temperament, Thomas and Chess [43] surveyed the evidence for genetic influences and concluded that they played an appreciable but by no means exclusive role. Environmental influences might accentuate, modify, or even change temperamental traits over time.

Carey [5] in his recent review reached essentially the same conclusion, and he called particular attention to the problem of assessing the consistency in temperament for a given infant (a matter also discussed by Rutter [36] and Thomas and Chess [43]). The general expectation is that if temperament is rooted in constitutional/genetic variables, there must be some continuity in its expression over the developmental history of the child.

But a variety of normal phenomena may confound efforts to demonstrate stability of temperament, not the least of which are varying rates of maturation of the underlying CNS structures and of age-linked behavioral competencies that may markedly alter the mode of expression for a given temperamental style. The problem (and the challenge) is one of determining when dissimilar behaviors over time reflect the same characteristic style, recognizing that the behavioral criteria must necessarily be age-specific, and therefore the criteria must coordinate with each other as homologies rather than exact replicas.

It is worth noting that there are now several longitudinal twin studies in progress that are examining the patterning and concordance of temperament variables for infant twins [69–72]. Aside from addressing the issues of continuity/discontinuity over ages, these studies may reveal whether the apparent changes in temperament occur in parallel for both members of a twin pair. The earlier quote by Manning [26] might be recalled here, since it relates to possible genetic discontinuities in behavior. Perhaps the discontinuities in temperament may also reveal an underlying patterning or synchrony for monozygotic twins, as was true for mental development.

MATURATION AND BEHAVIOR

The theme of maturation has been revived in several of the preceding papers after a period of virtual exclusion from developmental psychology, and it may be instructive to reconsider some of the earlier findings. Two of the classic twin studies contributed to the area—Gesell and Thompson's study [15] of twins raised in a nursing home from 2 weeks to 18 months of age; and McGraw's longer study [28], continuing until the twins were 6 years old. In both studies one twin was given special training and the other was not, being left simply to its own devices for self-initiated activity. The effects of special training were transient at best, particularly in relation to the standard species-typical activities such as grasping, crawling, creeping, and walking. McGraw [28] remarked that the major aspects of these phyletic activities had become determined during phylogeny to such an extent as to be resistant to alteration. She noted some greater effects of specialized training on more complex activities such as swimming, skating, and riding a tricycle, although the interpretation was clouded somewhat when the twins were later diagnosed as fraternal rather than identical.

Gesell's twins were clearly identical and thus provided a co-twin control for assessing the net benefits of special training, and the contrasting role of maturation in promoting behavioral competencies without special training. Gesell noted that there was a high degree of similarity in the twins' development, and the differences were of a small nature, even in the area of emotional behavior. He concluded [15:p 114]: "These findings point consistently to the preponderant importance of maturational factors in the determination of infant behavior pattern. . . . Although function enters into the growth, training does not transcend maturation."

MUNN AND CARMICHAEL ON MATURATION

Aside from these two case studies of twins, the behavioral development of children and its correlation with maturational status has been broadly surveyed in Munn [30,31] and Carmichael [6]. Both of these sources are useful for their very detailed coverage of the behaviors that may be studied in the human infant and for illustrating the nominal effects of special training or exercise in accelerating these behaviors. Munn's conclusions basically echo those of McGraw and Gesell, but he adds one of particular interest, namely that the efficacy of training or special exercise is directly proportional to the degree of maturation of the underlying mechanisms.

This latter point is significant not only for coordinating behavioral development with the steady advance in maturation of brain structures, but also for identifying a crucial dimension of individual differences. The differences in maturation rate have a profound influence on the degree of advancement or lag for individual children, and indeed there may be an uneven rate of progression within the same child for different behavioral capabilities [11].

THE BRAIN AND BEHAVIORAL DEVELOPMENT

Since the brain is the ultimate structure underwriting human behavioral development, it is instructive to consider the present evidence for the extraordinary precision and detail by which the various regions of the brain become progressively interconnected and rendered functional. Sperry, a premier contributor in this area, provided an eloquent overview and interpretation of his work [38,39], and then offered his conclusion that the growth of neural circuits is principally guided by indigenous chemical processes.

> The complicated nerve fiber circuits of the brain grow, assemble, and organize themselves through the use of intricate chemical codes under genetic control. The outgrowing fibers in the developing brain are guided by a kind of probing chemical touch system that leads them along exact pathways . . . [until they] connect with certain other neurons, often far distant, that have appropriate molecular labels [39:30–32].

Exactly how this precise wiring is coded in the DNA and then executed remains an unsolved problem [19]. There is no doubt, however, that the brain becomes wired in an extremely precise manner during development, and an excellent survey of how these connections become established and organized may be found in Cowan [9].

Equivalently precise wiring for the autonomic nervous system has been reported [73], with central neurons extending to highly specific peripheral sites; and it now appears that, in infant mammals, central pathways within the brain can be regenerated and accurately reconnected even after damage [22]. The authors reported that when the pyramidal tract axons were cut in infant hamsters, there was a massive regrowth of the severed axons to their appropriate terminal sites in the medulla and spinal cord. The results were interpreted as suggesting that CNS axons damaged early in life might regenerate in a functionally useful way.

The long-standing observation of greater recovery of function among the young after CNS injury [18] now appears to have a possible foundation in the regeneration of neural connections, and this in turn raises the fundamental question of how specific cells become committed to a certain fate, and how they retain the capability to duplicate again a previously executed pattern of growth.*

MATURATION AND CNS FUNCTIONING

In addition to the precise wiring accomplished in the central nervous system, the orderly progression of functions is intimately connected to the maturation of these neural structures. Goldman [16] has recently surveyed a large number of studies with reference to the maturation of the nervous system and its effect upon behavior. She notes that there is a strong interdependence of structure and function, even at the cellular level, and many cells do not attain fully mature status and become functional until long after they originate. She adds that the gradient of maturation is not necessarily synchronized for neurons of different types, nor for similar neurons located in different regions of the brain.

Goldman then turns to studies showing that certain cortical regions responsible for delayed-reaction responses and complex perceptual tasks only slowly mature, and that in some animals this process of maturation may extend over a period of 2 years or more. With humans, of course, the period is even further extended [8]. Other reviewed studies on visual deprivation and on cortical lesions inflicted at various ages all testify to intrinsic regenerative processes that affect the extent of deficit and degree of recovery.

Goldman's review [16] is very thorough and detailed, and her summary is worth quoting.

> Development is by definition a sequential process. One function of a stepwise maturational progression may be to regulate the order and impact of internal and external stimuli and experience on the developmental process itself. Thus . . . the maturational status of the organism provides a filter through

---

*The regeneration of neural connections is only one of several remarkable findings now emerging from developmental neurobiology. It has become apparent that many more neural cells are generated than ultimately survive, and these cells are eliminated by tightly programmed phases of cell death [9]. Further, there is a proliferation of synaptic connections for each neuron during early development, but the surplus connections are progressively eliminated until only a single neural connection remains [35]. A concise but wide-ranging summary of recent developments in this field may be found in Purves [74], and it illustrates the far-reaching effects of programmed biological events on the wiring of the brain and its regulation of behavior.

which only a subset [of stimuli] can be effective at particular
times [16:pp 70–71].

This review suggests a revised view of maturation that is closely coordinated with definable properties of the nervous system at every level
from the cell upward. The functioning of the brain is dependent not
just on the formation of cells or influx of experience—it is dependent
on the maturation of these structures, which involves growth in cell size,
myelination of fibers, proliferation of dendrites, and the exponential
gain in connections among cells and fibers [16,41].

Further, maturational processes are subject to wide and pervasive individual differences; and even within a given child, the time course of
development across behavioral systems may be partially disjunctive and
out of phase. These phenomena suggest a foundation in timed gene-
action systems that furnish a detailed timetable of emergent capabilities,
fixed in broad outline by the basic species program, but idiosyncratic in
detail for the individual.

CONCEPTS FROM DEVELOPMENTAL GENETICS

This final section will touch briefly on some recent advances in developmental genetics that seem to hold promise for a fuller understanding of the mechanisms underlying behavioral development. The focus
is upon gene action at the cellular level and its role in promoting the
differentiation by which a cell becomes committed to a particular function and then matures according to a set schedule.

Since all cells start with the same genetic material, it seems apparent
that only a limited portion of the gene complex is activated within each
cell, and this in turn is dictated by the timing of certain key regulatory
events. Related clusters of cells then construct the integrated components
of the central nervous system, and these several components interconnect
and become functional in accordance with intrinsic maturational schedules. The developmental progressions in behavior therefore represent
the end-product of an extraordinary collection of timed gene-action
systems that have their origin at the cellular level, and that in aggregate
dictate the rates of growth and maturation for the interlocking neural
systems that underwrite behavior.

How is the commitment of each cell to a particular function determined? Present evidence suggests that, in each cell, only the small subset
of genes needed to guide that cell's special behavior are activated, and
the remaining genes are inhibited or repressed [10]. At a prescribed

point in the developmental process, the target genes are activated that shape the cell into a particular form, and all other genes thereafter remain repressed.

Prior to the point of differentiation, the cell is virtually equipotential—it can be shifted to an alternate outcome if transposed to another site—but once differentiation has taken place, the cell is committed to a particular fate, and the repressed genes lose their effectiveness.

While there is some disagreement about whether these genes are irreversibly repressed or not [eg, 4], the major conclusion seems clear: As development proceeds, the developmental potential of each cell (ie, its ability to differentiate into a number of different phenotypes) is markedly restricted. Thus, a large portion of cells from developmentally advanced tissues have restricted potential, and the percentage of cells that retain unlimited potential progressively declines as development proceeds [4].

One intriguing speculation that the above conclusion suggests is a model for the greater recovery potential following CNS insult in younger organisms, whereby a larger number of cells might retain unlimited developmental potential and would subsequently be recruited to help restore a compromised function. As Goldman [16] has observed, the developing nervous system has a quantitatively greater capacity for reorganization than the mature nervous system; and both clinical and experimental data on brain injury and recovery of function seem to be emphatic on the same point [18: especially Chapter 9].

Perhaps there are distinctive gradients in the retention of developmental potential among the various cell clusters of the brain, and the recuperative potential of each cluster declines as the cells become differentiated and fixed into a specific state. A speculation might be that the evolutionarily more recent brain structures, and those that are slower to mature, are the ones with a higher retention of developmental potential in the cell cluster. It may also be that the strongly directional and self-correcting processes involved in canalization are ultimately dependent upon the retained potential of aggregate cell clusters to proceed towards their targeted end-states. Once a cell cluster has been given its direction by the target genes, the cluster moves persistently in that direction until the differentiating processes have run their course.

COMPARTMENTS OF DEVELOPMENT

How does the commitment of individual cells to a particular fate ultimately produce a highly differentiated organism? A detailed and lucid description of how gene-regulated developmental processes serve to construct the organism on a piece-by-piece basis has been published by Garcia-Bellido et al [14]. They note initially that the blueprint for accurate development is encoded in the DNA; then they remark that organisms seem to be made up of different but fundamentally homologous compartments.

The authors describe experiments in which each segment of an insect seems to result from the activity of a few founder cells that determine the actual structure to be formed, and then accomplish this by creating daughter cells that carry genetic information about where to locate and how to form. These cloned cells have a precisely defined destiny in the sense of contributing only to their home compartment, and they become marked by a distinctive genetic address that is subsequently passed along to their progeny.

> In summary, we suggest that each piece of the insect—a compartment made by a particular group of cells—is specified by a genetic address, in effect a binary zip code representing the decisions of key regulatory genes. The final binary code in an adult cell contains the history of the decisions made by the cell's ancestors [14:pp 107–108].

The authors then consider whether the same model might be applicable to higher organisms, and they close with the following query: "Do insects, mice and man all develop according to a similar genetic strategy, expressed in compartments?" (p 110). Acknowledging the rhetorical nature of the query, the implied answer would seem to be in the affirmative.

These studies bear witness to the extraordinary precision and detail of gene activity in regulating the course of development. Perhaps the above question might be paraphrased in the following terms: Is behavioral development guided by a genetic strategy analogous to that for biologic development? The answer would also seem to be yes, both at the species level and in the realm of individual differences. If, as Carmichael [6] says, behavior is structure in action, then it can hardly be divorced from the profound developmental processes by which the structures are formed.

The end-product—the phenotypic behavior of the human, cradle to grave—is distilled from the constant interplay of genetic material and the environmental surroundings. But the message, the conserved microfilm of evolution's choices, is preserved in the genotype, and it is progressively actualized throughout the life span. Perhaps an appreciation of this fact can help anchor the concepts in developmental psychology and lead to a more comprehensive model for assaying the determinants of behavior.

IMPLICATIONS FOR RESEARCH STRATEGY

What strategy for studying behavioral development would seem most appropriate from this standpoint? Clearly, if each child's development is characterized by distinctive episodes of spurt and lag—if, indeed, the steady progression of behavioral capabilities in any domain is subject to individual variations—then it would require detailed longitudinal data to document the collective pathways of development. Waddington's remark is worth recalling here, to the effect that a developmental process is one that involves progressive change as time passes, not one that simply persists. The phasing and scope of these progressive changes only become evident via repeated measurements on the same individual over time.

This strategy also puts a high premium on reliable data, so that the continuities and discontinuities in behavioral development may be confidently treated as genuine phenomena, and not as by-products of measurement error. It is a particular burden in early childhood, since standardized behavioral assessments are more the exception than the rule, but it is an absolute core requirement if we are to fully comprehend the progressions in development. Given the state of the art in behavioral assessment, a multimethod approach would be the preferred vehicle for securing a stable composite measure on each child.

Finally, if the continuities and discontinuities in behavior are to be examined for potential genetic influence, then the use of infant twins may be recommended as a vital first step. To the extent that monozygotic twins display synchronized pathways of development in significantly greater degree than dizygotic twins or sibling pairs, the role of genetic factors may be affirmed. In fact, the relative contribution of genetic and environmental factors to the pathways of development may be articulated by examining the patterns of convergence and divergence among matched pairs of infants. Ultimately, it is from such comparisons that the behavioral trajectories will be brought into coordination with the underlying foundation processes.

ACKNOWLEDGMENTS

Preparation of this paper was supported in part by research grants from the Office of Human Development (OCD 90-C-922) and the John

D. and Catherine T. MacArthur Foundation. A portion of this material was presented at the Henri Pieron Centennial, Paris 1981.

REFERENCES

1. Bateson, P. P. G. (1976). Rules and reciprocity in behavioral development. In Bateson P.P.G. and Hinde R.A. (eds): "Growing Points in Ethology." Cambridge: Cambridge University Press.
2. Bayley, N. (1955). On the growth of intelligence. *Amer Psychol.* 10:805–819.
3. Bell, R. Q. (1974). Contributions of human infants to caregiving and social interaction. In Lewis M. and Rosenblum L.A. (eds): "The Effect of the Infant on Its Caregiver." New York: Wiley, pp 1–20.
4. Caplan, A. I., Ordahl, C. P. (1978). Irreversible gene repression model for control of development. Science 201:120–130.
5. Carey, W. B. (1981). The Importance of Temperament-Environment Interaction for Child Health and Development. In Lewis M. and Rosenblum L.A. (eds): "The Uncommon Child." New York: Plenum, pp 31–55.
6. Carmichael, L. (1970). Onset and early development of behavior. In Mussen P.H. (ed): "Carmichael's Manual of Child Psychology," Vol. I. New York: John Wiley.
7. Caspari, E. (1971). Differentiation and pattern formation in the development of behavior. In Tobach E., Aronson L.R. and Shaw E. (eds): "The Biopsychology of Development." New York: Academic.
8. Conel, J. L. (1967). "The postnatal development of the human cerebral cortex," Vol 8. Cambridge: Harvard University Press.
9. Cowan, W. M. (1979). The development of the brain. Sci Am 241:112–133.
10. Davidson, E. H. (1976). "Gene Activity in Early Development," 2nd Ed. New York: Academic.
11. Eichorn, D. H. (1975). Asynchronizations in adolescent development. In Dragostin S.E. and Elder G.H. (eds): "Adolescence in the life cycle." Washington: Hemisphere Press.
12. Fishbein, H. D. (1976). "Evolution, Development, and Children's Learning." Pacific Palisades, Calif.: Goodyear Press.
13. Freedman, D. G. (1974). "Human Infancy: An Evolutionary Perspective." New York: Lawrence Erlbaum.
14. Garcia-Bellido, A., Lawrence, P. A., Morata, G. (1979). Compartments in animal development. Sci Am 241:102:110.
15. Gesell, A., Thompson, H. (1929). Learning and growth in identical infant twins. Gen Psychol Monogr 6:1–123.
16. Goldman, P. S. (1976). Maturation of the mammalian nervous system and the ontogeny of behavior. In Rosenblatt J.S., Hinde R.A., Shaw E. and Beer C. (eds): "Advances in the Study of Behavior," Vol 7. New York: Academic.
17. Gottesman, I. I. (1974). Developmental genetics and ontogenetic psychology: Overdue detente and propositions from a matchmaker. In Pick A.D. (ed): "Minnesota Symposia on Child Psychology," Vol 8. Minneapolis: University of Minnesota Press, pp 55–80.
18. Hecaen, H., Albert, M. L. (1979). "Human Neuropsychology." New York: John Wiley.
19. Hubel, D. H. (1979). The brain. Sci Am 241:44–53.
20. Hunt, J. McV. (1961). "Intelligence and Experience." New York: Ronald Press.
21. Hunt, J. McV. (1979). Psychological development: Early experience. Ann Rev Psychol 30:103–143.

22. Kalil, K., Reh, T. (1979). Regrowth of severed axons in the neonatal central nervous system: Establishment of normal connections. Science 205:1158–1161.
23. Kitchener, R. F. (1978). Epigenesis: The role of biological models in developmental psychology. Hum Dev 21:141–160.
24. Lewis, M., Rosenblum, L. A. (eds) (1974). "The Effect of the Infant on Its Caregiver." New York: Wiley.
25. Lorenz, K. (1972). The enmity between generations and its probable ethological causes. In Piers M.W. (ed): "Play and Development." New York: W. W. Norton.
26. Manning, A. (1976). The place of genetics in the study of behaviour. In Bateson P.P.G. and Hinde R.A. (eds): "Growing Points in Ethology." Cambridge: Cambridge University Press.
27. McClearn, G. E. (1970). Genetic influences on behavior and development. In Mussen P.H. (ed): "Carmichael's Manual of Child Psychology." Vol I. New York: John Wiley.
28. McGraw, M. B. (1935). "Growth: A Study of Johnny and Jimmy." New York: Appleton-Century.
29. Muller, K. J., Scott, S. A. (1979). Correct axonal regeneration after target-cell removal in the central nervous system of the leech. Science 206:87–89.
30. Munn, N. L. (1965). "The Evolution and Growth of Human Behavior," 2nd Ed: Boston: Houghton Mifflin.
31. Munn, N. L. (1974). "The Growth of Human Behavior," 3rd Ed: Boston: Houghton Mifflin.
32. Piaget, J. (1952). "The Origins of Intelligence in Children." New York: International Universities Press.
33. Piaget, J. (1971). "Biology and Knowledge." Chicago: University of Chicago Press.
34. Plomin, R., Rowe, D. C. (1977). A twin study of temperament in young children. J Psychol 97:107–113.
35. Purves, D., Lichtman, J. W. (1980). Elimination of synapses in the developing nervous septem. Science 210:153–157.
36. Rutter, M. (1970). Psychological development: Predictions from infancy. J Child Psychol Psychiatr 11:49–62.
37. Scarr-Salapatek, S. (1976). An evolutionary perspective in infant intelligence: Species patterns and individual variations. In Lewis M. (ed): "Origins of Intelligence." New York: Plenum.
38. Sperry, R. W. (1958). Developmental basis of behavior. In Roe A. and Simpson G.G. (eds): "Behavior and Evolution." New Haven: Yale University Press.
39. Sperry, R. W. (1971). How a developing brain gets itself properly wired for adaptive function. In Tobach E., Aronson L.R. and Shaw E. (eds): "The Biopsychology of Development." New York: Academic.
40. Super, C. M. (1980). Behavioral development in infancy. In Monroe R.L., Monroe R.H., and Whiting B.R. (eds): "Handbook of Cross-Cultural Human Development." New York: Garland Press.
41. Tanner, J. M. (1970). Physical growth. In Mussen P.H. (ed): "Carmichael's Manual of Child Psychology," Vol I. New York: John Wiley.
42. Thomas, A., Chess, S., Birch, H. G., Hertzig, M. E., Korn, S. (1963). "Behavioral Individuality in Early Childhood." New York: New York University Press.
43. Thomas, A., Chess, S. (1977). "Temperament and development." New York: Brunner/Mazel.
44. Torgersen, A. M., Kringlen, E. (1978). Genetic aspects of temperamental differences in infants. Am Acad Child Psychiatr 17:433–444.
45. Waddington, C. H. (1957). "The Strategy of Genes." London: Allen and Unwin.

46. Waddington, C. H. (1962). "New Patterns in Genetics and Development." New York: Columbia University Press.
47. Waddington, C. H. (1971). Concepts of development. In Tobach E., Aronson L.R. and Shaw E. (eds): "The Biopsychology of Development." New York: Academic.
48. Waddington, C. H. (1975). "The Evolution of an Evolutionist." Ithaca, NY: Cornell University Press.
49. Wilson, R. S. (1978). Synchronies in mental development: An epigenetic perspective. Science 202:939–948.
50. Wilson, R. S., Matheny, A. P. (1978). Determinants of temperament in infant twins: Issues in assessment. In: "JSAS Catalog of Selected Documents in Psychology," 1080, 10, MS # 1978.
51. Mayr, E. (1958). Behavior and systematics. In Roe A. and Simpson G.G. (eds): "Behavior and Evolution." New Haven: Yale University Press.
52. Mayr, E. (1978). Evolution. Sci Am 239:46–55.
53. Hess, E. H. (1970). Ethology and developmental psychology. In Mussen P.H. (ed): "Carmichael's Manual of Child Psychology," Vol I. New York: John Wiley.
54. Blurton Jones, N. (ed), (1972). "Ethological Studies of Child Behavior." Cambridge: Cambridge University Press.
55. Bateson, P. P. G., Hinde, R. A. (eds), (1976). "Growing Points in Ethology." Cambridge: Cambridge University Press.
56. McClearn, G. E. (1964). Genes and development. In Hoffman M.L. and Hoffman L.W. (eds): "Review of Child Development Research," Vol I. New York: Russell Sage Foundation.
57. Lindzey, G., Loehlin, J., Manosevitz, M., Thiessen, D. (1971). Behavioral genetics. Annu Rev Psychol 22:39–94.
58. Broadhurst, P. L., Fulker, D. W., Wilcock, J. (1974). Behavioral genetics. Ann Rev Psychol 25:389–415.
59. Scarr-Salapatek, S. (1975). Genetics and the development of intelligence. In Horowitz F.D. (ed): "Review of Child Development Research," Vol 4. Chicago: University of Chicago Press.
60. DeFries, J. C., Plomin, R. (1978). Behavioral genetics. Annu Rev Psychol 29:473–515.
61. Willerman, L. (1979). "The Psychology of Individual and Group Differences." San Francisco: W.H. Freeman.
62. Henderson, N. D. (1982). Human behavior genetics. Annu Rev Psychol 33:403–440.
63. Kagan, J. (1976). Resilience and continuity in psychological development. In Clarke A.M. and Clarke A.D.B. (eds): "Early Experience: Myth and Evidence." New York: Free Press, pp 97–121.
64. McCall, R. B., Eichorn, D. H., Hogarty, P. S. (1977). Transitions in early mental development. Monographs of the Society for Research in Child Development, Serial No. 171, 42:1–108.
65. Sameroff, A. J., Chandler, M. J. (1975). Reproductive risk and the continuum of caretaking casuality. In Horowitz F.D. (ed): "Review of Child Development Research," Vol 4. Chicago: University of Chicago Press.
66. Sroufe, L. A., Waters, E. (1977). Attachment as an organizational construct. Child Dev 48:1184–1199.
67. Mineka, S., Suomi, S. J. (1978). Social separation in monkeys. Psychol Bull 85:1376–1400.
68. Kohen-Raz, R. (1977). "Psychobiological Aspects of Cognitive Growth." New York: Academic Press.

69. Goldsmith, H. H., Gottesman, I. I. (1981). Origins of variation in behavioral style: A longitudinal study of temperament in young twins. Child Dev 52:91–103.
70. Plomin, R. (1981). Heredity and temperament: A comparison of twin data for self-report questionnaires, parental ratings, and objectively assessed behavior. In Gedda L., Parisi P. and Nance W.E. (eds): "Twin Research 3: Intelligence, Personality and Development." New York: Alan R. Liss.
71. Torgersen, A. M. (1982). Influence of genetic factors on temperament development in early childhood. In CIBA Symposium 89, "Temperamental Differences in Infants and Young Children." London: Pitman.
72. Wilson, R. S. (1982). Intrinsic determinants of temperament. In CIBA Foundation symposium 89, "Temperamental Differences in Infants and Young Children." London: Pitman, pp 121–140.
73. Bunge, R., Johnson, M., Ross, C. D. (1978). Nature and nurture in the development of the autonomic neuron. Science 199:1409–1416.
74. Purves, D. M. (1981). "Neuronal development and repair." Quincy, Mass: Grass Instrument Co, Bulletin #X854H81.

5

How People Make Their Own Environments: A Theory of Genotype → Environment Effects

Sandra Scarr and Kathleen McCartney

Yale University

We propose a theory of development in which experience is directed by genotypes. Genotypic differences are proposed to affect phenotypic differences, both directly and through experience, via 3 kinds of genotype → environment effects: a passive kind, through environments provided by biologically related parents; an evocative kind, through responses elicited by individuals from others; and an active kind, through the selection of different environments by different people. The theory adapts the 3 kinds of genotype-environment correlations proposed by Plomin, DeFries, and Loehlin in a developmental model that is used to explain results from studies of deprivation, intervention, twins, and families.

Reprinted with permission from *Child Development*, 1983, Vol. 54, 424–435. Copyright 1983 by the Society for Research in Child Development, Inc.

We thank Emily Cahan, Jerome Kagan, Katherine Nelson, Robert Plomin, and Theodore D. Wachs for their critical and helpful comments on several drafts of this paper. Their disagreements with us were stimulating and always constructive. Much of the family research reviewed here was done in collaboration with Richard A. Weinberg and supported by the W. T. Grant Foundation and the National Institute of Mental Health. The day-care studies have the collaboration of J. Conrad Schwarz, Susan Grajek, and Deborah Phillips and were supported by the W. T. Grant Foundation and the Bermuda Government.

INTRODUCTION

Theories of behavioral development have ranged from genetic determinism to naive environmentalism. Neither of these radical views nor interactionism has adequately explained the process of development or the role of experience in development. In this paper we propose a theory of environmental effects on human development that emphasizes the role of the genotype in determining not only which environments are experienced by individuals but also which environments individuals seek for themselves. To show how this theory addresses the process of development, the theory is used to account for seemingly anomalous findings for deprivation, adoption, twin, and intervention studies.

For the species, we claim that human experience and its effects on development depend primarily on the evolved nature of the human genome. In evolutionary theory the two essential concepts are selection and variation. Through selection the human genome has evolved to program human development. Phenotypic variation is the raw material on which selection works. Genetic variation must be associated with phenotypic variations, or there could be no evolution. It follows from evolutionary theory that individual differences depend in part on genotypic differences. We argue that genetic differences prompt differences in which environments are experienced and what effects they may have. In this view, the genotype, in both its species specificity and its individual variability, largely determines environmental effects on development, because the genotype determines the organism's responsiveness to environmental opportunities.

A theory of behavioral development must explain the origin of new psychological structures. Because there is no evidence that new adaptations can arise out of the environment without maturational changes in the organism, genotypes must be the source of new structures.

Maturational sequence is controlled primarily by the genetic program for development. As Gottlieb (1976) said, there is evidence for a role of environment in (1) maintaining existing structures and in (2) elaborating existing structures; however, there is no evidence that the environment has a role in (3) inducing new structures. In development, new adaptations or structures cannot arise out of experience per se.

The most widely accepted theories of development are vague about how new structures arise; for example, Piaget (1980) fails to make the connection between organism and environment clear in his references to interaction. Nor is development well described by maturation alone (see Connolly & Prechtl, 1981). Neither Gesell and Ilg (1943) nor contemporary nativists (e.g., Chomsky, 1980) appreciate the inextricable links of nature and nurture in a hierarchically organized system of development.

We suggest that the problem of new structures in development has been extraordinarily difficult because of a false parallel between genotype and environment, which, we argue, are not constructs at the same level of analysis. The dichotomy of nature and nurture has always been a bad one, not only for the oft-cited reasons that both are required for development, but because a false parallel arises between the two. We propose that development is indeed the result of nature *and* nurture but that genes drive experience. Genes are components in a system that organizes the organism to experience its world. The organism's abilities to experience the world change with development and are individually variable. A good theory of the environment can only be one in which experience is guided by genotypes that both push and restrain experiences.

Behavioral development depends on both a genetic program and a suitable environment for the expression of the human, species-typical program for development. Differences among people can arise from both genetic and environmental differences, but the process by which differences arise is better described as genotype → environment effects. Like Chomsky and Fodor (1980), we propose that the genotype is the driving force behind development, because, we argue, it is the discriminator of what environments are actually experienced. The genotype determines the *responsiveness* of the person to those environmental opportunities. Unlike Chomsky and Fodor, we do not think that development is precoded in the genes and merely emerges with maturation. Rather, we stress the role of the genotype in determining which environments are actually experienced and what effects they have on the developing person.

We distinguish here between environments to which a person is exposed and environments that are actively experienced or "grasped" by the person. As we all know, the relevance of environments changes with development. The toddler who has "caught on" to the idea that things have names and who demands the names for everything is experiencing a fundamentally different verbal environment from what she experienced before, even though her parents talked to her extensively in infancy. The young adolescent who played baseball with the boy next door and now finds herself hopelessly in love with him is experiencing her friend's companionship in a new way.

A model of genotypes and environments.—Figure 1 presents our model of behavioral development. In this model, the child's phenotype (P_c), or observable characteristics, is a function of both the child's genotype (G_c) and her rearing environment (E_c). There will be little disagreement on this. The parents' genotypes (G_p) determine the child's genotype, which in turn influences the child's phenotype. Again, there should be little controversy over this point. As in most developmental theories, transactions occur between the organism and the environment; here they are described by the correlation between phenotype and rearing environment. In most models, however, the source of this correlation is ambiguous. In this model, both the child's phenotype and rearing environment are influenced by the child's genotype. Because the child's genotype influences both the phenotype and the rearing environment, their correlation is a function of the genotype. The genotype is *conceptually prior* to both the phenotype and the rearing environment.

It is an unconventional shorthand to suggest that the child's genotype can directly affect the rearing environment. What we want to represent is developmental changes in the genetic program that prompt new experiences, before the full phenotype is developed. An example could be found in the development of productive speech; the child becomes attentive to the language environment receptively months before real words are produced. Our argument is that changes in what is "turned on" in the genotype affect an emerging phenotype both directly through maturation $(G_c$ to $P_c)$ and through prompting new experiences.

The model could just as well specify intermediate phenotypes, such as receptive language in the example of productive speech, but the *idea* that genetic differences (both developmental changes for an individual

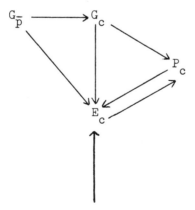

FIG. 1.—A model of behavioral development

over time and differences among individuals) affect experiential differences could be lost in a web of path diagrams. The model is designed to present our ideas, not for analysis of variance.

Also clouded by an endless regress of intermediate phenotypes would be the idea that the correlation or transaction between phenotype and environment is determined by developmental changes in the genotype. We recognize that this is not a popular position, but we propose it to account for data to be discussed in the final sections of the paper.

Thus, we intend the path from G_c to E_c to represent the idea that developmental changes in phenotypes are prompted both by changes in the effective genotype and by changes in the salience of environments, which are then correlated.

The path from the G_c to P_c represents maturation, which is controlled primarily by the genetic program. New structures arise out of maturation, from genotype to phenotype. Behavioral development is elaborated and maintained, in Gottlieb's sense, by the transactions of phenotype and environment, but it cannot arise de novo from this interaction. Thus, in this model, the course of development is a function of genetically controlled maturational sequences, although the rate of maturation can be affected by some environmental circumstances, such as the effects of nutrition on physical growth (Watson & Lowrey, 1967). Behavioral examples include cultural differences in rates of development through the sequence of cognitive stages described by Piaget and other theoretical sequences (see Nerlove & Snipper, 1981).

Separation of genetic and environmental effects on development.—The major problem with attempts to separate environmental from genetic effects and their combinations is that people evoke and select their own environments to a great extent. There may appear to be arbitrary events of fate, such as being hit by a truck (did you look carefully in both directions?), falling ill (genetic differences in susceptibility, or a life-style that lowers resistance to disease?), but even these may not be entirely divorced from personal characteristics that have some genetic variability. Please understand that we do not mean that one's environmental fate is *entirely* determined by one's genotype—only that some genotypes are more likely to receive and select certain environments than others. A theory that stresses either genetic or environmental differences per se cannot account for the processes by which people come to be the way they are. At any one point in time, behavioral differences may be analyzed into variances that can be attributed more or less to genetic and environmental sources (see Plomin, DeFries, & Loehlin, 1977; Scarr & Kidd, in press). A quantitative genetic approach to estimating variances, however, does not attempt to specify the processes by which individuals developed their phenotypes.

Genotype-environment correlations.—Plomin et al. (1977) have described a model of phenotype variation that estimates the amount of variance that arises from genetic and environmental differences. Genotype-environment correlation is a nonlinear component in the additive variance model, included to account for situations in which "genotypes are selectively exposed to different environments." They did not intend to describe developmental processes, as we are doing here. Rather, Plomin and his colleagues were responding to the question, How much of the variation in a phenotype is due to differences among genotypes, differences among environments, dominance effects, genotype-environment interactions, and genotype-environment correlations? Their model addresses sources of individual differences in a population of phenotypes at one point in time. By contrast, our use of the term, genotype → environment effects, is to describe developmental *processes* over time, not to estimate sources of variance in phenotypes. We seek to answer the questions, How do genotypes and environments *combine* to produce human development? and How do genetic and environmental differences *combine* to produce variation in development?

AN EVOLVING THEORY OF BEHAVIORAL DEVELOPMENT

Plomin et al. (1977) described three kinds of genotype-environment correlations that we believe form the basis for a developmental theory. The theory of genotype → environment effects we propose has three propositions:

1. The process by which children develop is best described by three kinds of genotype → environment effects: a *passive* kind, whereby the genetically related parents provide a rearing environment that is correlated with the genotype of the child (sometimes positively and sometimes negatively); an *evocative* kind, whereby the child receives responses from others that are influenced by his genotype; and an *active* kind that represents the child's selective attention to and learning from aspects of his environment that are influenced by his genotype and indirectly correlated with those of his biological relatives.

2. The relative importance of the three kinds of genotype → environment effects changes with development. The influence of the passive kind declines from infancy to adolescence, and the importance of the active kind increases over the same period.

3. The degree to which experience is influenced by individual gen-

otypes increases with development and with the shift from passive to active genotype → environment effects, as individuals select their own experiences.

The first, *passive* genotype → environment effects arise in biologically related families and render all of the research literature on parent-child socialization uninterpretable. Because parents provide both genes and environments for their biological offspring, the child's environment is necessarily correlated with her genes, because her genes are correlated with her parents' genes, and the parents' genes are correlated with the rearing environment they provide. It is impossible to know what about the parents' rearing environment for the child determines what about the child's behavior, because of the confounding effect of genetic transmission of the same characteristics from parent to child. Not only can we not interpret the direction of effects in parent-child interaction, as Bell (1968) argued, we also cannot interpret the *cause* of those effects in biologically related families.

An example of a positive kind of passive genotype-environment correlation can be found in reading; parents who read well and enjoy reading are likely to provide their children with books; thus, the children are more likely to be skilled readers who enjoy reading, both for genetic and environmental reasons. The children's rearing environment is positively correlated with the parents' genotypes and therefore with the children's genotypes as well.

An example of a negative passive genotype-environment correlation can also be found in reading. Parents who are skilled readers, faced with a child who is not learning to read well, may provide a more enriched reading environment for that child than for another who acquires reading skills quickly. The more enriched environment for the less able child represents a negative genotype → environment effect (see also Plomin et al., 1977). There is, thus, an unreliable, but not random, connection between genotypes and environments when parents provide the opportunities for experience.

The second kind of genotype → environment effect is called evocative because it represents the different responses that different genotypes evoke from the social and physical environments. Responses to the person further shape development in ways that correlate with the genotype. Examples of such evocative effects can be found in the research of Lytton (1980), the theory of Escalona (1968), and the review of Maccoby (1980). It is quite likely that smiley, active babies receive more social stimulation than sober, passive infants. In the intellectual area, cooperative, attentive preschoolers receive more pleasant and instructional interactions from the adults around them than uncooperative, distractible children. Individual differences in responses evoked can also be found in the physical world; for example, people who are skillful at electronics receive feedback of a sort very different from those who fail consistently at such tasks.

The third kind of genotype → environment effect is the active, niche-picking or niche-building sort. People seek out environments they find compatible and stimulating. We all select from the surrounding environment some aspects to which to respond, learn about, or ignore. Our selections are correlated with motivational, personality, and intellectual aspects of our genotypes. The active genotype → environment effect, we argue, is the most powerful connection between people and their environments and the most direct expression of the genotype in experience.

Examples of active genotype → environment effects can be found in the selective efforts of individuals in sports, scholarship, relationships—in life. Once experiences occur, they naturally lead to further experiences. We agree that phenotypes are elaborated and maintained by environments, but the impetus for the experience comes, we argue, from the genotype.

Developmental changes in genotype → environment effects.— The second proposition is that the relative importance of the three kinds of genotype → environment effects changes over development from infancy to adolescence. In infancy much of the environment that reaches the child is provided by adults. When those adults are genetically related to the child, the environment they provide in general is positively related to their own characteristics and their own genotypes. Although infants are active in structuring their experiences by selectively attending to what is offered, they cannot do as much seeking out and niche-building as older children; thus, passive genotype → environment effects are more important for infants and young children than they are for older children, who can extend their experiences beyond the family's influences and create their own environments to a much greater extent. Thus, the effects of passive genotype → environment effects wane when the child has many extrafamilial opportunities.

In addition, parents can provide environments that are negatively related to the child's genotype, as illustrated earlier in teaching reading. Although parents' genotypes usually affect the environment they provide for their biological offspring, it is sometimes positive and sometimes negative and therefore not as direct a product of the young child's genotype as later environments will be. Thus, as stated in proposition

3, genotype → environment effects increase with development, as active replace passive forms. Genotype → environment effects of the evocative sort persist throughout life, as we elicit responses from others based on many personal, genotype-related characteristics from appearance to personality and intellect. Those responses from others reinforce and extend the directions our development has taken. High intelligence and adaptive skills in children from very disadvantaged backgrounds, for example, evoke approval and support from school personnel who might otherwise despair of the child's chances in life (Garmezy, Note 1). In adulthood, personality and intellectual differences evoke different responses in others. Similarities in personal characteristics evoke similar responses from others, as shown in the case of identical twins reared apart (Bouchard, Note 2). These findings are also consistent with the third proposition.

A probabilistic model.—The concept of genotype → environment effects is emphasized in this emerging theory for three major reasons: the model results in a testable set of hypotheses for which disconfirmation would come from random association between genotypes and environments, it describes a developmental process, and it implies a *probabilistic* connection between a person and the environment. It is more likely that people with certain genotypes will receive certain kinds of parenting, evoke certain responses from others, and select certain aspects from the available environments; but nothing is rigidly determined. The idea of genetic differences, on the other hand, has seemed to imply to many that the person's developmental fate was preordained without regard to experience. This is absurd. By invoking the idea of genotype → environment effects, we hope to emphasize a probabilistic connection between genotypes and their environments. Although mismatches between the behaviors of parents and children certainly exist (see Nelson, 1973), we argue that on the average there are correlations of parents' characteristics and the rearing environment they provide.

Waddington (1962) postulated a probable but not determinant connection between genotypes and phenotypes through an epigenetic space, in which environmental events deflect the course of the developing phenotype. Figure 2 illustrates Waddington's theory of the probable relationship between genotypic and phenotypic differences. Note that a correlation remains between genotype and phenotype, even though one cannot specify in advance what environmental events will affect phenotypic development. To this conception, we add that genotypes shape many of their own experiences through evocative and active genotype → environment correlations.

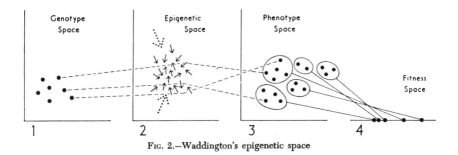

FIG. 2.—Waddington's epigenetic space

THE ROLE OF THE ENVIRONMENT REVISITED

If genotypes are the driving force behind development and the determinants of what environments are experienced, does this mean that environments themselves have no effects? Clearly, environments are necessary for development and have effects on the average levels of development, but they may or may not cause variations among individuals (McCall, 1981). We argue like McCall that nature has not left essential human development at the mercy of experiences that may or may not be encountered; rather, the only necessary experiences are ones that are generally available to the species. Differences in experience per se, therefore, cannot be the major cause of variation among individuals. The major features of human development are programmed genetically and require experiences that are encountered by the vast majority of humankind in the course of living. Phenotypic variation among individuals relies on experiential differences that are determined by genetic differences rather than on differences among environmental effects that occur randomly.

Imposed environments.—In developmental studies, we usually think of environments provided for a child, such as parental interaction, school curricula, and various experimental manipulations. In some cases there are passive and evocative genotype-environment correlations that go unrecognized, as in parent-child interaction and the selection of children into school curricula. In a few cases there may be no correlation of the child's genotype with the treatment afforded an experimental group of which she is a member. On the other hand, it is impossible to ignore the attention and learning characteristics the child brings to the situation, so that the effects of environmental manipulations are never entirely free of individual differences in genotypes. Development is not necessarily constrained by genotype-environment correlations, although most often genotypes and environments are correlated in the real world, so that in fact, if not in principle, there are such constraints.

Sometimes, the influence of genotypes on environments is diminished through unusual positive or negative interventions, so that the environments experienced are less driven by genotypes and may even be negatively related to genotypes, as in the passive, familial situation. Examples of this effect can be found in studies of deprivation, adoption, and day care. Studies of children reared in isolation (Clarke & Clarke, 1976) and children reared in unstimulating institutions (Dennis & Najarian, 1951; Hunt, 1961, 1980) have demonstrated the adverse effects of deprived environments on many aspects of development. Such studies usually address average responses to these poor environments. In any case, studies of environments that are so extreme as to be outside of the normal range of rearing environments for the species have few implications for environmental variation that the vast majority of human children experience.

In contrast to the extremely poor environments in the deprivation literature, the adoption studies include only rearing environments in the range of adequate to very good. The evidence from studies of biologically related and adoptive families that vary in socioeconomic status from working to upper middle class is that most people experience what Scarr and Weinberg (1978) have called "functionally-equivalent" environments. That is, the large array of individual differences among children and late adolescents adopted in infancy were not related to differences among their family environments—the same array of environmental differences that were and usually are associated with behavioral differences among children born to such families (Scarr, 1981; Scarr & Kidd, in press; Scarr & Weinberg, 1976, 1977, 1978). On the average, however, adopted children profit from their enriched environments, and they score above average on IQ and school achievement tests and on measures of personal adjustment.

Negative genotype-environment correlations.—Environments provided to children that are negatively related to their genotypes can have dramatic effects on average levels of development. Extrafamilial interventions that provide unusual enrichments or deprivations can alter the developmental levels of children from those that would be predicted by their family backgrounds and estimated genotypes. Intervention theories predict these main effects (Caldwell & Richmond, 1968; Hunt, 1980).

Enriched day-care environments have been shown to enhance intellectual development of children from disadvantaged backgrounds (Ramey & Haskins, 1981; McCartney, Note 3). Similarly, less stimulating day-care environments can hamper children's intellectual and social development, even if they come from more advantaged families (McCartney, Scarr, Phillips, Grajek, & Schwarz, 1981; McCartney, Note 3).

These are, however, rather rare opportunities, or lack of same, providing negatively correlated experiences for genotypes. In the usual course of development beyond early childhood, individuals select and evoke experiences that are directly influenced by their genotypes and therefore positively correlated with their own phenotypic characteristics.

Environmental effects on averages versus individuals.—One must distinguish environmental events that on the average enhance or delay development for all children from those that account for *variation* among children. There can be "main effects" that account for variation among groups that are naturally or experimentally treated in different ways. Within the groups of children there still remain enormous individual differences, some of which arise in response to the treatment. It is rare that the variation *between* groups approaches the magnitude of differences *within* groups, as represented in the pervasive overlapping distributions of scores. In developmental psychology, we have usually been satisfied if the treatment observed or implemented produced a statistically reliable difference between groups, but we have rarely examined the sources of differential responsiveness within the groups.

Most often, the same treatments that alter the average performance of a group seem to have similar effects on most members of the group. Otherwise, we would find a great deal of variance in genotype-environment interactions; that is, what's sauce for the goose would be poison for the gander. For the kinds of deprivation or interventions studied most often in developmental psychology, the main effects seem not to change the rank orders of children affected. The main effects are real, but they are also small by comparison to the range of individual variation within groups so treated or not. Some children may be more responsive than others to the treatment, but we doubt that there are many situations in which disordinal interactions are the rule. Very few children lose developmental points by participating in Headstart or gain by being severely neglected in infancy. (Cronbach & Snow, 1977) and genotype-environment interactions (Erlenmeyer-Kimling, 1972) have not produced dramatic or reliable results.

In studies of adoptive and biologically related families, the correlation of children's IQ scores with the educational level of biological parents is about .35, whether or not the parents rear their children (Scarr & Weinberg, in this issue). Adopted children on the average have higher

IQ scores than their biological parents as a result of the influence of their above-average adoptive parents. Taken together, these findings support the claim that treatments can have main effects without overcoming genetic differences in children's responsiveness to those environments. Adopted children have IQ scores above those of their biological parents, yet the *correlations* of adopted children are higher with their biological than adoptive parents (Scarr & Weinberg, 1977, 1978, in this issue). The average effects of treatments, such as adoption, seem to increase the mean IQ scores, but they do not seem to affect the rank order of the children's scores with respect to their biological parents, and it is on rank orders, not means that correlations depend. These results imply that the effect of adoptive families is to increase the scores of adopted children above those which would be predicted by their biological parents, but not to alter radically the rank order of individual differences among children they rear. And so it is, we think, with most treatments.

ANSWERING QUESTIONS FROM PREVIOUS RESEARCH ON TWINS AND FAMILIES

Neither extreme genetic determinism nor naive environmentalism can account for seemingly anomalous findings from research on twins and families. Three puzzling questions remain, the first of which concerns the *process* by which monozygotic (MZ) twins come to be more similar than dizygotic (DZ) twins, and biological siblings more similar than adopted siblings on all measurable characteristics, at least by the end of adolescence (Scarr & Weinberg, 1978). The second question concerns the declining similarities between DZ twins and adopted siblings from infancy to adolescence. The third question arises from the unexpected similarities between identical twins reared in different homes.

A theory of genotype-environment correlation can account for these findings by pointing to the degree of genetic resemblance and the degree of similarity in the environments that would be experienced by the co-twins and sibs.

Genetic resemblance determines environmental similarity.—The expected degree of environmental similarity for a pair of relatives can be thought of as the product of a person's own genotype $\rightarrow$ environment path and the genetic correlation of the pair. Figure 3 presents a model of the relationship between genotypes and environments for pairs of relatives who vary in genetic relatedness. G_1 and G_2 symbolize the two genotypes, E_1 and E_2 their respective environments. The similarity in the two en-

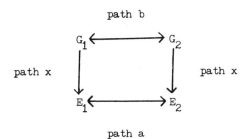

path b

path x   path x

path a

FIG. 3.—A model of environmental similarity based on genetic resemblance.

vironments (path *a*) is the product of the coefficient of each genotype with its own environment (path *x*) and the genetic correlation of the pair (path *b*). On the assumption that individuals' environments are equally influenced by their own genotypes, the similarity in the environments of two individuals becomes a function of their genetic correlation.

This model can be used to answer question 1 concerning the process by which MZ twins come to be more similar than DZ twins and biological siblings more similar than adopted siblings. For identical twins, for whom $b = 1.00$, the relationship of one twin's environment with the other's genotype is the same as the correlation of the twin's environment with her own genotype. Thus, one would certainly predict what is often observed: that the hobbies, food preferences, choices of friends, academic achievements, and so forth of the MZ twins are very similar (Scarr & Carter-Saltzman, 1980). Kamin (1974) proposed that all of this environmental similarity is imposed on MZ co-twins because they look so much alike. Theories of genetic resemblance do not speak to how close resemblances arise. We propose that the home environments provided by the parents, the responses that the co-twins evoke from others, and the active choices they make in their environments lead to striking similarities through genotypically determined correlations in their learning histories.

The same explanation applies, of course, to the greater resemblance of biological than adopted siblings. The environment of one biological sib is correlated to the genotype of the other as one-half the coefficient of the sibling's environment to her own genotype, because $b = 0.50$, as described in Figure 3. The same is true for DZ twins. There is a very small genetic correlation for intelligence between adopted siblings in most studies that arises from selective placement of the offspring of similar mothers in the same adoptive home. More important for this theory, however, is the selective placement of adopted children to match the intellectual characteristics of the adoptive parents. This practice allows adoptive parents to create a positive, passive genotype-environment correlation for their adopted children in early childhood, when the theory asserts that this kind of correlation is most important. In fact, the selective placement estimates from studies by Scarr and Weinberg (1977) can account for most of the resemblance between adoptive parents and their children. In addition, adoptive parents, like their biological counterparts, can provide negative genotype-environment correlations that assure that their several children will not differ too much on important skills, such as reading.

Changing similarities among siblings.—The second question left unanswered by previous research concerned the declining similarities of dizygotic twins and adopted siblings from infancy to adolescence. It is clear from Matheny, Wilson, Dolan, and Krantz's (1981) longitudinal study of MZ and DZ twins that the DZ correlations for intelligence of .60–.75 are higher than genetic theory would predict in infancy and early childhood. For school age and older twins, DZ correlations were the usual .55. Similarly, the intelligence correlations of a sample of late adolescent adopted siblings were zero, compared to the .25–.39 correlations of the samples of adopted children in early to middle childhood (Scarr & Weinberg, 1978).

Neither environmental nor genetic theories can effectively address these data. How can it be that the longer you live with someone, the less like them you become? One could evoke some ad hoc environmental theory about sibling relationships becoming more competitive, or "deidentified," but that would not account for the continued, moderate intellectual resemblance of biological siblings. Genetic theory has, of course, nothing to say about decreasing twin resemblance or any resemblance among young adoptees.

The theory put forward here predicts that the relative importance of passive versus active genotype-environment correlations changes with age. Recall that passive genotype-environment correlations are created by parents who provide children with both genes and environments, which are then correlated. Certainly in the case of DZ twins, whose prenatal environment was shared and whose earliest years are spent being treated in most of the same ways at the same time by the same parents, the passive genotype → environment effect is greater than that for ordinary sibs. Biological and adopted siblings do not, of course, share the same developmental environments at the same time because they differ in age. The passive genotype-environment correlation still operates for siblings, because they have the same parents, but to a lesser extent than for twins. (See Table 1.)

Monozygotic twin correlations for intellectual competence do not decline when active genotype-environment correlations outweigh the importance of the passive ones, because MZ co-twins typically select highly correlated environments anyway. Dizygotic pairs, on the other hand, are no more genetically related than sibs, so that as the intense similarity of their early home environments gives way to their own choices, they select environments that are less similar than their previous environments and about as similar as those of ordinary sibs.

Adopted sibs, on the other hand, move from an early environment, in which mother may have produced similarity, to environments of their own choosing. Because their genotypes are hardly correlated at all, neither are their chosen environmental niches. Thus, by late adolescence, adopted siblings do not resemble each other in intelligence, personality, interests, or other phenotypic characteristics (Grotevant, Scarr, & Weinberg, 1977; Scarr, Webber, Weinberg, & Wittig, 1981; Scarr & Weinberg, 1978).

Biological siblings' early environments, like those of adopted children, lead to trait similarity as a result of passive genotype → environmental effects. As biological siblings move into the larger world and begin to make active choices, their niches remain moderately correlated because their genotypes remain moderately correlated. There is no marked shift in intellectual resemblance of biological sibs as the process of active genotype → environment influence replaces the passive one.

Identical twins reared apart.—The third question concerned the unexpected degree of resemblance between identical twins reared mostly apart. With the theory of genotype → environment effects, their resemblance is not surprising. Given opportunities to attend selectively to and choose from varied opportunities, identical genotypes are expected to make similar choices. They are also expected to evoke similar re-

TABLE 1

The Similarity of Co-twin's and Sibling's Genotypes and Environments Due To:

| | Genetic Correlation | Correlations in the Environments of Related Pairs | |
		Passive Genotype → Environment Effects in Early Development	Active Genotype → Environment Effects in Early Development
MZ twins	1.00	High	High
DZ twins	.52	High	Moderate
Biological siblings	.52	Moderate	Moderate
Adopted siblings	.01	Moderate	Low

sponses from others and from their physical environments. The fact that they were reared in different homes and different communities is not important; differences in their development could arise only if the experiential opportunities of one or both were very restricted, so that similar choices could not have been made. According to previous studies (Juel-Nielsen, 1980; Newman, Freeman, & Holzinger, 1937; Shields, 1962) and the recent research of Bouchard and colleagues at the University of Minnesota (Bouchard, Note 2), the most dissimilar pairs of MZs reared apart are those in which one was severely restricted in environmental opportunity. Extreme deprivation or unusual enrichment can diminish the influence of genotype and environment and therefore lessen the resemblance of identical twins reared apart.

RESEARCH STRATEGIES

The theory we propose can be tested in several ways and prove unable to account for results. First, studies of parental treatment of more than one child would be informative about passive genotype → environment effects. In general, we expect the rearing environment provided for the children in a family to differ in ways that are related to each child's characteristics. Do parents treat all of their children alike, as so many studies of one child per family seem to imply? Can parents be authoritative with one child and permissive with another? Our theory predicts that parents will respond to individual differences in their children, in keeping with Lytton's (1980) research on families with twins. If parent treatment of their children is not related to children's talents, interests, and personalities, the theory is wrong.

Second, studies of responses that individuals evoke from others would test our ideas about evocative genotype → environment effects. The social psychology literature in attractiveness (Bersheid & Walster, 1974; Mursteid, 1972), for example, would seem to support our view that some personal characteristics evoke differential responses from others. Similarly, teachers' responses to children with high versus low intelligence, hyperactivity versus acceptable levels of energy, and so forth provide some evidence for our theory. If others do not respond differentially to individual characteristics for which there is genetic variability, then the theory is wrong.

Third, active niche-building is being studied by the Laboratory of Comparative Human Cognition in their naturalistic observations of children's adaptations to problem-solving situations (Cole & The Laboratory of Comparative Human Cognition, Note 4). Our theory predicts that children select and build niches that are correlated with their talents, interests, and personality characteristics. If not, the theory is wrong.

Fourth, longitudinal studies of adopted children, such as the ongoing work of Plomin and colleagues, can provide valuable evidence of the changing influences of family environments on children. The theory predicts that children's characteristics will be more related to characteristics of the adoptive parents and other adopted siblings in earlier than later development. If adopted children are as similar to their adoptive parents and each other in late adolescence as they were in early childhood, that aspect of the theory is wrong.

Fifth, studies of older adolescents and adults who were adopted in infancy and others who were born into their families can provide evidence on the long-term effects of passive genotype → environment effects within families. Both evocative and active kinds of genotype → environmental effects can be traced through the similarities and dissimilarities of the two kinds of siblings.

In these ways, and others, the theory can be tested. It can fail to account for results obtained, or it can account for the diverse results more adequately than other theories Given the various results of family studies presented in this paper, we believe that its predictions will be fulfilled. At least, we hope it will encourage more developmentalists to study more than one child per family, genetically unrelated families, and individual differences in experience.

SUMMARY

In summary, the theory of genotype → environment correlations proposed here describes the usual course of human development in terms of three kinds of genotype-environment correlations that posit cooperative efforts of the nature-nurture team, directed by the genetic quarterback. Both genes and environments are constituents in the developmental system, but they have different roles. Genes direct the course of human experience, but experiential opportunities are also necessary for development to occur. Individual differences can arise from restrictions in environmental opportunities to experience what the genotype would find compatible. With a rich array of opportunities, however, most differences among people arise from genetically determined differences in the experiences to which they are attracted and which they evoke from their environments.

The theory also accounts for individual differences in responsiveness to environments—differences that are not primarily interactions of genotypes and environments but roughly linear combinations that are better described as genotype-environment correlations. In addition, the theory accounts for seemingly anomalous results from previous research on twins and families.

Most important, the theory addresses the issue of process. Rather than presenting a static view of individual differences through variance allocation, this theory hypothesizes processes by which genotypes and environments combine across development to make us both human and unique.

REFERENCE NOTES

1. Garmezy, N. (1981, August). *The case for the single case in experimental-developmental psychology*. Paper presented at the annual meeting of the American Psychological Association, Los Angeles.
2. Bouchard, T. (1981, August). *The Minnesota study of twins reared apart: Description and preliminary findings*. Paper presented at the annual meeting of the American Psychological Association.
3. McCartney, K. (1982). *The effect of quality of day care environment upon children's language development*. Unpublished doctoral dissertation, Yale University.
4. Cole, M., & The Laboratory of Comparative Human Cognition (1980). *Niche-picking*. Unpublished manuscript, University of California, San Diego.

REFERENCES

Bell, R. Q. (1968). A reinterpretation of the direction of effects in studies of socialization. *Psychological Review, 75*, 81–95.

Bersheid, E., & Walster, E. (1974). Physical attractiveness. In L. Berkowitz (Ed.), *Advances in experimental social psychology*. New York: Academic Press.

Caldwell, B. M., & Richmond, I. (1968). The Children's Center in Syracuse. In L. Dittman (Ed.), *Early child: The new perspectives*. New York: Atherton.

Chomsky, N. (1980). On cognitive structures and their development: A reply to Piaget. In M. Piattelli-Palmarini (Ed.), *Language and learning: The debate between Jean Piaget and Noam Chomsky*. Cambridge, Mass.: Harvard University Press.

Chomsky, N., & Fodor, J. (1980). Statement of the paradox. In M. Piattelli-Palmarini (Ed.), *Language and learning: The debate between Jean Piaget and Noam Chomsky*. Cambridge, Mass.: Harvard University Press.

Clarke, A. M., & Clarke, A. D. B. (1976). *Early experience: Myth and evidence*. New York: Free Press.

Connolly, K. J., & Prechtl, H. F. R. (Eds.) (1981). *Maturation and development: Biological and psychological perspectives*. Philadelphia: Lippincott.

Cronbach, L. J., & Snow, R. E. (1977). *Attitudes and instructional methods*. New York: Irvington.

Dennis, W., & Najarian, P. (1951). Infant development under environmental handicap. *Psychological Monographs, 71*(7, Whole No. 436).

Erlenmeyer-Kimling, L. (1972). Gene-environment interactions and the variability of behavior. In L. Ehrman, G. Omenn, & E. Caspair (Eds.), *Genetics, environment and behavior.* New York: Academic Press.

Escalona, S. C. (1968). *The roots of individuality.* Chicago: Aldine.

Gesell, A., & Ilg, F. L. (1943). *Infant and child in the culture of today.* New York: Harper & Bros.

Gottlieb, G. (1976). The role of experience in the development of behavior in the nervous system. In G. Gottlieb (Ed.), *Studies in the development of behavior and the nervous system.* Vol. **3**. *Development and neural and behavioral specificity.* New York: Academic Press.

Grotevant, H. D., Scarr, S., & Weinberg, R. A. (1977). Patterns of interest similarity in adoptive and biological families. *Journal of Personality and Social Psychology,* **35**, 667–676.

Hunt, J. McV. (1961). *Intelligence and experience.* New York: Ronald.

Hunt, J. McV. (1980). *Early psychological development and experience.* Worcester, Mass.: Clark University Press.

Juel-Nielsen, N. (1980). *Individual and environment: Monozygotic twins reared apart.* New York: International Universities Press.

Kamin, L. J. (1974). *The science and politics of IQ.* Potomac, Md.: Erlbaum.

Lytton, H. (1980). *Parent-child interaction: The socialization process observed in twin and single families.* New York: Plenum.

McCall, R. B. (1981). Nature-nurture and the two realms of development: A proposed integration with respect to mental development. *Child Development,* **52**, 1–12.

McCartney, K., Scarr, S., Phillips, D., Grajek, S., & Schwarz, J. C. (1981). Environmental differences among day care centers and their effects on children's development. In E. F. Zigler & E. W. Gordon (Eds.), *Day care: Scientific and social policy issues.* Boston: Auburn House.

Maccoby, E. E. (1980). *Social development.* New York: Harcourt, Brace, Jovanovich.

Matheny, A. P., Jr., Wilson, R. S., Dolan, A. B., & Krantz, J. Z. (1981). Behavioral contrasts in twinships: Stability and patterns of differences in childhood. *Child Development,* **52**, 579–598.

Murstein, B. I. (1972). Physical attractiveness and marital choice. *Journal of Personality and Social Psychology,* **22**, 8–12.

Nelson, K. (1973). Structure and strategy in learning to talk. *Monographs of the Society for Research in Child Development,* **38**(1–2, Serial No. 149).

Nerlove, S. B., & Snipper, A. S. (1981). Cognitive consequences of cultural opportunity. In R. H. Munroe, R. L. Munroe, & B. B. Whiting (Eds.), *Handbook of cross-cultural human development.* New York: Garland.

Newman, H. G., Freeman, F. N., & Holzinger, K. J. (1937). *Twins: A study of heredity and environment.* Chicago: University of Chicago Press.

Piaget, J. (1980). The psychogenesis of knowledge and its epistemological significance. In M. Piattelli-Palmarini (Ed.), *Language and learning: The debate between Jean Piaget and Noam Chomsky.* Cambridge, Mass.: Harvard University Press.

Plomin, R., DeFries, J. C., & Loehlin, J. C. (1977). Genotype-environment interaction and correlation in the analysis of human behavior. *Psychological Bulletin,* **84**, 309–322.

Ramey, C. T., & Haskins, R. (1981). The modification of intelligence through early experience. *Intelligence,* **5**, 5–19.

Scarr, S. (1981). *IQ: Race, social class and individual differences, new studies of old problems.* Hillsdale, N.J.: Erlbaum.

Scarr, S., & Carter-Saltzman, L. (1980). Twin method: Defense of a critical assumption. *Behavior Genetics,* **9**, 527–542.

Scarr, S., & Kidd, K. K. Behavior genetics. In M. Haith & J. Campos (Eds.), *Manual of child psychology: Infancy and the biology of development.* (Vol. **2**). New York: Wiley, in press.

Scarr, S., Webber, P. L., Weinberg, R. A., & Wittig, M. A. (1981). Personality resemblance among adolescents and their parents in biologically-related and adoptive families. *Journal of Personality and Social Psychology,* **40,** 885–898.

Scarr, S., & Weinberg, R. A. (1976). IQ test performance of black children adopted by white families. *American Psychologist,* **31,** 726–739.

Scarr, S., & Weinberg, R. A. (1977). Intellectual similarities within families of both adopted and biological children. *Intelligence,* **1**(2), 170–191.

Scarr, S., & Weinberg, R. A. (1978). The influence of "family background" on intellectual attainment. *American Sociological Review,* **43,** 674–692.

Scarr, S., & Weinberg, R. A. The Minnesota adoption studies: Genetic differences and malleability. *Child Development,* in this issue.

Scarr-Salapatek, S. (1976). An evolutionary perspective on infant intelligence. In M. Lewis (Ed.), *Origins of intelligence: Infancy and early childhood.* N.Y.: Plenum.

Shields, J. (1962). *Monozygotic twins brought up apart and brought up together.* London: Oxford University Press.

Waddington, C. H. (1962). *New patterns in genetics and development.* New York: Columbia University Press.

Watson, E. H., & Lowrey, G. H. (1967). *Growth and development of children.* Chicago: Year Book Medical Publishers.

PART II: HEREDITY-ENVIRONMENT
INTERACTION

6

Environmental Effects on Intelligence: The Forgotten Realm of Discontinuous Nonshared Within-Family Factors

Robert B. McCall

Boys Town Center, Boys Town, Nebraska

The author argues that environmental variation that occurs within families but is not shared by siblings—nonshared within-family environmental variation—is a major influence on general mental performance and has largely been ignored. Data are presented from longitudinal studies that reveal that intraindividual variation over age in IQ accounts for as much or more variability than has been estimated to be the nonshared within-family environmental variation in IQ. Given these results, the author speculates that such factors may account for 15%–25% of all variability in IQ and 30%–50% of environmental variability in IQ. The implications of this type of environmental factor are considered from conceptual and methodological perspectives.

Reprinted with permission from *Child Development*, 1983, Vol. 54, 408–415. Copyright 1983 by the Society for Research in Child Development, Inc.

These analyses were begun while I was a staff member at Fels Research Institute, and permission to include the Fels data was graciously granted by Beatrice Lacey, acting scientific director at Fels. The Berkeley data were generously provided by Drs. Nancy Bayley and Dorothy Eichorn, Institute of Human Development, University of California, Berkeley. I am indebted to these individuals and to the many researchers, assistants, participants, and funding sources who made these data possible. I also appreciate the considerable guidance and thought provided by John C. Loehlin on an earlier draft of this manuscript.

119

The environmental factors that contribute to a child's intelligence typically are said to include what might be called the "general intellectual climate of the home." Psychologists would list parental encouragement for achievement, responsiveness of parents to the child's overtures, stimulating toys or books, educational opportunities, parents who value and model intellectual activities and accomplishments, and so forth. Note that most of these factors are characteristics that distinguish the general environment of one family from another, and they might be expected to influence all children within a family to approximately the same extent. As a result they are called "between-family environmental factors."

Without question, between-family environmental factors are influential (e.g., Freeberg & Payne, 1967; McCall, 1979), but they are not the only kind of environmental circumstance that contributes to mental performance. Recently, Rowe and Plomin (1981) have argued that the traditional emphasis on between-family factors may be too great, not only with respect to the development of intelligence but to a variety of personality and psychopathological characteristics as well. Within-family environmental factors, they argue, are also important.

Within-family factors are largely *not shared* by siblings and thus tend to make them different from one another. Rowe and Plomin (1981) review the available literature and suggest that half the variance of general mental performance (i.e., typically IQ) is environmental and half of that environmental variation is within-family and not shared by siblings. Such factors might include sibling interactions, differential treatment of siblings by parents, birth order and spacing, cohort differences, illness and separation, and nonfamily members specific to individual children (e.g., peers, teachers). One might add to this list environmental events that impinge on all family members (e.g., relocation, divorce, neighbors, death of relatives) but that have different effects on individual family members because of differences in their ages, personalities, genetic dispositions, and other factors.

What emerges is a provocative, perhaps alarming, hypothesis: We have ignored an entire class of environmental factors—nonshared within-family factors—which may account for 25% of all variation in IQ and at least as much of the environmental variation as the between-family factors that have been the focus of attention in the last few decades.

But nonshared within-family factors can be broken down further into two general types. One class includes factors that exert a continuing influence over one child versus another within a family. Let us call them "continuous nonshared within-family environmental factors." For example, being a firstborn male may be associated with a continuing pattern of parental favoritism for intellectual pursuits, and the child may always look to parents, rather than peers, as stronger models for achievement. By definition, these continuous factors should contribute a constant amount to mental performance over age.

A second class of nonshared environmental factors are those circumstances that occur at one age or another. Obviously they do not influence mental performance before that point but may exert a temporary or permanent influence thereafter. These are discontinuous nonshared within-family environmental factors. For example, moving into a new school district, finding success as a high school athlete, or the development of parent-child alienation in adolescence are not present throughout a child's life but may contribute to intellectual performance when they occur and for varying periods of time thereafter.

These latter factors—discontinuous nonshared within-family environmental factors—and their reflection in intraindividual developmental changes in mental performance are the focus of this paper. My argument is that variation in IQ reflects *relative* changes in rank within a group on an omnibus test of mental performance; it does not reflect absolute increases in mental skill or knowledge or changes in those attributes not represented on the IQ test. Yet such variation is large, it does not seem to be predominantly random error, and it does not seem to be associated with the emergence of genetic trends, at least not with developmental genetic trends that are shared by siblings. Therefore, this source of variation deserves much more conceptual and empirical attention than it has received.

THE EXTENT OF INTRAINDIVIDUAL DEVELOPMENTAL VARIATION IN IQ

The first point of my argument is that developmental variation in IQ within individuals occurs to a much greater extent than is commonly recognized. One reason for this erroneous impression is that individual differences in IQ are perhaps the most developmentally stable of any behavioral trait we have measured, especially following age 6 when year-to-year correlations typically exceed .85 (e.g., Bayley, 1949).

But such correlations are deceiving. For example, McCall, Appelbaum, and Hogarty (1973) showed that for the Fels Research Institute sample, which reveals similarly high age-to-age correlations, a substantial amount of intraindividual variation in IQ is present nevertheless. Specifically, the average range of IQ test performance between 2½ and 17 years of age was 28.5 IQ points. Moreover, one in seven subjects displayed shifts of more than 40 points, and one individual recorded an increase of 74

IQ points during childhood and adolescence. It will be helpful to quantify, replicate, and explain this intraindividual developmental variation more thoroughly within the Fels and the Berkeley Growth Study samples.

The Fels Longitudinal Study

Subjects.—Two samples of children from the Fels Longitudinal Study were examined (see Sontag, Baker, & Nelson, 1958, for a description of the entire sample). These children come from a variety of home backgrounds and have above-average IQ (approximate Binet IQ of 117, depending on age) but normal variability (SD = 16.9).

The "sibling sample" consisted of 114 children used previously to study similarity in IQ change among siblings (McCall, 1970, 1972). It contained 48 males and 66 females from 46 families. IQ tests, mostly Binet and Wechsler, were given at 14 ages beginning at age 3 and continuing every 6 months until age 6 and every year thereafter through age 12. Details of the sample and missing data are presented in McCall (1970).

The "Binet sample" consisted of 80 individuals (37 of which were also in the sibling sample) who had relatively complete IQ data between 2½ and 17 years of age using only the Binet IQ test. These subjects were from 56 different families, and the data consisted of a maximum of 17 IQ tests given every 6 months until age 6, every year until age 12, and at 14, 15, and 17 years of age. Details of this sample and missing data are reported in McCall et al. (1973).

Results.—All data were converted to standard scores (mean = 0, SD = 1) separately for each type of IQ test at each age on the basis of all the children in the Fels sample (average $N = 151$). This had the effect of making the tests statistically comparable and of removing any general age trends or effects of secular changes and repeated testing. Then the standard deviation was computed separately for each subject over his or her set of childhood scores. In the case of these Fels data, only actual IQ measurements were used; all data points that were filled artificially for the purpose of previous analyses were omitted in these calculations.

For the sibling sample, the average intraindividual standard deviation of the standardized IQ scores was .47 for each sex (median standard deviations were comparable). For the Binet sample, the average standard deviation was also .47. Thus, this estimate was probably not influenced by the length of the childhood period, particular IQ tests, or the degree of family representation in the sample (although the two groups of subjects, the assessment ages, and the type of tests overlapped considerably).

Since the mean standard deviation over subjects at single ages for the tests used in these calculations was approximately 16.5, the average intraindividual standard deviation of .47 was equivalent to a standard deviation of approximately 7.8 IQ points. It should be remembered that standardizing scores before calculating removed any intraindividual developmental variation associated with any general age trend that might be present in this sample (McCall et al., 1973). Therefore, this estimate may be viewed as conservative.

The Berkeley Growth Study

Subjects.—Subjects from the Berkeley Growth Study sample were selected if they had no more than four missing mental assessments either between 18 and 60 months or between 6 and 36 years of age. Twenty-two boys and 19 girls qualified. Details of the Berkeley Growth Study sample and testing schedule can be found in Bayley (1949). All test scores were standardized (0,1) within the entire Berkeley sample before all analyses.

Results.—Data were analyzed in three ways. In the replication analysis, assessments from the Berkeley schedule were selected to correspond as closely as possible to those in the Binet sample of the Fels study. Fifteen IQ tests were included, specifically at 30, 36, 42, 48, 54, and 60 months and 6, 7, 8, 9, 10, 11, 12, 14, and 17 years of age.

In contrast to the Fels study, in which the analyses were restricted to actual scores, linearly interpolated-extrapolated data (see McCall et al., 1973) were included in all the analyses of the Berkeley study. An examination of this practice indicated quite clearly that use of the filled data points resulted in a smaller standard deviation within individuals than would be the case if only actual data points were used. In the entire sample of 41 subjects by 15 possible assessments (615 possible individual testings), only 16 were missing for this analysis. Twenty-six of the 41 subjects had no missing data at all.

The mean intraindividualized standard deviation for standardized IQ over age was .51 for boys and .52 for girls (median standard deviations were comparable). Since the average standard deviation over subjects for tests at separate ages included in this analysis was approximately 19.1 (if deviation IQs are used; Pinneau, 1961), the individual variation was equivalent to a standard deviation of 9.7 (boys) to 9.9 (girls) IQ points. This is even higher than the 7.8 found for the comparable analysis of the Fels data.

The amount of change can be expressed another way. The average range of scores for an individual over age was 1.83 standardized units. Given a standard deviation of 16 IQ points, this is a personal average range of 29.3 IQ points. However, the average variance in deviation IQ scores at a single age for the Berkeley sample was estimated to be 19.1 for this set of scores, which yields an average range of 35 points. The first estimate is nearly identical to the individual range of 28.5 IQ points for Fels subjects, and the second is substantially above it. Depending on which estimate one picks, between 32% and 71% of Berkeley subjects displayed a personal developmental range of 30 or more points of IQ change over age (Fels: 33%), 17% to 22% changed more than 40 points (Fels: 14%), and one subject shifted between 65 and 78 IQ points (Fels: 74). Thus, developmental variation in the Berkeley samples is at least as great, and probably greater, than in the Fels group, perhaps in part because Berkeley subjects score at higher levels (approximately 124 vs. 117) where individual items are worth more months of mental age.

A second analysis, the preschool analysis, included 11 assessments made between 18 and 60 months of age, specifically at 18, 21, 24, 27, 30, 33, 36, 42, 48, 54, and 60 months. Since the same subjects were involved, approximately the same amount of missing data existed for these assessments as for the replication analysis. The average intraindividual standard deviation for these 11 assessments made between 1½ and 5 years of age was .58 for boys and .66 for girls. The median over both sexes was .60. In terms of deviation IQ, the average standard deviation over subjects for tests in this period was approximately 16.7, so the intraindividual standard deviation of .60 is equivalent to 10 IQ points.

In the third analysis, the child-adult analysis, assessments were restricted to those given between 6 and 36 years, specifically at 6, 7, 8, 9, 10, 11, 12, 13, 14, 15, 16, 17, 18, 21, 26, and 36 years. The average intraindividual standard deviation for these 16 IQ assessments was .35 for both boys and girls. The average standard deviation over subjects for tests in this period was approximately 18.8 deviation IQ points, so the intraindividual variation for scores at age 6 and thereafter was approximately 6.6 IQ points.

Thus, age-to-age variation appears substantially greater during the preschool years than during childhood and adulthood. The amount of this difference associated with real plasticity in human mental abilities and the amount associated with greater measurement error and unreliability in the early years is open to debate at present.

Causes of Intraindividual Developmental Variation

Change in IQ over age could reflect one or more phenomena: (*a*) gene-based developmental trends, (*b*) the emergence of greater genetic control over IQ with development, (*c*) random temporary environmental fluctuations and test error, (*d*) changes in the nature of what is being measured on the IQ test, and (*e*) discontinuous within-family environmental influences. Consider these possibilities in turn.

Gene-based developmental trends.—If variability over age reflected gene-based developmental trends, one would expect siblings to be similar in their developmental pattern. This possibility has been evaluated for the sibling sample from the Fels study analyzed above (McCall, 1970, 1972). No greater similarity in IQ change was found for siblings (or for parent-child pairs) than for unrelated pairs, although siblings and parent-child pairs were more similar in their average IQ over all ages. Thus, kinship was related to similarity in general level of IQ performance but not to similarity in pattern of intraindividual developmental change.

Of course, sibling comparisons are not the most sensitive method of revealing genetic trends, so it is possible that some genetic similarity in the pattern of age-to-age changes occurs (Wilson, 1973, 1978; but for a counterargument, see McCall, 1979). Nevertheless, the fact that siblings are not more similar to one another than unrelated children in the Fels data does suggest that, even if gene-based developmental trends are present, they are not a strong force in this sample. The bulk of intraindividual variation must be nongenetic.

This lack of similarity in pattern of change among siblings also suggests that the intraindividual variation observed here mirrors nonshared and discontinuous factors. Of course, a single event that occurs in secular time would influence two children at different ages and contribute to different patterns of change for siblings even if that event had the same effect on both children. But when siblings were matched for calendar year rather than age, their patterns of IQ over age did not become more similar, and the degree of similarity was not related to the extent of birth spacing (McCall, 1970). Therefore, it would appear that the general intellectual climate of the home and, perhaps, major events that impinge on an entire family are not strong, direct contributors to sibling similarity in intraindividual developmental variation in IQ.

Increasing genetic control.—If the genetic contribution to test performance and IQ change increased over age, there should be greater sibling similarity later in childhood than earlier. The Berkeley data suggest greater intraindividual variation prior to age 5½ than later, which might reflect early temporary environmental variation. Greater stability later could derive from a greater genetic contribution (Honzik, 1957).

But the Fels data do not substantiate this interpretation. For example, correlations for siblings and for parent-child pairs for the Fels sample (McCall, 1970) do not show a consistently increasing pattern across age in the way that parent-child similarity has been reported previously (Honzik, 1957). However, the Fels correlations were for tests given at different points in calendar time but at the same ages. Furthermore, the sibling r's begin at .54 at 42 months and remain relatively constant thereafter. Same-age parent-child r's begin at .36 at 42 months and range unsystematically between .17 and .50 thereafter. It appears for this sample that whatever genetic influence is present has been established by 42 months, when pair members were assessed at identical ages.

More to the point, however, when pattern of IQ change among siblings was restricted to the preschool years (3–6 years) and separately to the school years (6–13 years), siblings were not found to be more similar to one another than unrelated children during either age segment (McCall, 1972).

Again, there is some ambiguity in the data, but it seems safe to conclude that for the Fels sample, at least, changing genetic influences through the childhood period do not seem to exert a marked influence on changes in IQ test performance. Having said that, however, it should be pointed out that the possible genetic influences that are being minimized by these arguments are genetic main effects. It is still possible for changes in mental performance to be associated with genetic-environment interactions. That is, an environmental event or opportunity (e.g., a stimulating math teacher) may have greater influence on one sibling versus another sibling because it matches a genetic disposition (e.g., math ability) present in one but not the other child.

These arguments, then, suggest that intraindividual variation in IQ is not genetic in the sense of main effects, not shared by siblings, and discontinuous.

Error of measurement.—The variation may be nongenetic, but it could be random error. If the variability of an individual's performance over age was simply a reflection of temporary environmental effects or random test error, the patterns of IQ change over age should consist of irregular fluctuations about a constant value. This is true for some subjects. But reports of individual IQ curves for the Fels samples reported above show that individual variation tends to consist of non-random, simple linear or quadratic trends of sizable proportions spanning the entire childhood period (McCall, 1970, 1972; McCall et al., 1973; Sontag et al., 1958).

For example, in the Fels sibling sample, 65% displayed a significant (.05) monotonic, bitonic, or tritonic individual nonparametric trend. One member of 84% of the sibling pairs and both members of 46% of the pairs had significant trends, suggesting that the lack of sibling correspondence was not simply the expected lack of similarity for random variation (McCall, 1970).

Therefore, while there is apparent random fluctuation about a line in some individual plots of IQ change over age, there is a trend in a substantial percentage of the cases.

Changes in the test.—Still, the changes may not reflect systematic environmental events but systematic changes in the nature of the test. Assessing this possibility is more difficult, but consider the following arguments.

First, any general shifts in the entire sample associated with changes in the nature of the tests or repeated testing would have been removed by the standardization procedure. Second, secular change and cohort effects are not likely to be strong, because the results from Fels and Berkeley were similar in showing substantial developmental change, although the data were collected very differently in this regard. (Berkeley is a single cohort, whereas Fels sampled continuously over several decades.) Third, the Guilford (1967) and Meeker (1969) subtest scores, which presumably reflect different mental operations, contents, and products, were calculated at each age for the Fels-Binet sample. The relative potential contribution of these subtests to the total IQ score does not vary after age 3½ for these subjects. Moreover, if the age trends for each of these subtest scores are plotted, they are all nearly coincident with the developmental pattern of general IQ (see McCall et al., 1973, for details and limitations of this analysis). Fourth, in other studies from the Fels project (Sontag et al., 1958), children characterized by marked increases or decreases in IQ did not differ in their ability to pass some types of items than others.

Of course, it is difficult to determine that the mental processes governing performance on a test at one age are the same as those influencing performance at another age, even if the name of the test, the type of item, or the actual items are the same at the two ages. However, the data presented for this sample suggest that the individual variability described here is not an obvious reflection of gross changes in the nature of the IQ test.

Within-family environmental factors.—Very little data are available to assess directly the contribution of within-family environmental factors of any kind. In an analysis of types of IQ change, McCall et al. (1973) showed that parental attempts to accelerate a child's development and the severity of punishments they administered were related to the type of IQ change displayed by that child. However, these home variables were averaged over the relevant age period, so they do not demonstrate concomitant changes in environmental events and in IQ. Studies that attempt to show a relationship between naturalistic environmental change and performance change are needed badly.

How Big an Effect?

It is never safe to converge on an explanation by default, but it is a reasonable hypothesis that a substantial portion of the intraindividual variation of 8–10 IQ points between 2½ and 17 years described here is discontinuous nonshared within-family environmental or genetic-environmental interaction variation. How much of the observed developmental variation is systematically related to such factors cannot be determined precisely for these data, but the following exercise provides a speculative perspective on the size of this effect.

Rowe and Plomin's (1981) summary indicated that 50% of the variation in IQ for a given group of subjects at a single age is nongenetic, presumably environmental. Moreover, half of this environmental variation is within-family and not shared by siblings. Assuming a standard deviation of 16 for an IQ test given at a single age, 25% of the total variance of 16^2 (or 256) is 64, the square root of which is 8. Therefore, given Rowe and Plomin's estimates, the nonshared within-family environmental standard deviation at a single age is 8 points. This estimate is quite consistent with the 7.8–10 SD obtained here.

But to suggest that the intraindividual variation data presented here replicate the Rowe and Plomin estimate is a bit glib. We have not really considered the role of unreliability in assessing the size of the intraindividual variation. This is a major problem because, even if the IQ test is considered to have a reliability of .90 or .95, substantial change in IQ resulting from unreliability is possible within developmental patterns that span up to 30 years and involve as many as 17 IQ testings. On the other hand, as argued above, if such changes were predominantly random error, why did 65% of the subjects in one sample display relatively simple, consistent patterns of change across several ages? And how does one discriminate between lack of test-retest reliability and meaningful individual differences in developmental pattern? It seems prudent, then, to suggest that the true nonshared within-family environmental variation is somewhat less than 25% of all IQ variance, perhaps between 15% and 25%, and perhaps 30%–50% of environmental variation, although the lower estimates are guesses at this point. In any case, it is a nontrivial component.

Discontinuous variation.—Notice that Rowe and Plomin's SD of 8 could be composed of continuous or discontinuous nonshared within-family environmental variation. Accepting that most of developmental change observed here is indeed discontinuous nonshared within-family environmental variation and not primarily associated with other factors, as I have argued, then the vast bulk of Rowe and Plomin's nonshared within-family environmental variance reflects discontinuous environmental circumstances that affect different children within the same family in different ways or to different extents and at different ages.

Take the argument from another perspective. Even when we declare that the "general intellectual climate of the home" is important to mental development, do we seriously propose that such factors only, or even mainly, operate in a continuous manner (i.e., contribute a constant increment or decrement to performance over all ages) or are shared among siblings (i.e., affect all siblings equally and at the same ages)? I think not. To suggest that such factors are continuous denies the obvious fact that the infant, child, and adolescent require different types of potentially enriching environmental circumstances (e.g., responsive toys, then a rich and responsive verbal model, then stimulating teachers and educational opportunity). To suggest that such factors are mostly shared and mainly distinguish between families, not between siblings within families, is to minimize the potential influence of sibling rivalry, peers, differential parental interaction with their children, shifts in location and schools, divorce, and a host of other changing or isolated events.

Of course, general factors influence mental performance. But many so-called general factors are really general labels for a changing set of functional events (e.g., "parental encouragement of achievement" is expressed behaviorally very differently by the same parent to the infant, child, and adolescent). To expect the organism, but not the nurturing environment, to develop and change or to expect the human organism not to be susceptible to or benefit from momentary or unique opportunities oversimplifies the nature of mental development and the plasticity and adaptability of the human species.

Admittedly, I have stepped on several mossy stones on the path to this conclusion, and, sadly, we have little direct evidence (except for special enrichment programs) that changes in naturalistic environmental events are associated with changes in mental performance. But if I am allowed to speculate, then the heuristic implication of this exercise is clear: We have been toiling in only half the garden in our attempt to explain the environmental contribution to tested intelligence.

Example.—What kind of discontinuous nonshared within-family environmental events might influence a child's mental performance? In addition to Rowe and Plomin's list, McCall et al. (1973) proposed the following hypothetical case. Suppose a family with 16-year-old and 9-year-old boys visits the Space Center in Florida. The experience might have no effect whatsoever on the older child, who is heavily committed to basketball and dating. However, the younger boy, while showing aptitude in mathematics, has never really blossomed academically. He finds the Space Center fascinating. When he returns home he discovers his neighbor is a pilot, who shows the youngster about planes and takes him up for a ride. This ignites the child's interest in aviation. A unit on flight in a science class later that year reinforces it, and the child shows a marked increase in mental performance with this surge in motivation.

Notice that the events of visiting the Space Center, having a pilot as a neighbor, and a class unit on aviation either impinged on or influenced one but not the other child. Moreover, if the youngster did not have a latent aptitude in mathematics, genetic or otherwise, or if the trip had been taken when he was younger or much older, these experiences might not have had the same effect. In short, environmental events that relate to a child's interests and aptitudes at the time may constitute a crucial class of environmental influences on general mental performance.

Methodological issue.—But if discontinuous nonshared within-family environmental factors that are uniquely matched with a child's aptitudes and interests at the time are a major influence on mental development, does this not excise the issue out of the body of science? The proposition is really that major contributors to mental development are idiosyncratic and therefore outside science, which seeks general laws.

The premise, while overstated, has some validity, but the conclusion is false. We can study these factors, but we must be more developmental and multivariate in both independent and dependent variables, and we must mix experimental interventions with attention to individual differences (McCall, 1977, 1981). We can describe concomitant changes in environmental events and mental performance. We can define sets of environmental variables and hypothesize that the *set* will be effective in influencing behavior even though individual variables may be effective for some but not other subjects. We can deliberately create a cafeteria of environmental offerings and experimentally cross them with subjects differing in relevant aptitudes and motivations, hypothesizing that matches will be more effective than nonmatches. We can observe how subjects select their own matched or unmatched opportunities in naturalistic contexts (e.g., school course offerings) and the outcomes. We can define the independent variable, not in terms of its specific overt characteristics but in terms of whether it is matched or not matched with the aptitudes and interests of subjects and replicate the design over different domains of specific environmental events.

The task is still within the realm of science, but it will be more difficult and complicated. We need to abandon our arm's-length approach and get closer to our subjects and their families and friends. We must be more developmental and multivariate on both independent and dependent sides of the research equation. And we should consider individual differences within our experimental designs.

REFERENCES

Bayley, N. (1949). Consistency and variability in the growth of intelligence from birth to eighteen years. *Journal of Genetic Psychology*, **75**, 165–196.

Freeberg, N. E., & Payne, D. T. (1967). Parental influence on cognitive development in early childhood: A review. *Child Development*, **38**, 65–88.

Guilford, J. P. (1967). *The nature of human intelligence*. New York: McGraw-Hill.

Honzik, M. P. (1957). Developmental studies of parent-child resemblance in intelligence. *Child Development*, **28**, 215–228.

McCall, R. B. (1970). IQ pattern over age: Comparisons among siblings and parent-child pairs. *Science*, **170**, 644–648.

McCall, R. B. (1972). Similarity in IQ profile among related pairs: Infancy and childhood. *Proceedings of the 80th Annual Convention of the American Psychological Association*, **7**, 79–80. (Summary)

McCall, R. B. (1977). Challenges to a science of developmental psychology. *Child Development*, **48**, 333–344.

McCall, R. B. (1979). The development of intellectual functioning in infancy and the prediction of later IQ. In J. D. Osofsky (Ed.), *Handbook of infant development*. New York: Wiley.

McCall, R. B. (1981). Nature-nurture and the two realms of development: A proposed integration with respect to mental development. *Child Development*, **52**, 1–12.

McCall, R. B., Appelbaum, M. I., & Hogarty, P. S. (1973). Developmental changes in mental performance. *Monographs of the Society for Research in Child Development*, **38**(3, Serial No. 150).

Meeker, M. N. (1969). *The structure of intellect: Its interpretation and uses*. Columbus, Ohio: Merrill.

Pinneau, S. R. (1961). *Changes in intelligence quotient: Infancy to maturity*. New York: Houghton-Mifflin.

Rowe, D. C., & Plomin, R. (1981). The importance of nonshared (E_1) environmental influences in behavioral development. *Developmental Psychology*, **17**, 517–531.

Sontag, L. W., Baker, C. T., & Nelson, V. L. (1958). Mental growth and personality development: A longitudinal study. *Monographs of the Society for Research in Child Development, 23*(2, Serial No. 68).

Wilson, R. S. (1973). Testing infant intelligence. *Science, 182,* 734–737.

Wilson, R. S. (1978). Synchronies in mental development: An epigenetic perspective. *Science, 202,* 939–948.

7

Sex Chromosomal Anomalies: Prospective Studies in Children

Arthur Robinson, Bruce Bender, Joyce Borelli, Mary Puck, and James Salbenblatt

National Jewish Hospital and Research Center/National Asthma Center, Denver

This report represents a summary of the current status of a prospective study of 51 children with sex chromosomal aneuploidy (SCA). The children were identified in an unbiased fashion during the years 1964–1974, and their growth and development have been documented in order to define the natural history of individuals with SCA. Siblings are similarly followed as a partial control for environmental and other genetic influences. These children and adolescents have developmental patterns which, although within normal limits, in general are below the mean for their ages. The mosaics are more similar to their siblings than the pure karyotypes. The significant variability in the phenotypes of propositi is stressed. The frequent diagnosis of SCA prenatally makes the definition of prognosis for the different karyotypes of even increased importance.

Reprinted with permission from *Behavior Genetics*, 1983, Vol. 13, No. 4, 321–329. Copyright 1983 Plenum Publishing Corporation.

This research was supported by Grant 5R01–HD10032 from the U.S. Public Health Service; Grant RR–69 from the General Clinical Research Centers Program of the Division of Research Resources, National Institutes of Health; and The Genetic Foundation. An earlier version of this article was presented at the Behavior Genetics Association Meeting, Fort Collins, Colorado, June 1982.

INTRODUCTION

One of the amazing facts to emerge since Tjio and Levan first determined that the normal human karyotype contained 46 chromosomes (Tjio and Levan, 1956) has been the large amount of fetal wastage and serious human disease associated with aberrations of the karyotype. It is estimated that at least 5% of all conceptuses and about 1/200 newborns have gross chromosomal abnormalities, a majority of which is produced by the process of nondisjunction and at least half of which produce serious developmental disease (Hook, 1981).

In an attempt to determine possible causes of nondisjunction, we started an epidemiological study in 1964 utilizing a sex chromatin (Barr body) examination of the amniotic membrane. Between 1964 and 1974 we screened 40,000 consecutive births at two Denver hospitals for individuals with numerical abnormalities of the X chromosome. This method had the advantage of permitting the examination of every consecutive birth, no matter what the viability or prematurity of the baby. Only the last 15,641 newborns were also screened for the Y chromatin, since the techniques for obtaining this information from the transected umbilical cord were developed only in 1970 (Greensher et al., 1971).

We asked the following questions.

1. What is the natural history of the various sex chromosome aberrations affecting newborns ascertained in an unbiased fashion? The increased prevalence of these conditions in selected populations of aberrant individuals (mostly adults) with psychosis, psychopathy, mental retardation, and sterility suggests that these chromosomally affected newborns, the majority of whom are phenotypically normal, represent a group at risk in later life.

2. Can one identify early in life those individuals who are at particular risk and by early intervention (anticipatory guidance) prevent or ameliorate the seemingly irreversible manifestations which may affect adolescents and adults with these conditions?

After 10 years, the epidemiological screening study was stopped in 1974. Interesting and statistically significant seasonal and annual differences in the birth of children with sex chromosomal aneuploidy were found (Robinson et al., 1969). As a result of the study we identified SCA newborns, most of whom would otherwise not have been diagnosed early in life. Our continuing primary goal since then has been to define as precisely as possible the long-term prognosis of this group and to establish the nature of any disabilities.

METHODS

The various aneuploid groups (45,X,47,XXX,47,XXY, and 47,XYY) as well as sex chromosome mosaics are being followed. A major effort is being made to evaluate the impact of family environment on the propositi. To this end we call our project a "family development study" and are following the siblings as one form of control for some of the environmental and genetic influences which may affect them as well as the propositi. We are also trying to evaluate the impact of the study itself on the propositi and their parents ("self-fulfilling prophecy"). In the original screening program, 68 newborns with SCA were identified in this unbiased fashion. Seven of these (11%) died in the neonatal period (Robinson, 1974). Fifty-one of the remaining 61 (now 8–18 years of age) are still cooperating in the program. We now have a total case load of 177 children including prenatally diagnosed additional propositi and siblings (Table I). In this group there are six propositae with monosomy X karyotypes (45,X) and three with partial monosomy X. Since both of the latter groups have strikingly similar cognitive profiles, we have lumped them together.

During the first year of life the children were seen quarterly and after

TABLE I
Case Load

Karyotype	Newborn series				Prenatal diagnostic series			
	No. propositi	Age range (years)	No. sibs	Age range (years)	No. propositi	Age range (years)	No. sibs	Age range (years)
47, XXY	16	6–16	39	1–26	3	0–2	12	5–20
47, XXX	11	9–16	23	5–31				
45, X	6	7–15	15	6–21				
46, XXq-	2	9–13	3	9–15				
45, X/46, Xr(X)	1	8	1	11				
47, XYY	4	7–9	5	1–11	1	1		
46, XY/47, XXY	2	7–15	5	5–20				
45, X/46, XX/47, XXX	1	15	1	11				
45, X/46, XX	5	10–14	10	2–16				
46, XX/47, XXX	2	8–16	6	1–17				
45, X/47, XXX	1	9	2	12–18				
Totals	51		110		4		12	

that annually in order to measure their physical, intellectual, emotional, and behavioral development in comparison to that of their siblings. Their parents were informed of the research project at the time of diagnosis (either at birth or at the 18th week of gestation). In return for their cooperation in the study, we offer them support, information, and early attention to those developmental problems to which these children are prone. School and home visits are made when appropriate. The evaluating staff includes a developmental pediatrician, a child psychiatrist, a psychiatric social worker, a clinical psychologist, a speech pathologist, and a physical therapist. In general, this has not been a blind study except for language evaluations, motor evaluations, and the current psychiatric evaluations of adolescent propositi and siblings.

RESULTS AND DISCUSSION

In this paper we are summarizing our results to date. These are of particular importance because of the paucity of information on the developmental progress of children with SCA identified in an unbiased fashion. With the advent of genetic amniocentesis, these data have increasing relevance. Detailed data on these studies are to be found in previous publications (Puck *et al.*, 1975; Tennes *et al.*, 1975, 1977; Robinson *et al.*, 1979; Salbenblatt *et al.*, 1981; Webber *et al.*, 1982; Pennington *et al.*, 1982; Bender *et al.*, 1983).

Physical Development

The physical findings are not particularly remarkable. In general, the 47,XXY boys and 47,XXX girls are significantly taller than their siblings, and the 45,X girls are significantly smaller than their siblings. Head circumferences are within normal limits but tend to skew below the average. Male adolescents have a low testicular volume. Essential hypertension and serous otitis media are frequent in 45,X girls (Robinson *et al.*, 1982).

Neuromuscular maturational lags have been found, but because of the inherent difficulties in quantifying these impressions we have begun to utilize the Bruininks-Oseretsky Test of Motor Proficiency with its age appropriate standards (Bruininks, 1978). Thus far, these tests have matched our clinical impressions as follows:

The 47,XXY boys have delayed neuromuscular maturation with visual-motor and sensory integration problems, balance and equilibrium difficulties, and hypotonia, all more marked in propositi than in siblings.

The 47,XXX girls had some early problems in motor development, including late onset of walking. Qualitatively, the gross and fine motor coordination is below that of their siblings, with evidence of visual-motor and sensory perceptual integration difficulty.

The 45,X girls, as has been reported before (Shaffer, 1962), show decreased perceptual awareness of the body in space, with some impulsivity and distractibility evident.

The mosaic children approximate their siblings in growth and development much more closely than the children with pure karyotypes.

Intellectual Development

Intelligence is generally within normal limits, with a predominance of scores in the lower part of the scale.

Intelligence testing (Wechsler Preschool and Primary Scale of Intelligence) at 5 years of age indicated a generalized cognitive deficit in the 47,XXX girls, a generalized and a specific perceptual deficit in the 45,X (monosomy X) girls and the partial monosomy X girls (who in our sample have similar cognitive profiles), and a specific verbal deficit in 47,XXY boys relative to siblings. The mosaic group did not differ from the control group on any of the IQ measures (Table II).

TABLE II
Mean IQ Scores

	Full	Verbal	Performance
45, X and partial X monosomy			
(N = 9)			
$\bar{X}$	87.1*	93.4	82.6*
SD	(19.7)	(24.5)	(12.3)
47, XXX			
(N = 11)			
$\bar{X}$	86.6*	85.2*	88.6*
SD	(15.3)	(16.0)	(16.3)
47, XXY			
(N = 13)			
$\bar{X}$	94.9	89.2*	101.8
SD	(17.2)	(18.8)	(14.7)
Mosaics			
(N = 8)			
$\bar{X}$	103.3	101.9	104.0
SD	(18.3)	(16.2)	(18.2)
Siblings			
(N = 17)			
$\bar{X}$	111.2	113.4	106.8
SD	(14.8)	(15.2)	(14.2)

*Significantly different from sibs ($P < 0.05$).

Language Development

Forty-one of the propositi and 31 sibling controls received a comprehensive speech and language evaluation administered blindly by a speech and language pathologist. The SCA children have significantly more mild to severe language disorders than siblings in the areas of auditory processing, receptive language, expressive language, and overall language skills. The ratings indicate that 47,XXY boys and 47,XXX girls are at a greater risk for problems in the development of speech and language skills than their siblings. Similar, but not statistically significant findings were noted in the 45,X group. The mosaic children were the most similar to their siblings (Table III).

Learning Disorders

An overview of school intervention for learning disorders (repetition of a grade, assignment to a special-education program) revealed that two-thirds of SCA children exhibited a learning disorder, with one-fifth of siblings ($P < 0.05$) (Table III). Again, the mosaics were consistently the least severely affected in comparison to siblings. Thus, it may be concluded that children with a "pure" sex chromosome anomaly are at an increased risk for learning problems.

The learning problems may be karyotype specific. In particular, the 45,X girls, even at age 5 years, showed a decreased mean performance IQ and later a significantly increased incidence of handwriting problems, whereas the 47,XXY males at the age of 5 years had a decreased mean

TABLE III
Language and Learning Disorders

	Language disorder		Learning disorder	
	Present	Absent	Present	Absent
45, X and partial X monosomy	6	2	6	3
47, XXX	7	2	9	2
47, XXY	13	1	9	5
47, XYY	4	0	3	1
Totals	30	5	27	11
Mosaics	3	3	3	7
Siblings	14	17	4	16

verbal IQ. In addition, 5 of 14 of these boys had an increased incidence of specific reading delay, whereas none was found in the 20 other propositi. The 47,XXX girls have experienced consistently more difficulty with all academic subjects than their siblings.

Emotional Development

The two groups, propositi and siblings, do not show marked differences in the incidence of diagnosed psychopathology in childhood. However, when the children were rated by our assessment team on a three-level scale of emotional development reflecting quality of family and peer relationships, self-esteem, maturity, and personal happiness (1 = good, 2 = adequate, 3 = poor), the propositi with the exception of the mosaics presented a picture of poorer emotional development than did the siblings closest in age. Most striking, the risk for emotional dysfunction for propositi increased more rapidly than for siblings as the family stress factor increased (Fig. 1) (1 = little stress and 3 = great stress), reflecting a heightened vulnerability to adverse environment

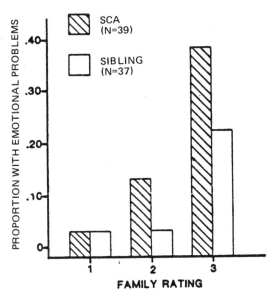

Fig. 1. Emotional dysfunction of propositi with "pure" SCA compared to siblings. Family environmental ratings (1 = high, 2 = average, 3 = low) are based on assessments of socioeconomic status, parenting skills, and adverse stress conditions (e.g., divorce, death, crime) affecting all family members.

among pure karyotype propositi. This emotional vulnerability is not limited to any specific karyotype group. However, great variability has been observed, including seven families with a sibling significantly more disturbed than the propositus.

Impact of Study on Participating Families

Because there is a difference of opinion among those studying sex-chromosome variations as to whether parents should be informed of the diagnosis as soon as it is confirmed or at some arbitrarily set later date, we are asking each family if in retrospect they would have preferred not to know the diagnosis or if they would rather have learned it later. The response to these questions was emphatic in all of the 44 families thus far questioned: "We wanted to know—we have a right to know." This response confirms our observation that participating families need to feel that their adaptive skills are valued and essential to their maximal participation in the care of their child and in the study. There is no question that the diagnosis and the study have a profound impact on the families which stresses their adaptive capacity. Their trust in and continuing commitment to the study supports their ability to cope and follow recommendations.

The doctrine of self-fulfilling prophecy has been invoked by some (Beckwith and King, 1974) as a reason for concealing these diagnoses from families on the assumption that knowledge of the existence of risk for deviance from normal development creates a self-defeating emotional climate of parental rejection. On the contrary, we feel that only if parents and physicians are fully informed of the diagnosis can the most appropriate anticipatory guidance be given. We stress the absence of complete genetic determinism and the need for vigorous attempts to provide a supportive environment.

We have not felt that a double blind study was ethically feasible, and hence the effects of anticipatory guidance cannot be measured. It is of interest to note, however, that the mosaic children with a milder genetic lesion but treated exactly like the "pure" karyotype have uniformly been much more like their siblings than the probands without mosaicism. Finally, we find it impressive that studies done in six other centers[1] using somewhat different methods, often without informing parents or following closely, are reporting similar findings (Stewart, 1982).

---

[1] Ratcliffe *et al.* (Edinburgh, Scotland), Nielsen *et al.* (Aarhus, Denmark), Stewart *et al.* (Toronto, Canada), Walzer *et al.* (Boston, Mass.), Hamerton *et al.* Winnipeg, Canada), and Leonard *et al.* (New Haven, Conn.).

In short, there is no evidence in our study,with the kind of support the families receive, that the original early communication has been harmful. It is our feeling that much more harm is caused by the inaccurate information that is being dispersed because of lack of knowledge of the prognosis of these conditions.

CONCLUSION

This prospective study is still continuing. We are impressed by the tremendous variability of the phenotypic expression of sex chromosomal aneuploidies and are encouraged that "anticipatory guidance" can modify the ultimate prognosis of these individuals—at least until adolescence. We are currently starting an intensive investigation of the impact on families of early knowledge of the likelihood of a child being infertile during adulthood.

The importance of data being obtained from prospective studies on individuals with sex chromosome aneuploidy ascertained in an unbiased fashion has increased, since these diagnoses are now being made *in utero.*

REFERENCES

Beckwith, J. and King, J. (1974). The XYY syndrome: A dangerous myth. *New Sci.* **64**:474–476.

Bender, B., Fry, E., Pennington, B., Puck, M., Salbenblatt, J. and Robinson, A. (1983). Speech and language development in 41 children with sex chromosome anomalies. *Pediatrics,* **71**:262–267.

Bruininks, R. H. (1978). *Bruininks-Oseretsky Test of Motor Proficiency Examiner's Manual.* American Guidance Service, Minnesota.

Greensher, A., Gersh, R., Peakman, D., and Robinson, A. (1971). Screening of newborn infants for abnormalities of the Y chromosome. *J. Pediatr.* **79**:305–306.

Hook, E. B. (1981). Prevalence of chromosome abnormalities during human gestation and implications for studies of environmental mutagens. *Lancet* **2**:169–172.

Pennington, B. F., Bender, B., Puck, M., Salbenblatt, J., and Robinson, A. (1982). Learning disabilities in children with sex chromosome anomalies. *Child Devel.* **53**:1182–1192.

Puck, M., Tennes, K., Frankenburg, W., Bryant, K., and Robinson, A. (1975). Early childhood development of four boys with 47,XXY karyotype. *Clin. Genet.* **7**:8–20.

Robinson, A. (1974). Neonatal deaths and sex chromosome anomalies. *Lancet* **1**:1223.

Robinson, A., Goad, W. B., Puck, T. T., and Harris, J. (1969). Studies on chromosomal nondisjunction in man. III. *Am. J. Hum. Genet.* **21**:466–485.

Robinson, A., Puck, M., Pennington, B., Borelli, J., and Hudson, M. (1979). Abnormalities of the sex chromosomes: A prospective study on randomly identified children. In Robinson, A., Lubs, H., and Bergsma, D. (eds.), *Sex Chromosome Aneuploidy: Prospective Studies in Children,* Birth Defects: Original Article Series, Alan R. Liss, New York, Vol. 15(1), pp. 203–241.

Robinson, A., Bender, B. G., Borelli, J., Puck, M. H., Salbenblatt, J., and Webber, M. L. (1982). Sex chromosomal abnormalities (SCA): A prospective and longitudinal study of newborns identified in an unbiased manner. In Stewart, D. A. (ed.), *Children With Sex Chromosome Aneuploidy: Follow-Up Studies*, Birth Defects: Original Article Series, Alan R. Liss, New York, Vol. 18(4), pp. 7–39.

Salbenblatt, J. A., Bender, B. G., Puck, M. H., Robinson, A., and Webber, M. L. (1981). Development of eight pubertal males with 47,XXY karyotype. *Clin. Genet.* **20**:141–146.

Shaffer, J. W. (1962). A specific deficit observed in gonadal aplasia (Turner's syndrome). *J. Clin. Psychol.* **18**:403–406.

Stewart, D. A. (ed.) (1982). *Children With Sex Chromosome Aneuploidy: Follow-Up Studies*, Birth Defects: Original Article Series, Vol. 18, No. 4, Alan R. Liss, New York.

Tennes, K., Puck, M., Bryant, K., Frankenburg, W., and Robinson, A. (1975). A developmental study of girls with trisomy X. *Am. J. Hum. Genet.* **27**:71–80.

Tennes, K., Puck, M., Orfanakis, D., and Robinson. A. (1977). The early childhood development of 17 boys with sex chromosome anomalies. A prospective study. *Pediatrics* **59**:574–583.

Tjio, J. H., and Levan, A. (1956). The chromosome number in man. *Hereditas* **42**:1–6.

Webber, M. L., Puck, M. H., Maresh, M. M., Goad, W. B., and Robinson, A. (1982). Skeletal maturation of children with sex chromosome abnormalities. *Pediatr. Res.* **16**:343–346.

Part III

FAMILY STUDIES

The crucial role played by the family system in the child's developmental course has by now been documented in a host of studies. (Of course, "crucial role" does not in any way imply "exclusive role," as it seems to do for some enthusiastic advocates of family therapy.) What is now needed to enrich our understanding of the family's influence are data on the significance of cultural differences in different family groups, the specific effects of sex differences at various age periods and on different types of families, and the influence of special factors in the family or child or both. The papers in this section address a number of these important issues.

McDermott and his associates, in their report on "Cultural Variations in Family Attitudes and Their Implications for Therapy," compare the cultural values of two groups of American families in Hawaii, one Japanese, the other Caucasian. The samples, drawn from nonclinical populations, avoid the danger of generalizing from pathological family units. Significant differences between the two groups were found and are presented. Such findings may appear obvious, but it is the discussion of their implications for therapy that gives this paper its special value. The authors spell out in detail the need to pay serious attention to a family's cultural values and attitudes if a "goodness of fit" between the therapist's goals and the specific family patterns is to be achieved.

In the second paper, the same group of investigators identify certain important differences between adolescent boys and girls in the context of their families, whether Japanese-American or Caucasian. Their findings support the work of Gilligan on psychological differences between the sexes, and they emphasize the implications for a differential approach to adolescent boys and girls, whether in the family itself or in a psychotherapeutic setting.

The issue of whether it would be harmful to children for their mothers to work outside the home continues to bedevil many parents of young children. We ourselves continue to be amazed at how many mental health professionals continue to ignore the impressive body of research literature on this subject, which uniformly have found no harm due to maternal employment as such. Instead of reassuring young women who are fearful that their desire for children will conflict with their continuing the careers they have worked so hard to build, and providing practical advice on managing these dual responsibilities, such professionals only magnify and intensify the conflicts of such troubled young women. The paper by Zimmerman and Bernstein not only adds to the consensus of the research literature on the lack of harm of maternal employment, but documents this finding in families representing a variety of types of living units.

Finally, the paper by Meadow and her associates reports a careful study which finds that deaf children of deaf parents show the development of secure attachment behavior comparable to children with normal hearing. Their finding is in sharp contrast to one from another center, which found serious deficiencies in their emotional development, a report which has agitated and worried many mothers of deaf children. Meadows and her associates point out the serious methodological weaknesses of this other study, at the same time that they do not minimize the special developmental complexities created by deafness.

8

Cultural Variations in Family Attitudes and Their Implications for Therapy

John F. McDermott, Jr., Walter F. Char,
Albert B. Robillard, Jing Hsu, Wen-Shing Tseng,
and Geoffrey C. Ashton

University of Hawaii School of Medicine, Honolulu

A volunteer sample of 158 American families (Japanese and Caucasian) with adolescent offspring was surveyed for family attitudes and values. Ethnic differences between parents were statistically significant in areas reflecting cognitive versus emotional expression and group versus individual orientation. Implications for family assessment and therapy are discussed.

In recent decades the family has become a new "unit" for therapeutic intervention. The treatment of a child within his or her natural social context seems logical enough. However, integration of this approach into the field of child psychiatry has not been without struggle (McDermott and Char, 1974).

Part of this difficulty is inherent in the family therapy movement itself, with its many separate "schools" having their own competing conceptual frameworks. From these have evolved a wide array of strategic interventions, from the psychodynamic (Ackerman, 1958; Boszormenyi-

Reprinted with permission from the *Journal of the American Academy of Child Psychiatry*, 1983, Vol. 22, No. 5, 454–458. Copyright 1983 by the American Academy of Child Psychiatry.

Supported by a grant from the Davies Charitable Trust. The authors thank Joy Ashton for assistance in collecting and assembling the data.

Nagy, 1981; Framo, 1970; Lidz, 1963, 1976; Meissner, 1978; Paul and Paul, 1975), communication and experiential (Satir, 1964, 1972; Whitaker and Keith, 1981), family systems theory and differentiation (Bowen, 1978), behavioral (Liberman, 1970; Patterson et al., 1975), strategic (Haley, 1967, 1970, 1973, 1976, 1980; Selvini Palozzoli et al., 1978) to the currently most popular structural approach (Aponte and Van Deusen, 1981; Minuchin 1974; Minuchin et al., 1967) which focuses on restructuring the family hierarchy and coalitions to correct the distorted boundaries of "enmeshed" and "disengaged" families at either end of a spectrum of family functioning.

Perhaps the explosion of so many varied approaches and theoretical frameworks of family psychopathology reflects the lack of a solid empirical data base of family functioning. To a large extent, theory has evolved from practice in dealing with dysfunctional families, not from the study of well-functioning ones. It has largely been based on the intuitive assumptions of clinicians who have generalized about normal family functioning from their work with those troubled families coming to the clinic. When certain family "styles" have been found among these troubled families, a cause and effect relationship often has been assumed and the style of family functioning has become the target for change. (Only recently have more solid data for evaluation of family competence emerged [Beavers, 1977; Epstein et al., 1978; Lewis et al., 1976] utilizing "average" families from the community who have not been assessed clinically.)

Socioeconomic and cultural variables affecting family functioning have not been well studied in this atmosphere of generalization from the pathological to the normal. Indeed the need for careful scrutiny of these variations has sometimes been dismissed. Minuchin (1974) presented interviews with families from different cultures to illustrate how problems *transcend* cultural differences. Yet it would be useful to consider culture as an independent variable in the study of normal, well-functioning families so that varying "cultural styles" might be separated from notions of psychopathology. Certainly the dimensions of family functioning which Minuchin's structural family therapy stresses, the family hierarchy and nature of the parental coalition, as well as degree of differentiation of family members from each other are highly related to culture. Knowledge of these variations is not only important to differentiate family style from family psychopathology, but also has implications for matching clinical approaches which "fit" with the particular family style. For example, one of the most controversial questions in the issue of indications and contraindications for family therapy (Mc-

Dermott, 1981) focuses on adolescents. In selectively choosing family therapy for youngsters in this critical developmental phase, knowledge about family values and attitudes among the various individuals in the family may be very useful.

PURPOSE

Our purpose in this report is to compare family attitudes between a nonclinical sample of families of two major ethnic groups— Americans of Japanese ancestry (Japanese) and Americans of European ancestry (Caucasian) who have teenage children. We wish to determine whether there are different attitudes about family functioning which have implications for clinical practice, i.e., that families can be assessed, not just for psychopathology, but for their basic style which is the way they prefer to deal with problems. If so, we suggest that the therapeutic approach can be shaped to *fit* this style rather than the style seen as just another dimension in need of change.

DESCRIPTION OF PROJECT

An interdisciplinary team of investigators at the University of Hawaii School of Medicine is conducting a large-scale study of family functioning, inspecting the interaction of ethnicity in a cross-section of families from the community. The aim of the study is to investigate families of different ethnic backgrounds to determine variations in family functioning (and the functioning of the individuals making them up) which should be considered in working with troubled families who come to the clinic. The first step in this investigation was to administer a questionnaire to nuclear family units, asking mothers, fathers, daughters and sons to react by disagreeing or agreeing to a number of statements about attitudes about ideal family functioning. The questionnaire was composed of 25 items and was administered to 407 families representing several ethnic groups. They were largely a middle-class volunteer research population drawn from the Hawaii Family Study of Cognition (Ashton et al., 1979). The respondents were asked to interpret each statement on the questionnaire in terms of their notion of an ideal family. They were told by written instruction that there were no right or wrong answers, only their opinions, and that was what was desired in the form of a response to each question. Questionnaires were to be filled out individually. Each respondent was asked to react to a statement along a continuum, extending from "strongly disagree" to "strongly agree."

Along each continuum there were five choices, each indicating the degree of relative agreement or disagreement. Using analysis of variance we were able to assess significant differences across the distribution of means for each item by sex, ethnicity, and generation.

The focus of this report is on the two major ethnic groups, the 84 Caucasian and the 74 Japanese families which were intact and had at least two unmarried children between the ages of 13 and 20. There were 121 Japanese and 126 Caucasian teenagers, 129 boys and 118 girls, falling within the imposed age-range constraints irrespective of position within the sibship. In this report, we will examine the questionnaire data to determine whether and how ethnicity significantly affected the responses of parents to these statements.

In another report (McDermott et al., 1983), we have discussed the surprising lack of ethnic difference in family attitudes among Japanese and Caucasian adolescent offspring in this sample. Cultural assimilation could account for this. On the other hand, it may be that adolescents, at least middle-class adolescents, have a common experience that binds them more closely by age than culture. However, sex-linked differences were striking and found girls of both ethnic groups seeking closeness and emotional expression within the family, and boys seeking separation and privacy. Generational differences found parents on the side of the clear lines of authority, family obligations and closeness compared to their adolescent sons and daughters, parents stressing openness, while teenagers emphasized the wish for privacy of thoughts and feelings. It is suggested that these generational differences validate the notion that the adolescent experience of psychologically separating from parents requires at least internal challenge to the family hierarchies and rules of childhood which are held longer by parents than their youngsters. However, the degree of separation/individuation and the route taken to achieve independence and maturity may differ markedly between boys and girls.

RESULTS

While we have reported no significant differences in family values between the Japanese and Caucasian adolescents, there *are* distinct differences between their parents (see Table 1). Japanese parents showed stronger agreement than Caucasian parents that important family decisions should involve discussion among its members ($p < 0.035$). This was born out even more strongly in their conviction that when important decisions are to be made, every family member should participate (p

TABLE 1

Analysis of Variance: Comparison of Japanese Parents with Caucasian Parents

			Deviation from Mean	
Question	Main Effects[a]	Mean Score	Japanese parents	Caucasian parents
Family members should openly acknowledge their affection for each other	<0.001	4.19	−0.25	0.20
Every member of the family has a right to keep certain thoughts and feelings private	<0.001	4.49	−0.13	0.11
Important family decisions should involve discussion among its members	<0.035	4.35	0.06	−0.05
When important decisions are to be made, every family member should participate	<0.001	3.93	0.13	−0.10
It is all right for a member of the family to cry openly when sad or upset	<0.001	4.21	−0.19	0.16
Children over the age of seven should be allowed to know about unpleasant events in the family or community	<0.001	3.72	−0.16	0.13
Family members should share their deepest thoughts with one another	<0.001	3.04	0.18	−0.14

[a] Probability levels.

< 0.001). They also held more strongly than their Caucasian counterparts that family members should share their deepest thoughts with one another (p < 0.001). On the other hand, Caucasian parents differed significantly from Japanese parents in their beliefs that family members should openly acknowledge their affection for each other (p < 0.001) and be able to cry openly when sad or upset (p < 0.001), yet at the same time promoting the right of the individual to keep certain thoughts and feelings private (p < 0.001). They also stood out from Japanese parents in their belief that youngsters should be allowed to know about unpleasant events in the family (p < 0.001).

DISCUSSION

These findings that there are significant differences in parental beliefs between Japanese and Caucasian parents in families who have not come for clinical assessment may have implications for a family "style" of functioning which should be considered in therapy with troubled families. Japanese families appear more oriented toward collective action, cognitive approaches, and task orientation. Caucasian parents favor sharing affective expression. Consistent with this, they may be less likely to shield their youngsters from unpleasantness in the family which might arouse such affective expression. Caucasian parents favor both the right to expression and the right to privacy, while Japanese parents value a sharing of the deepest level of thoughts among family members. In summary, there appears to be a strong tendency for Caucasians, in contrast to the Japanese, to emphasize affective life (versus cognitive) and the individual (versus the group).

What are the implications of these findings both for functional and dysfunctional families? First of all, we should consider that on most of the 25 questions there was basic agreement, or at least no significant disagreement, between the parents in these two different ethnic groups with very different family traditions. This, of course, may reflect the commonly held belief that Japanese-Americans have shown a very high rate of assimilation into American society (Montero, 1981). Yet in spite of this assimilation or change in behavioral pattern, certain traditional values and attitudes remain firmly embedded in the family and emerge as significant differences from those of their Caucasian counterparts. Indeed, for generations (Yamamoto, 1938), traditional family relationships among Japanese have been considered to exclude emotional display as bad form, and even Japanese language forms have restrictive words for affective expression. Even today, Hsu (1982) finds that Asian families support each other in practical behaviors rather than through emotional expression. In any event, these findings suggest that differing family attitudes, when deeply rooted in racial or ethnic tradition, reflect family styles of functioning which should be considered and respected. Indeed, they may even be utilized in therapeutic approaches to families with problems.

For example, with Japanese families, a cognitive, task-oriented problem solving approach might be adopted by the therapist, one in which the parents are viewed as in charge, but are oriented toward listening to the opinions of their youngsters and considering them in problem solving through negotiation and compromise. To expect open democratic discussion of emotion or affective experience by individuals in these families may be unrealistic or even antitherapeutic. But during the working out of "tasks," affects will most likely be seen, subtly expressed and worked out in the background. On the other hand, the same therapist might approach Caucasian families who value affective expression with a "focus on feelings" as an avenue, consistent with the usual family style, for the resolution of conflict (concentrating on affects closest to the surface). Here it may also be that the "content" of these conflicts will emerge by itself if the affective route is chosen. Naturally, these illustrations are generalizations not to be applied automatically to families without individual assessment. Flexibility is needed. A sensitive clinician will find the proper balance between affective and cognitive approaches, combining and shifting back and forth between them.

Consider another clinical implication found in our data. Certain correlations may suggest potential family problems. For example, the previously cited generational difference in which teenagers, regardless of ethnic group, strongly differ from their parents in their wish for privacy of thoughts and feelings, may clash with our Japanese parents' position that family members should share their deepest thoughts with one another, or the Caucasian parents' conviction that family members should openly acknowledge positive and negative feelings. Caucasian parents, on the other hand, differed from Japanese parents in their belief that every family member has a right to keep certain thoughts and feelings private, and in this way overlap with the values of their adolescent children and may be less likely to clash with them or find it more easily negotiable. Just how parental attitudes compare or contrast with those of their adolescent children must be explored with each family individually in considering family or individually oriented sessions or the best combination. But comparing parental attitudes in this study with adolescent boy and girl differences found in the previous study (McDermott et al., 1983) suggests that the stated willingness of girls from both ethnic groups to struggle with emotional issues within the family presents a better "fit" for family therapy for them than for their brothers.

In any case, being alert to these issues may be important for child psychiatrists who treat families with adolescent children and promote specific assessment of them. For this study has presented only expressed attitudes, how families *say* they function, not how they actually behave. It is obvious that statistical data do not describe individual families and cannot be applied as stereotypes to individual clinical cases. There is no substitute for individual assessment of family style. We suggest that this can and should be done as part of a clinical assessment of families (regardless of ethnicity or social class) in order to establish a "profile" of family members and to identify conflict and potential conflict areas, as well as the family style. One can, in many cases, then adapt a therapeutic approach to fit their own particular preference. Assessing family style may be considered analogous to the screening of patients before surgery. A baseline level of physiological and biochemical functioning is established in the workup, not only to suggest surgical approaches, but also to identify other potential problems to be encountered. It may be that such an assessment of all members of the family at the time of intake will not only identify the extent and nature of generational differences, but also differences in values between the parents themselves, as well as other members of the family.

CONCLUSION

A study of family attitudes among a nonclinical sample of Japanese and Caucasian families elicited significant differences between Japanese and Caucasian parents suggesting that the Japanese were more likely to emphasize collective action, cognitive approaches, and task orientation, while the Caucasian emphasis was on affective expression and individual differences. These variations may suggest different "routes" for clinicians to follow in approaching families, especially those of different ethnic background. They also suggest that a baseline assessment of family values for all family members at intake may be useful prior to initiating family therapy.

These findings will be tested carefully to understand them more fully. They are being investigated through interviews, psychological tests, and videotaped family interactions. Our hope is that meaningful comparison of actual family behaviors with the preferences expressed in the questionnaire will sharpen our understanding of variations in family functioning.

REFERENCES

Ackerman, N. W. (1958). *The Psychodynamics of Family Life.* New York: Basic Books.

Aponte, H., & Van Deusen, J. (1981). Structural family therapy. In *Handbook of Family Therapy,* ed. A. Gurman. New York: Brunner/Mazel.

Ashton, G. C., Polovina, J. J. & Vandenberg, S. G. (1979). Segregation analysis of family data for 15 tests of cognitive ability. *Behavioral Genet.,* 9:329–347.

Beavers, W. R. (1977). *Psychotherapy and Growth: A Family Systems Perspective.* New York: Brunner/Mazel.

Boszormenyi-Nagy, I. (1981). Contextual family therapy. In: *Handbook of Family Therapy,* ed. A. Gurman. New York: Brunner/Mazel.

Bowen, M. (1978). Theory in the practice of psychotherapy. In: *Family Therapy in Clinical Practice.* New York: Aronson.

Epstein, N. B., Bishop, D. S. & Levin, S. (1978). The McMaster model of family functioning. *J. Marriage Family Counseling,* 4:19–31.

Framo, J. (1970). Symptoms from a family transactional viewpoint. In: *Family Therapy in Transition,* ed. N. Ackerman. Boston: Little, Brown.

Haley, J. (1967). Toward a theory of pathological systems. In: *Family Therapy and Disturbed Families,* ed. I. Boszormenyi-Nagy & G. Zuk. Palo Alto: Science & Behavior Books.

——— (1970). Approaches to family therapy. *Int. J. Psychiat.,* 9:233–242.

——— (1973). *Uncommon Therapy: The Psychiatric Techniques of Milton H. Erickson, M.D.* New York: Norton.

——— (1976). *Problem-Solving Therapy: New Strategies for Effective Family Therapy.* San Francisco: Jossey-Bass.

——— (1980). *Leaving home.* New York: McGraw-Hill.

Hsu, J. (1982). The Chinese family: relations, problems, and therapy. Unpublished manuscript presented at the Conference on Chinese Culture and Mental Health at East-West Center, Honolulu, Hawaii, March 1–7.

Lewis, J. M., Beavers, W. R., Gossett, J. T. & Phillips, V. A. (1976). *No Single Thread: Psychological Health in Family Systems.* New York: Brunner/Mazel.

Liberman, R. (1970). Behavioral approaches to family and couple therapy. *Amer. J. Orthopsychiat.,* 40:106–118.

Lidz, T. (1963). *The Family and Human Adaptation.* New York: International Universities Press.

——— (1976). *The Person* (rev. ed.) New York: Basic Books.

McDermott, J. F. (1981). Indications for family therapy: question or non-question? *This Journal,* 20:409–419.

——— & Char, W. F. (1974). The undeclared war between child and family therapy. *This Journal,* 13:422–436.

——— Robillard, A. B., Char, W. F., Hsu, J., Tseng, W. S. & Ashton, G. C. (1983). Further development of the concept of adolescence: differences between boys and girls in the context of their families. *Amer. J. Psychiat.* (in press).

Meissner, W. W. (1978). The conceptualization of marital and family dynamics from a psychoanalytic perspective. In: *Marriage and Marital Therapy,* ed. T. Paolino & B. McCrady. New York: Brunner/Mazel.

Minuchin, S. (1974). *Families and Family Therapy.* Cambridge: Harvard University Press.

——— Mantalvo, B., Guerney, G., Rosman, B. & Schumer, F. (1967). *Families of the Slums.* New York: Basic Books.

Montero, D. (1981). The Japanese Americans: changing patterns of assimilation over three generations. *Amer. Sociological Rev.,* 46:829–839.

Patterson, G. R., Reid, J. B., Jones, R. R. & Conger, R. E. (1975). *A Social Learning Approach to Family Intervention*. Eugene, Oregon: Castalia.

Paul, N. L. & Paul, B. B. (1975). *A Marital Puzzle: Transgenerational Analysis in Marriage*. New York: Norton.

Satir, V. (1964). *Conjoint Family Therapy*. Palo Alto, Calif.: Science & Behavior Books.

――― (1972). *Peoplemaking*. Palo Alto, Calif.: Science & Behavior Books.

Selvini Palazzoli, M., Boscolo, L., Cecchin, G. & Prata, G. (1978). *Paradox and Counterparadox*. New York: Aronson.

Whitaker, C. & Keith, D. (1981). Functional family therapy. In: *Handbook of Family Therapy*, ed. A. Gurman. New York: Brunner/Mazel.

Yamamoto, M. (1938). Cultural conflicts and accommodations of the first and second generation Japanese. *Social Process in Hawaii*, 4:4–48.

PART III: FAMILY STUDIES

9

Reexamining the Concept of Adolescence: Differences Between Adolescent Boys and Girls in the Context of Their Families

John F. McDermott, Jr., Albert B. Robillard, Walter F. Char, Jing Hsu, Wen-Shing Tseng, and Geoffrey C. Ashton

University of Hawaii School of Medicine, Honolulu

As part of a larger study on family functioning, the authors administered a questionnaire on individual attitudes toward family values to 158 Japanese-American and Caucasian families. Differences between the generations on questions of authority and responsibility were predictable; few differences were found between ethnic groups. However, differences were striking between adolescent boys and girls, regardless of ethnicity: Girls valued family affiliation, closeness, and emotional expression significantly more highly than did boys. The authors emphasize the need for families to value girls' needs for closeness and emotional expression as highly as boys' needs for independence and self-differentiation. They suggest that the concept of separation-individuation as the major goal of adolescence be reexamined.

Reprinted with permission from the *American Journal of Psychiatry*, 1983, Vol. 140, 1318–1322. Copyright 1983 by the American Psychiatric Association.

Supported by a grant from the Davies Charitable Trust. The authors thank Joy Ashton for assistance in collecting and assembling the data.

Adolescence is but one stage in the human life cycle, but since it serves as a transition between childhood and adulthood, it is fraught with problems. More has been written about adolescence, yet less may be known about it than about any other stage of life. Until very recently assumptions about "normative" adolescent psychosocial phenomena have been based largely on psychiatrists' clinical experience with emotionally disturbed teenagers. Throughout this century, clinicians have described adolescence as a time when the personality is severely strained and inner turmoil inevitably results (1–4). Anna Freud (5) pointed out that the principal task of the adolescent is one of separation from the family and development of individuality and that this cannot be accomplished without upheaval. Erik Erikson (6) described the major task of adolescence as the establishment of a stable identity through a necessary questioning of values that will produce conflict with parents, rebellion and anger, and lack of communication with adults.

Generalizations about normal adolescent growth and development went unchallenged, except for some studies of college students (7–9), until the monumental studies of Offer (10–12) and Vaillant (13, 14) in the 1970s. Vaillant presented longitudinal studies and Offer an intensive survey of normal adolescent males. Offer found that about one-quarter of his sample progressed smoothly through adolescence and developed values similar to those of their parents, while a second group developed by spurts with periodic turmoil, and a third group experienced the turmoil previously thought to characterize all adolescents.

While others, such as King (15), have since also disagreed with the inevitability of turmoil, subsequent studies of normal adolescents do not suggest the absence of struggle. A report by the Group for the Advancement of Psychiatry (16) noted that intergenerational struggle may vary from group to group. The fact that Offer found struggle in a minority of his male subjects may be related to cultural factors as well as to sex. But even though Offer and associates' recent studies (17) are more comprehensive, our current understanding of the process of normal adolescence is based primarily on studies of middle-class Caucasian boys; few, if any, studies have included girls or minority groups. Studies of these populations may greatly expand our understanding of this stage of life.

An interdisciplinary team of investigators at the University of Hawaii is conducting a large-scale study of family functioning by observing the interaction of an ethnic cross section of families in the community. The first step in this investigation was to administer a questionnaire to intact nuclear family units in which family members were asked to agree or disagree with a number of statements about family values. Our objective was to establish a baseline so that the values and attitudes articulated could be compared with actual behaviors in subsequent videotaped family interactions and individual interviews. Our sample was drawn from a largely middle-class population of Chinese-American, Japanese-American, Caucasian, and part-Hawaiian families who had volunteered as research subjects in a previous study with the university's department of genetics, the Hawaii Family Study of Cognition (18).

Our purpose in this paper is to present the questionnaire data and to discuss how ethnicity, generation, and sex affected responses of family members.

METHOD

We administered a 25-item questionnaire to 407 families representing the various ethnic groups. The family members were asked to respond to each statement in terms of their notion of an ideal family. The written instructions said that there were no right or wrong answers and that we wanted their opinions. Questionnaires were to be filled out individually. Subjects were asked to respond to each statement on a 5-point scale extending from 1, strongly disagree, to 5, strongly agree. Using analysis of variance, we were able to assess significant differences across the distribution of means for each item by sex, ethnicity, and generation.

The focus of this report is on the two major ethnic groups, the 84 Caucasian and 74 Japanese-American families who had at least two unmarried children between the ages of 13 and 20. There were 121 Japanese-American and 126 Caucasian teenagers (a total of 129 boys and 118 girls) falling within the imposed age constraints. All families were intact, with a total of 158 fathers and 158 mothers.

Most of the sample were in their late teens, and the ages of the boys and girls were comparable. In all cases in which significant differences are reported in the sample of 13- to 20-year-olds, the differences between groups were also significant by year, with significance increasing with increasing age, except for questions 17 and 20, in which an inverse relationship existed between age and the strength of significance of difference between boys and girls.

RESULTS

General differences between parents and their adolescent offspring were as one might predict. Differences between Caucasian and Japanese-

American adolescents about family values were fewer than one might expect, while differences between boys and girls, regardless of ethnic or cultural background, were most striking.

Generational Differences

Mothers and fathers showed stronger agreement than their adolescent offspring that there should be a clear line of authority within the family, with no one questioning who is in charge (Table 1). They also held more strongly to the beliefs that the family should eat together once a day, that everyone should do the jobs he or she is supposed to do, and that family members should prefer to be with each other rather than with outsiders. Parents also differed significantly from their offspring in believing that children should always be open and honest with parents, that family members should know how each one feels about most things, and that they should share their deepest thoughts with one another.

Adolescents, on the other hand, agreed significantly more strongly than their parents that every member of the family has a right to keep certain thoughts and feelings private but that family members should let each other know when they are angry at each other. They also differed with their parents in believing that adults should be able to admit their mistakes to their children.

These generational differences are not unexpected. They validate the notion that the adolescent experience of psychologically separating from parents to achieve independence and maturity requires at least an internal challenge to the authority hierarchies and family rules of childhood. Perhaps this challenge is best reflected in the adolescent's need for more privacy of thoughts and feelings. The data do not tell us whether adolescents experience this separation as an external or inner struggle, only that there is a split from traditional parental values among both Caucasian and Japanese-American adolescents. It is likely that the way parents deal with these adolescent needs (such as understanding them, gradually loosening ties, and expanding limits and privacy, versus insisting on conformity and the intrusive sharing of all thoughts and feelings) will shape the way in which they are expressed. The adolescent's response may vary from a smooth progression toward independence to defiance or passivity. The danger in the last two behaviors is that they may persist as significant personality traits.

TABLE 1. Significant Differences Between Parents and Adolescents on Questionnaire on Individual Attitudes Toward Family Values[a]

Question	Combined Mean Score	SD		p[b]
		Parents (N=316)	Children (N=247)	
Every member of the family has a right to keep certain thoughts and feelings private.	4.53	4.49	4.56	<.048
Family members should prefer to be with each other rather than with outsiders.	2.68	2.77	2.61	<.001
Adults should be able to admit their mistakes to their children.	4.41	4.36	4.45	<.009
When there is work to be done, each member should go about it in his or her own way.	3.36	3.30	3.41	<.031
Each family member should do the jobs that he or she is supposed to do.	4.23	4.28	4.19	<.016
There should be a clear line of authority within the family, and no question about who is in charge.	3.57	3.71	3.46	<.001
A family should eat together at least once a day.	3.92	4.10	3.77	<.001
Older children should have more privileges than younger ones.	3.49	3.59	3.41	<.001
When family members are angry at each other they should let the others know.	3.71	3.61	3.79	<.001
Children should be honest and open with parents.	4.40	4.49	4.33	<.001
Family members should know how they each feel about most things.	3.90	4.02	3.81	<.001
Family members should share their deepest thoughts with one another.	2.98	3.04	2.93	<.026
On weekends children over 7 or 8 years of age should be allowed to watch whatever they choose on television.	2.21	2.01	2.37	<.001
Boys should have more privileges than girls.	1.70	1.63	1.75	<.011

[a]Responses given on a scale of 1=strongly disagree to 5=strongly agree.
[b]p values for significance of difference between parents' SD and childrens' SD derived by analysis of variance for main effects.

Ethnic Differences

Only two items, both on child rearing, generated significant differences between the Japanese-American and Caucasian adolescents. Caucasian adolescents held a significantly stronger belief that older children should have more privileges than younger, while Japanese-American adolescents were more convinced that youngsters over age 7 or 8 should be able to watch whatever television programs they choose on weekends. At first glance this difference might appear paradoxical, given the commonly held stereotype of Asian-American families as being hierarchically oriented. Indeed, the more "permissive" attitude of Japanese-American adolescents may reflect the wish that things had been different for them. But it may also reflect a general tendency in Asian-American families to indulge the younger children.

The absence of any other significant differences between these ethnic groups may be important. Perhaps adolescents, or at least middle-class adolescents of any cultural background, have a common experience that binds them more closely than their culture does. Our preliminary findings on offspring over 20 years of age in these same families suggest that ethnic differences reappear more strongly in Japanese-American and Caucasian young adults. Thus, adolescence may be an experience, at least in American middle-class youngsters, that is so powerful in itself that it overrides cultural differences.

Sex Differences

The most striking differences we found were sex related (Table 2). Significant differences were found between adolescent boys and girls regardless of ethnic group. Girls expressed a stronger conviction than boys that all members of the family should help each other and that each family member should do the jobs that he or she is supposed to do. They also stated more strongly that family members should openly acknowledge their affection for each other, be open and honest with their parents, and be able to cry openly when sad or upset. They also stated that the family should eat together at least once a day and do something together regularly.

In summary, we found that compared with boys, girls stand firmly for strong interrelationships and obligations within the family, affectional ties, and open expression of emotion. These findings are not unexpected and support old notions that girls find family and other relationships more important than do boys, who are working more actively to break

TABLE 2. Significant Differences Between Adolescent Boys and Girls on Questionnaire on Individual Attitudes Toward Family Values[a]

Question	Combined Mean Score	SD Boys (N=129)	SD Girls (N=118)	p[b]
A family should do something together regularly.	4.14	4.04	4.24	<.029
Every member of the family should help each other.	4.45	4.33	4.58	<.002
Family members should openly acknowledge their affection for each other.	3.99	3.82	4.17	<.001
Each family member should do the jobs that he or she is supposed to do.	4.22	4.07	4.37	<.001
All family members should share in doing the household chores.	4.27	4.11	4.45	<.001
It is all right for a member of the family to cry openly when sad or upset.	4.09	3.91	4.29	<.001
A family should eat together at least once a day.	3.75	3.63	3.88	<.026
Children should be honest and open with parents.	4.23	4.14	4.32	<.038
Boys should have more privileges than girls.	1.99	2.40	1.54	<.001

[a]Responses given on a scale of 1=strongly disagree to 5=strongly agree.
[b]p values for significance of difference between boys' and girls' SD derived by analysis of variance for main effects.

away and substitute experiences in the outside world for family experiences.

DISCUSSION

Our findings suggest that adolescent boys and girls differ significantly both in the rate and degree of, and the way in which they handle, separation from the nuclear family. Daughters in our study appeared to be struggling for their individuality within the family. They sought open affection and expression of emotion among family members as an emotional vehicle for defining themselves. They wanted the whole family to eat together at least once a day and to have regular group activities. A family meal or activity is an occasion that tends to promote close interactions and discussion of personal thoughts and feelings. If boys prefer less openness than their sisters, it might be expected that they would not want to participate in family activities that spotlight a range of family interrelationships, either positive or negative.

It would appear that parents' views on family closeness, sense of responsibility, and emotional sharing tend to overlap more with their daughters' than with their sons'. Does this phenomenon stifle or facilitate the girls' drive toward maturation? Do boys, who express less need for these family values during adolescence, have more or less difficulty achieving a balance between independence and interdependence than their sisters, whose wish to struggle with these issues within the family is supported by their parents? Does a family characterized by distance and detachment between members run a high risk for a daughter's adolescent process, while one that emphasizes closeness and interdependence runs a high risk for problems with sons? We will address these questions in an intensive study involving observation of actual family interactions, along with individual interviews and psychological assessment of family members.

The limitations of our method must be recognized. Questionnaire data are subjective self-descriptions, not objective descriptions of behavior. Thus, the context in which the individual functions is inherent (and essential) in survey research. Furthermore, our sample was limited to middle-class families, and we did not consider ordinal position within the family or separate individuals in early, middle, or late adolescence for purposes of analysis.

Therefore our findings thus far must be considered with caution. They represent only group or general trends and do not apply to all adolescent boys and girls. Nor would we suggest that one preferred style is better than the other; they are simply different. Even though daughters may share the same goal of individuation, they seem to desire more emotional support and affection within the family context than their brothers in achieving it. This finding appears to hold today in spite of the social forces that have encouraged independence for girls during the past two decades.

In any event, our findings suggest that these differences should be recognized. Those who consider the differences innate might suggest flexibility by the family to allow physical separation for boys and the opportunity for their sisters to work out their separation within the family. The girls' wish for emotional openness can be encouraged in a way that might be viewed as intrusiveness by their brothers. Those who consider these differences to represent sexual stereotypes that are socially formed might suggest an opposite approach—that of encouraging boys and girls to explore the parts of themselves that have been subdued.

Furthermore, there are practical implications. Recognition of these differences is important to promote developmental progress as well as parent-child interactions during this critical stage of life. For example, parents who find their adolescent sons avoiding the family meal, picking at their food, and "eating and running" need not feel there is something wrong with the boys because their sisters prefer to sit and talk. Instead, parents can permit (but not force) emotional expression and interaction and act as a buffer between the different styles expressed by the two sexes. Adolescent sons need not be considered withdrawn because they keep feelings to themselves, nor need their sisters be labeled emotional because they are more open with them.

CONCLUSIONS

Our findings challenge the notion that adolescent boys and girls have the same family experience. The variations suggest that they may have different routes in achieving the common goal of maturity. In this respect, our results support those of Gilligan (19), who compared the "connected person" who emphasizes physical and emotional care for others and a marked concern for the survival of relationships with the "separate person" who considers relationships in terms of reciprocity between separate individuals and who operates by a system of rules that has been worked out without consideration of the other person's feelings. Gilligan studied girls and found that they view themselves predominantly as "connected," which Gilligan says simply means that they speak "in a different voice," not a better one or a worse one.

If society favors the separate mode over the connected one, it is a problem we all must address. In this context our profession may have a special responsibility—to reexamine the concept of separation-individuation as the major goal of adolescence. We need not consider the complete differentiation of the self from the family to be the ideal goal. Individuals who retain strong ties and an orientation to relationships may be more, rather than less, mature than those who separate more completely from the family. Some developmentalists have long held that maturity follows a spectrum from dependence to independence. Yet various points along this spectrum, such as interdependence, may be more functional than an end point of independence. And, of course, both dependence and independence may not only exist together but each may be a necessary condition for the other's expression.

Our findings are being further investigated through interviews, psychological tests, and videotaped family interactions. Our hope is that meaningful comparisons between actual family behaviors and the individual expressed preferences reported here will sharpen our understanding of normal variations in the adolescent stage of the life cycle, a process that ends with physical separation from one's family but which contains varying degrees of psychological differentiation.

REFERENCES

1. Hall, G. S. (1904). Adolescence: Its Psychology and Its Relations to Physiology, Anthropology, Sociology, Sex, Crime, Religion and Education. New York, Appleton-Century-Crofts.
2. Blos, P. (1962). On Adolescence: A Psychoanalytic Interpretation. New York, Free Press.
3. Masterson, J. (1967). The Psychiatric Dilemma of Adolescence. Boston, Little, Brown and Co.
4. Weiner, I., Del Gaudio, A. (1976). Psychopathology in adolescents: an epidemiological study. Arch Gen Psychiatry 33:187–194.
5. Freud, A. (1971). Adolescence as a developmental disturbance, in The Writings of Anna Freud, vol 7. New York, International Universities Press.
6. Erikson, E. (1950). Childhood and Society. New York, WW Norton & Co.
7. Silber, E., Hamburg, D. A., Coelho, G. V., et al. (1961). Adaptive behavior in competent adolescents: coping with the anticipation of college. Arch Gen Psychiatry 5:354–365.
8. Silber, E., Coelho, G. V., Murphey, E. B., et al. (1961). Competent adolescents coping with college decisions. Arch Gen Psychiatry 5:517–527.
9. Grinker, R. (1962). "Mentally healthy" young males (homoclites): a study. Arch Gen Psychiatry 6:405–453.
10. Offer, D. (1969). The Psychological World of the Teenager: A Study of Normal Adolescent Boys. New York, Basic Books.
11. Offer, D., Offer, J. (1975). From Teenage to Young Manhood: A Psychological Study. New York, Basic Books.

12. Offer, D. (1980). Normal adolescent development in Comprehensive Textbook of Psychiatry, 3rd ed, vol 3. Edited by Kaplan H, Freedman A, Sadock B. Baltimore, Williams & Wilkins Co.

13. Vaillant, G. E. (1974). The natural history of male psychological health, II: some antecedents of healthy adult adjustment. Arch Gen Psychiatry 31:15–22.

14. Vaillant, G. E. (1975). The natural history of male psychological health, III: empirical dimensions of mental health. Arch Gen Psychiatry 32:420–426.

15. King, S. (1972). Coping and growth in adolescents. Semin Psychiatry 5:355–366.

16. Power and Authority in Adolescents: The Origins and Resolutions of Intergenerational Conflict (1978). Group Adv Psychiatry [Rep] 101.

17. Offer, D., Ostrov, E., Howard, K. I. (1981). The Adolescent: A Psychological Self-Portrait. New York, Basic Books.

18. Ashton, G. C., Polovina, J. J., Vandenberg, S. G. (1979). Segregation analysis of family data for 15 tests of cognitive ability. Behav Genet 9:329–347.

19. Gilligan, C (1982). In a Different Voice. Cambridge, Harvard University Press.

10

Parental Work Patterns in Alternative Families: Influence on Child Development

Irla Lee Zimmerman and Maurine Bernstein

Neuropsychiatric Institute, University of California at Los Angeles

The increasing return to work by mothers of young children was documented for matching samples of mothers in families representing traditional marriages, single-mother units, social-contract relationships, and communal living groups. No evidence was found of negative effects on children's social, emotional, and cognitive development attributable to maternal absence due to employment.

Children of today are growing up with less and less full-time maternal care: working mothers have become the norm rather than the exception. A new mother's early return to work has a number of implications for her child. There is a reduction in the amount of mothering time available to the child and a substitution of alternative caretakers, which could affect the attachment between mother and child or subject the child to shifting, unstable attachment figures. The decreased interaction between mother and child reduces the mother's role as early "educator"; unless the caretaker is equally concerned and competent, important learning periods in a child's life may be short-changed.

At the same time maternal employment may offer the child a chance

---

Reprinted with permission from the *American Journal of Orthopsychiatry*, 1983, Vol. 53, No. 3, 418–425. Copyright 1983 by the American Orthopsychiatric Association, Inc.

Presented at the 1982 annual meeting of the American Orthopsychiatric Association in San Francisco.

to explore a wider world, to relate to other adult figures, to socialize with peers at an early age, to do more things for himself or herself, perhaps to have less supervision and restriction. Likewise, maternal employment presents different role models to the child; with both mother and father having jobs and sharing roles, sex-role stereotypes begin to fade.

An increasing number of studies have explored the effects of maternal employment on children. In recent reviews of research literature, such as those of Etaugh,[9] Hohenshil, Hummel and Maddy-Bernstein,[14] and Hoffman,[12,13] the authors concluded that maternal employment *per se* has limited influence on the development of the young child and that such factors as family circumstances may be more critical than actual employment status. At the same time, it is acknowledged[11,12] that before conclusions can be generalized, more information is needed on the impact of maternal employment on infants.

The Family Styles Project offers a unique opportunity to explore these issues. The role of family circumstances, assumed by Hoffman[12,13] and Etaugh[9] to be critical, can be studied in the various life styles. In addition, the influence of maternal employment on infants, and the sequential effect of maternal employment during the preschool years can be explored in our longitudinal data. One more factor, the ability level of the mothers, which may well relate to job opportunities, satisfactions, and income level, can be compared with their children's progress.

This study covers the effects of maternal employment on infants, toddlers, and preschoolers. The mothers and children involved represented families from traditional marriages, single-mother units, social-contract relationships, and communal living groups. In these settings, the effects of family circumstances making up the support systems (presence or absence of a husband, mate, or living group), maternal ability (intelligence level of the mother), and employment choice (not working, working part-time, working full-time) could be explored as these variables impinged upon the child's life at one year, three years, and six years of age.

PATTERNS OF MATERNAL WORK BY LIFE STYLE

Information regarding the time period at which each mother returned to work following the birth of her child, and the amount of work (part-time or full-time) she engaged in was collected periodically throughout the first six years of her child's life. This was grouped into time periods: work during the first year, work during the birth-to-two-year time period, the two-to-four-year time period, the four-to-six-year time period, and a final score totaling the amount of work through the entire six-year period.

The control group of traditionally married mothers was characteristic of much of the United States population in their work patterns. Almost 70% remained at home during the first year of their child's life. However, by the end of the child's second year, more than half of the traditionally married women were working at least part-time. By four years, two-thirds were working at least part-time, but by six years this dropped to 43%, perhaps reflecting the economic downturn. Nevertheless the 43% of the traditional mothers who worked part-time or full-time during this preschool time period is identical to the percentage of employed traditionally married mothers of preschoolers reported in the 1979 census.

Classically, single mothers are the most frequently employed mothers of young children. In our sample, 62% remained at home during the first year of their child's life, comparable to the traditional mothers (69%). In fact, 20% of both traditional and single mothers worked full-time during the first year. At each succeeding time period, however, more single mothers entered the job market, so that by the fourth year, 75% were working part- or full-time. However, the single mother showed the same drop in employment at the four-to-six-year time period as seen by traditional mothers (62%), almost identical to the 1979 single mother census findings (60%). Overall, more single mothers were employed, particularly full-time, than were mothers in any other group, but their work patterns are closer to those of the traditionally married control group than to the other alternative mothers.

Social-contract mothers were least apt to work either part- or full-time at one year, or by the end of the second year. Most of those who were employed worked only part-time. The same pattern of part-time rather than full-time work characterized social-contract mothers during the next two time periods, although by the end of six years 26% worked full-time, similar to the traditional mothers. In all, only 4% of the social-contract mothers had continuously worked full-time, significantly less than either traditional marrieds or single mothers.

Of all the life styles, more communal living group mothers chose to work part-time, and were not apt to work full-time. At no time period did more than 9% work full-time. In all, only 2% of the communal group mothers had worked full-time since their children's birth, and thus resembled the work pattern of the social-contract mothers. However, 59% had worked part-time, more than any other group, a consistent pattern from the birth of their first child. Again, they were significantly different from the traditional marrieds and single mothers with respect to employment patterns.

To summarize, traditional mothers in this study show the same work pattern as the traditional mother population reported in the 1979 census, with 43% working part- or full-time by the preschool period. Single mothers were most likely to work full-time at each stage of their children's lives, again showing the same work pattern as that of single mothers in the 1979 census, with 62% working by the preschool period. In contrast, the alternative social-contract and communal living group mothers were characterized by rarely working full-time, preferring part-time work.

Another factor that influences the child's development and must be considered when reviewing the impact of a working mother is the mother's ability level. The GAT-B, a standard test of intelligence, was administered to each mother as part of our assessment procedures. The scores were converted to a Wechsler-type IQ (mean 100, SD 15) to be consistent with the results obtained with the WISC-R administered to the children at age six.

To reiterate, the mothers in this study were white, between the ages of 18 and 35, and from families of origin that were predominantly middle class. The sample as a whole was well educated; almost a third had graduated from college with a BA or higher degree, and only 9% had failed to finish high school. While, as a group, the traditionally married controls were better educated, the ability level of all the mothers was above average (GAT-B[20] for mothers who were not working was 109, for those working part-time it was 113, and for those engaged in full-time work it was 114). While these differences were not significant, the direction of difference, that is, increasing intelligence of those who worked part- and full-time, was identical for all life styles. At each time period, as more mothers returned to work, the trend continued: mothers working full-time functioned intellectually at a slightly higher level than those working part-time, who in turn slightly surpassed those who chose not to work.

RESULTS

This study sought to determine the effect of maternal employment on the cognitive, social, and emotional development of the child. The children were observed and tested at the UCLA office at three critical periods: at age one, at age three, and again at six years. Results of the test batteries were analyzed by original life style, the mothers' time of entry into the work force, whether she worked part- or full-time, and her ability level (GAT-B).

One-Year Measures

When the children were one year old, their development was assessed on the Bayley Scales of Infant Development.[3] Development was above average on the mental scale (MDI mean 110), and almost identical for all life styles (ranging 109–110). These results parallel closely the estimated general aptitude of their mothers (GAT-B mean 111). When these findings were considered in terms of the amount of work engaged in by the mother, differences were minimal, averaging 110 for children whose mothers remained at home or worked part-time, and 112 for those whose mothers worked full-time. When mothers' ability level was parceled out, results remained the same. In other words, the children were functioning above average, and this was true regardless of life style, maternal ability, or extent of mothers' employment.

At one year, children are considered at the height of attachment to their mothers. At this point, the child is most aware of the mother as a source of comfort, and as a secure base from which to explore the environment. Using the Ainsworth Strange Situation Test,[2] attachment was measured, then analyzed by life style, ability level, and work patterns of the mothers. The sample as a whole showed 76% firmly attached, 15% insecure avoidant, and 10% insecure anxious, results similar to those reported by Ainsworth *et al*[1] for middle-class samples. No differences were attributable to life style. When considered in terms of mothers working or not working in the first year, infants of mothers who worked full- or part-time were as likely to be as securely attached to their mothers as were infants whose mothers stayed home.

Three-Year Measures

At age three, the children were subjected to a battery of cognitive, emotional, and social measures, using such tests as the Stanford-Binet,[18] which at age three measures a variety of perceptual motor tasks intermingled with verbal items.[16] Also measured was receptive language (Peabody Picture Vocabulary Test, PPVT[6]), which might mirror the environmental linguistic setting in which the child was raised. Attachment, previously assessed at age one, was again assessed using the Strange Situation Test. However, at age three, this seems to elicit the child's ability to accept separation without distress, to explore and play without mother being present, rather than classical attachment per se.

Results of the three-year battery revealed the children to be functioning intellectually at the average level (Binet mean IQ 103 = 15), with identical receptive language skills (PPVT 103 = 15). Life-style differences were minimal, with no more than a three-point difference between the lowest (single mothers, 101) and the highest group (communal group, 104), in terms of intellectual competence. Receptive language was also not significantly different, although, again, children of single mothers scored lowest (98), with the other groups all but identical, and traditional mothers' children scoring highest (104). When these measures are compared by the mothers' work patterns during the first two years, children of traditional mothers, single mothers, and social-contract mothers all showed no differences attributable to maternal work patterns. However, communal living group children whose mothers were not working scored significantly lower than those whose mothers were employed.

At age three, attachment measures reveal more than half of the children (57%) to be independent and capable of tolerating mothers' brief absences without any distress. Just over a third (39%) showed the close attachment characteristic of age one (distress at separation, immediate relief at reunion), while acute distress was rare (4%). Again, children did not differ significantly by either life-style or by the mothers' work patterns.

Six-Year Measures

A battery of tests was administered to the children during the office visit at six years. At this age the children were capable of doing a wide variety of tasks that would reveal aspects of their emotional, social, and cognitive development and specific competencies.

The WISC-R,[21] administered first, was followed by drawing and story-telling tasks. Since the battery was lengthy, play time and a lunch break were imperative. However, the so-called play time was utilized as an unstructured session with a clinician present, and the child's play was observed and rated by an outside psychologist through a one-way mirror, thus adding assessment material from someone who was not cognizant of either the life-style or work pattern of the child's mother.

Some of the tests were adopted for obvious reasons, such as measures of reading skills (Peabody Individual Achievement test, PIAT[7]), visual motor development (Primary Visual Motor Test[10]), and creativity.[19] Others, such as the Children's Apperception Test,[4] presented opportunities to assess the child's perception of family interactions and parental and child roles. The battery also included the Two Houses Test,[17] which provided clues to family relationships and how the child comprehended his or her role in a complex living group or a reconstituted family. A measure of moral judgment[5] provided insight into a child's understanding of rules of behavior. An unsolvable puzzle (Puzzle Barrier[5]) revealed aspects of the child's achievement orientation and persistence. The child's conception of appropriate sex-role behavior was also assessed (Sex Role Learning Index, SRLI[8]), as was a measure of field independence (Children's Embedded Figures Test, CEFT[22]).

Needless to say, in such a long testing session, many aspects of the child's abilities and temperament were observed, giving us an in-depth view of the cognitive, emotional, and social strengths and weaknesses that the child had developed by age six.

When all these measures were analyzed for life-style differences, these proved to be few, and presumably attributable to chance. The effects of maternal employment were more equivocal, with differences varying from one life-style to another. For instance, intelligence (WISC-R) averaged 114 for the sample as a whole, or just above the mothers' level of functioning. For all life-styles, scores tended to be higher for children with working mothers, but this did not reach significance for traditional or single-mother children, while differences were significant for both social-contract and communal living group children.

Studies of children of working mothers have suggested that one aspect of mothers working has been their children's less traditional sex-role concepts, in that they may observe smaller differences in male and female roles.[15] Emphasis on sexual egalitarianism has also been characteristic of alternative life styles. Therefore we measured the child's conception of sex roles. On the SRLI, the types of activities that children believed to be appropriate for both males and females, rather than exclusively one or the other, were assessed using an array of 20 tasks such as washing dishes, using a hammer, teaching, or being a doctor. We speculated that children whose parents stressed egalitarianism, or whose mothers worked, would be more apt to see tasks as appropriate for both males and females. Taken as a whole, there were no differences in the number of tasks that children accepted as appropriate for both males and females: approximately one-fourth of the roles were considered as appropriate to both sexes. Considered by extent of mothers' work, only one of the four life-styles revealed significant differences: children of mothers in communal living groups who worked part- or full-time were much more apt to see tasks as appropriate to both than did those whose mothers remained home during the first six years.

Maternal Support

To test the hypothesis that a working mother would perhaps be seen as unavailable and failing to provide for her child's needs, stories from the Children's Apperception Test[4] were analyzed in terms of support offered by the maternal figure. Scores ranged from "no support" (for example, the mother hen refused to feed the chicks) to "support" (the chicks are being given dinner). Among the children, 33% to 45% described the mother figure as totally supportive, with minimal differences attributable to life-style. There were no work pattern differences for three of the four life-styles. However, children of single mothers who worked in the first two years significantly more often ($p < .004$) described the maternal figure as unsupportive than did those whose mothers remained at home with their children. The same reaction continued when children of mothers working through the next time period (2–4) were considered. Only when results for children of parents working at the preschool period (4–6) were considered did differences fail to reach significance.

Field Independence

Field independence, assessed on the Children's Embedded Figures Test (CEFT[22]), a measure of the ability of the child to detect a pattern embedded in a concealing picture, has been hypothesized as relating to independence of thought, self determinism, intellectual curiosity, and a sense of separate identity. These are characteristics prized by some alternative families, such as the social-contract group, and rejected by others (specifically, the creedal group). However, children of working mothers might also be hypothesized as developing increasing field independence.

Life-style differences did not appear on the CEFT, nor were maternal work patterns significant for three of the four life-styles. However, for all life-styles, CEFT scores tended to be highest for children whose mothers worked full-time. And in the case of social-contract children, there was a significant increase in scores of children whose mothers worked full-time (102 *vs* 126, $p < .01$).

CONCLUSIONS

The increasing return to work by mothers of young children is a reality of the 1970s and 1980s which our sample of 200 young mothers whose children were born in the mid-seventies clearly substantiates. The fact that our control group of traditionally married mothers exactly match the work pattern of traditionally married mothers in the 1979 census, just as the single mothers exactly match the same group in the 1979 census, allows us to conclude that the Family Life Styles mothers are representative of the United States population as a whole.

Mothers appear to be returning to work in increasing numbers from as early as several weeks after the birth of their children, with 13% working full-time by the end of the first year. In-depth comparisons of children's functioning at various age levels revealed few differences attributable to life-style, no matter when the child was assessed. However, by ages three and six there were a few differences relating to the extent of mothers' work. These were not in the expected direction; in almost all cases, the mother who spent more time at work had a child who functioned at a higher level.

In summary, when the work patterns of 200 mothers were compared to a variety of measures of their children's social, emotional, and cognitive development, there was no evidence of negative effects traceable to maternal absence due to their employment. When the maternal ability level was controlled, children of working mothers tended to do slightly better on cognitive measures, to show no deficits in attachment to their mothers, to perceive the mothers as equally supportive, and to have less traditional sex-role perceptions. Since more and more mothers seem to be returning to the work force in the child's early years, the findings reported are a good omen for children of today.

REFERENCES

1. Ainsworth, M. et al. (1978). Patterns of Attachment. Erlbaum, Hillsdale, N.J.
2. Ainsworth, M. and Wittig, B. (1974). Attachment and exploratory behavior of one-year-olds in a strange situation. In Determinants of Infant Behavior. Vol. IV. M. Ainsworth et al. eds. London University Press, London.
3. Bayley, N. (1969). Bayley Scales of Infant Development. Psychological Corp., New York.
4. Bellach, L. and Bellach, S. (1978). Children's Apperception Test (CAT) C.P.S. Inc., New York.
5. Block, J. and Block, J. H. (1974). Ego development and the provenance of thought. Progress Report, NIMH.

6. Dunn, L. (1965). Peabody Picture Vocabulary Test (PPVT). American Guidance Service. Circle Pines, Minn.
7. Dunn, L. and Markwardt, F. (1970). Peabody Individual Achievement Test (PIAT). American Guidance Service. Circle Pines, Minn.
8. Edelbrock, C. and Sugawara, A. (undated). The Sex Role Learning Index (SRLI) Manual. Oregon State University, Corvallis, Ore.
9. Etaugh, C. (1974). Effects of maternal employment on children: a review of recent research. Merrill-Palmer Quart. 19–20:71–98.
10. Haworth, M. The Primary Visual Motor Test. Grune and Stratton, New York.
11. Hock, E. (1978). Working and nonworking mothers with infants: perceptions of their careers, their infants' needs, and satisfaction with mothering. Devlpm. Psychol. 14:37–43.
12. Hoffman, L. (1974). Effects of maternal employment on the child: a review of the research. Devlpm. Psychol. 10:204–228.
13. Hoffman, L. (1980). The effects of maternal employment on the academic attitudes and performance of school-aged children. Devlpm. Psychol. 9:319–335.
14. Hohenshil, T., Hummel, D. and Maddy-Bernstein, C. (1980). The impact of work patterns upon family development. Schl Psychol. Rev. 9:312–318.
15. Miller, S. (1975). Effects of maternal employment on sex role perception, interests, and self esteem in kindergarten girls. Devlpm. Psychol. 11:405–406.
16. Sattler, J. (1974). Assessment of Children's Intelligence (Rev. Ed.). W.B. Saunders, Philadelphia.
17. Szyrynski, V. (1963). Investigation of family dynamics with the "Two Houses Technique." Psychosomatics 4:68–72.
18. Terman, L. and Merrill, M. (1972). Stanford Binet Intelligence Scale. Form L-M. Houghton Mifflin, Boston.
19. Torrance, E. (1979). Thinking Creatively in Action and Movement: Manual. Georgia Studies of Creative Behavior, Athens, Ga.
20. U.S. Dept. of Labor Manpower Administration. (1970). Manual for the USES: General Aptitude Test Battery. U.S. Government Printing Office, Washington, D.C.
21. Wechsler, D. (1974). Wechsler Intelligence Scale for Children-Revised (WISC-R). Psychological Corp., New York.
22. Witkin, H. et al. (1971). A Manual for Embedded Figures Test (CEFT). Consulting Psychologists Press, Palo Alto, Calif.

11

Attachment Behavior of Deaf Children with Deaf Parents

Kathryn P. Meadow, Mark T. Greenberg, and Carol Erting

Gallaudet College, Washington, D.C.

Seventeen deaf children, all of whom have two deaf parents, were videotaped. Analyses of their behaviors indicated that they are comparable to children with normal hearing who have participated in research projects in the past. They are neither precocious nor are they delayed in their development of secure attachment to and independence from primary caregivers. Thus, children younger than age 3 were unwilling to consent to the parent's departure from the room and were distressed by the separation. Most of the children between ages 3 and 5 reached agreement about the plan for separation; only 1 showed distress while alone, and all were sociable upon reunion. Findings are compared with those of previous studies, and suggestions made for explanations of differences which emphasize the importance of the sociolinguistic environment for optimal development of deaf children.

Following the seminal work of Bowlby (1969) and of Ainsworth and her colleagues (1973, 1978), a great deal of research has accumulated describing the development of attachment in children to their mothers.

Reprinted with permission from the *Journal of the American Academy of Child Psychiatry*, 1983, Vol. 22, No. 1, 23–28. Copyright 1983 by the American Academy of Child Psychiatry.

We wish to express our appreciation to the families and to the teachers in the Preschool at the Kendall Demonstration Elementary School of Gallaudet College. At the time the data were collected, Dr. Robert Davila was Dean at KDES. We would like to acknowledge the generous support of Dr. Davila, and of Dr. Michael Deninger, currently Dean of KDES.

This has been, in fact, a primary interest of psychiatrists and psychologists for the past 15–20 years. Similarly, there has been an increasing, although much less extensive, interest in the personality development and characteristics of deaf persons. Beginning with the Heiders (1941) and Levine (1956), important series of studies have been conducted by groups at the New York Psychiatric Institute (Altshuler, 1974; Altshuler et al., 1976; Rainer et al., 1969), Michael Reese Hospital (Grinker, 1969; Mindel and Vernon, 1971), and the University of California, San Francisco (Schlesinger, 1978, 1979a; Schlesinger and Meadow, 1972). These studies have contributed a great deal to our knowledge of the influence of profound childhood deafness on personality development. However, until the publication of Greenberg's data (Greenberg and Marvin, 1979), no research report has appeared in the literature linking deafness to attachment theory. Greenberg reported attachment/separation data on 28 profoundly deaf preschool children, all of whom had hearing mothers and fathers.

The purpose of this paper is to report similar research data collected from 17 profoundly deaf preschool children, all of whom have deaf mothers and fathers. Hearing status of the parents of deaf children is a critical factor in determining the paths their development will take. Many studies have demonstrated the higher educational achievement levels of deaf children of deaf parents in comparison with deaf children of hearing parents (Brasel and Quigley, 1977; Meadow, 1968a; Stuckless and Birch, 1966; Vernon and Koh, 1970), and their more positive social and behavioral adjustment (Harris, 1978; Meadow, 1969; Meadow et al., 1981; Stokoe and Battison, 1981). These findings have been replicated with numerous populations despite the consistently lower educational and occupational status of deaf parents compared with the hearing population, and their more limited access to parent education and to mental health facilities (Schein, 1979).

The Office of Demographic Studies at Gallaudet College has reported that 3% of deaf children participating in their Annual Survey of Hearing Impaired Children and Youth have two deaf parents. An additional 6% of these children have one deaf parent (Rawlings and Jensema, 1977). So, despite the rarity of deaf child/deaf parent families, they comprise a theoretically interesting and important group because deaf families are capable of communication (in sign language) with their deaf children from infancy onward and because deaf parents find the diagnosis of deafness less traumatic than do hearing parents (Meadow, 1967). Even those hearing families who are willing to learn sign language face delays related to the diagnosis of deafness (Meadow, 1968b; Spradley and

Spradley, 1978), to the acquisition of a new language mode, and to internal and external conflicts about the acceptability of signed communication (Moores, 1978; Winefield, 1981).

Summary of Attachment Theory

Four phases or stages of attachment have been delineated during the child's first 4 years of life. The first two phases occur in early infancy and are marked by differential responsiveness to one or to a few caregivers on the part of an infant (Bowlby, 1969). During phase III, which begins at approximately 8 months of age, young children actively seek proximity to specific caregivers and often show distress at separation from these significant others. Three general types of behavior have been enumerated as characteristic of phase III: secure, avoidant and ambivalent (Ainsworth et al., 1978). During the later part of phase III, after the age of 2, most children do not show acute distress when they are separated from their mothers for brief periods of time (Maccoby and Feldman, 1972). Until some time after their third birthday, however, they usually seek proximity to the significant caregiver upon reunion (Marvin, 1977). Phase IV has been characterized by Bowlby (1969) as showing the ability of the child and the mother to come to an agreement (or partnership) about the mother's plan to separate from the child and to return. As this development progresses, the child becomes less dependent on the mother for constant presence and support. Marvin (1972, 1977) found that by the age of 4 most children were capable of achieving the phase IV partnership with their mothers in a laboratory situation. However, he found all 2-year-olds as well as 75% of children at the third birthday demonstrating phase III attachment patterns.

Because of the delay in language acquisition among most deaf children, and the supposed lessened abilities of these children to reach verbal agreement with their mothers or to understand the mother's explanation for her leave-taking, Greenberg and Marvin (1979) hypothesized that their deaf subjects would be delayed in their achievement of the phase IV (partnership) attachment pattern. However, they found that deafness *per se* did not lead to such a delay; instead, a strong relationship was found between the deaf child's communicative competence and attainment of the phase IV pattern.

METHOD

Subjects

The research group consisted of 17 deaf children, all of whom had two deaf or hard-of-hearing parents. The children came from 14 different families (that is, 3 families had 2 children who each participated in the study). Table 1 presents demographic information separately for the children, divided into younger (12 to 35 months) and older (36 to 60 months) groups. All parents routinely utilized either simultaneous communication (voice plus manual signing) or manual communication without voice (American Sign Language or Sign English) in everyday interaction with their children. In 13 of the 14 families, the mother was

TABLE 1
Demographic Information—Seventeen Deaf Children by Age

Characteristic	Age	
	Younger than 3 Years (N = 10)	3 Years or Older (N = 7)
Mean age (in months)	21.7	44.7
Age range (in months)	12–33	36–40
Mean hearing loss (dB, speech range, unaided)[a]	97 dB	100 dB
Sex		
Male	5	2
Female	5	5
Mothers' education		
High school graduate	—	1
Some college	10	6
Fathers' education		
High school graduate	1	2
Some college	9	5
Hearing status of grandparents: One or both sets of grandparents deaf	8	6
Fathers' occupation:		
Student or unemployed	1	1
Blue collar	1	3
White collar	7	3
Not available	1	—

[a]Hearing loss information not available for one child in each age grouping.

the primary caregiver. In 1 family the father filled this role, and he participated in the videotaping of his 2 children. All the families were intact at the time the videotaping was carried out. All children were enrolled in the preschool program of the Kendall Demonstration Elementary School, PreCollege Programs, Gallaudet College. None had been identified as having handicaps in addition to deafness.

Procedure

Each parent-child dyad was videotaped in a 30-minute sequence consisting of three segments (see Meadow et al., 1981). During the first 8 minutes, parents and children engaged in free play and shared simple refreshments. The room was approximately 3.5 by 4.5 meters and contained two chairs, two tables, and a large variety of toys. Fruit juice and cups were placed on one of the tables; cookies were "hidden" in a coffee can placed with the toys. During the free play segment, parents read a letter telling the child where the cookies were hidden. The separation segment began after 8 minutes when the parent was given a signal to leave the room. The parents were told that they could explain as much as they wished regarding their departure. The reunion segment began when the parent returned after the child had been alone for 3 minutes.

Coding

Attachment behavior was classified by means of a two-step data reduction process following Greenberg and Marvin (1979). First, the children were classified into categories describing the outcome of preseparation planning, separation behavior, and reunion behavior.

Preseparation planning began at the point where the parent first communicated that he/she was leaving the room, and ended when he/she actually went out the door:
1. Agrees with parent's departure—any verbal or nonverbal indication that the child was willing for the parent to leave;
2. Disagrees with parent's departure—any verbal or nonverbal indication that the child was not willing for the parent to leave, or that the child expects/insists on accompanying the parent;
3. No response to parent's departure—the child may or may not watch the parent during the explanation or leave-taking, but neither agrees nor disagrees with the parent's action. In cases where parents gave no explanation, no planning was possible and the child was also scored as "no response."

Separation activities of the children were also categorized in three ways:
1. Play/manipulatory toy exploration without any search or distress;
2. Play and search—toy play accompanied by occasional search behaviors such as calling parent, looking at, or approaching the door;
3. Distress and search—active attempts to reach parent by crying, angry, aggressive behavior or pounding on the door, unaccompanied by sustained play.

Reunion activities were coded during the first 30 seconds after the parent returned to the room:
1. Approach—the child moves within arm's reach of the parent within 15 seconds after she/he returns. Parent's approaching the child was not coded even though it resulted in proximity;
2. Sociable—although child did not approach the parent, he or she either greeted the parent with a smile or engaged in pleasant communication or interaction with him/her in the context of play within 30 seconds;
3. Avoidance—the child ignores the parent after reunion, that is, fails to acknowledge the parent's return by greeting, smiling, or responding to the parent's communications;
4. Resistance—the child shows angry/aggressive behavior, communicates negative affect, or resists contact with the parent; avoidance and resistance may both be accompanied by gaze aversion.

The second step of data reduction was classification of each child in phase III or phase IV of Bowlby's attachment model (Marvin, 1977). Children were classified in phase III if they displayed the proximity-based patterns characteristic of younger children (Ainsworth, 1973; Waters, 1978). Variations of phase III patterns included approaching, avoiding, or resisting the parent upon reunion regardless of preseparation agreement or disagreement. Children were classified in a phase IV partnership if they (1) agreed to the departure-reunion plan, (2) played during separation with no distress (with or without search), and (3) responded with social behavior without approach upon reunion.

Coder Agreement

All videotapes were coded independently by two raters. Estimates of agreement were computed as the number of agreements divided by the number of agreements plus the number of disagreements. Coder agreement equaled 94% for the preseparation categories, 100% for separation categories, 94% for reunion categories, and 88% for the attachment phase classification.

RESULTS

Table 2 shows the distribution attachment behaviors for the two age groups (younger and older than 3 years). Similar to findings of young hearing children (Weinraub and Lewis, 1977), only one child under the age of 3 years gave a verbal or nonverbal consent to the parent's plan for departure. While these younger children were alone, they were affected noticeably by the separation, with 50% becoming distressed (crying and calling for mother). Separations of 4 of the 5 distressed children were terminated early (i.e., before the prescribed 3 minutes had expired). Upon reunion, the majority of the younger children sought proximity to their caregivers and were sociable, while 2 (20%) showed avoidant or resistant patterns. These findings for both separation and reunion are comparable to those of hearing children (Ainsworth et al., 1978; Maccoby and Feldman, 1972). As Table 2 indicates, all of the children under the age of 3 displayed phase III patterns, which is in

TABLE 2

Classifications of Attachment Pattern/Phase by Age

	Age	
Sequence	Younger than 3 Years (N = 10)	3 years or Older (N = 7)
Preseparation planning		
Agree	1	5
Disagree	0	0
No response	9	2
Behavior while alone		
Play	0	3
Play and search	5	3
Distress	5	1
Reunion		
Sociable without proximity-seeking	2	6
Sociable with proximity-seeking	6	1
Avoidance or resistant behavior	2	0
Attachment phase		
Phase III		
Secure	8	2
Avoidance or resistant	2	0
Phase IV		
Goal-corrected partnership	0	5

precise agreement with Marvin's (1977) data on hearing children. Of these children, 20% showed anxious or insecure attachments, which is a similar but somewhat lower percentage than that reported for hearing children (Ainsworth et al., 1978; Waters, 1978).

Of the children ages 3 and older, 5 (71%) reached agreement with their parents regarding the plan for separation and reunion, only 1 showed distress while alone, and all were sociable upon reunion with only 1 child seeking proximity. Once again, findings are almost identical with those of Maccoby and Feldman (1972) and Marvin (1977) in documenting both the increased communication regarding separation, the absence of distress while alone, and the presence of sociable behavior without proximity-seeking upon reunion in children who had reached their third birthday. As Table 2 indicates, 5 (71%) of the older deaf children were classified in the more advanced phase IV partnership pattern which is an almost identical finding with Marvin's data on hearing 4-year-olds (75% of children in that age group had achieved the partnership phase).

DISCUSSION

The findings reported above indicate that the deaf children of deaf parents who participated in our study are comparable to children with normal hearing who have participated in research projects in the past. They are neither precocious nor delayed in their development of secure attachment with and independence from their caregivers. These findings are similar to data on the social interaction of deaf children and deaf parents that we have reported previously (Meadow et al., 1981). That earlier report compared three groups of deaf children with hearing children. That is, deaf children and deaf mothers performed in a similar manner to that of hearing children and hearing mothers; both of these groups exhibited interaction that was more complex and more mature than that of deaf children with hearing parents. In terms of attachment behavior, deaf children of deaf parents in this study performed in a manner that was similar to that of deaf children of hearing parents when the children had high communicative ability (Greenberg and Marvin, 1979).

These three sets of findings are in vivid and startling contrast to those reported by Galenson and her colleagues (1979). Based on clinical observations of four deaf children and their deaf mothers, they conclude:

All the deaf mothers had introduced early self-bottle feeding by 2 or 3 months, with the bottle first propped and later held by the baby . . . any . . . attempts at self-feeding solids were firmly discouraged, even well into the second year of life [p. 132] . . . during the second year . . . severe separation anxiety appeared and persisted. The clinging to the mother was of course aggravated by the deaf child's need to keep his mother in view in order to maintain contact with her . . . The severe separation anxiety suggested that there was considerable difficulty in the establishment of a stable maternal mental representation . . . The phase of autonomy in these deaf infants lagged well behind that of the hearing child, and its form and shape were unusually distorted [p. 135] . . . [there was] delay in developing the usual type of transitional object attachment to blankets or teddy bears during the first 16 months . . . [the deaf mothers'] emotional attachment failed to provide the requisite dependability for the child's optimal development [p. 136].

In our previous paper (Meadow et al., 1981), we speculated about possible reasons for the discrepancies between our conclusions and those of the Galenson group. These may be summarized in the context of the attachment data as well:

The Galenson data were collected in New York at a school that has long been known as a center for oral-only education, whereas data on deaf mothers and deaf children reported in this paper were collected at a preschool on the campus of Gallaudet College which is associated with the support of American Sign Language and Sign English. Since sign language was forbidden in the New York preschool, it is difficult to know how the deaf parents communicated either with their children or with the hearing researchers, and this might well have influenced both the kinds of observations that were made and the comfort that the deaf mothers displayed toward their deaf children. A second and probably more cogent explanation of differences in the two sets of observations could be that the deaf parents who enrolled themselves and their deaf children in an educational program where their preferred communicative mode was unwelcome are a self-selected unrepresentative group. Most deaf families prefer to send their deaf children to schools where sign language is used; those who follow a different pathway may comprise a subgroup that "identifies with the oppressors" (Schlesinger, 1979b).

The influence of the sociolinguistic environment is becoming recognized as a major factor in deaf education (Erting, 1978; Meadow, 1980).

The notion that the deaf parents in the New York group and those in the Gallaudet group may come from two distinct populations is supported by the following information: (a) 1 of 4 Lexington children had deaf grandparents compared to 14 of 17 Gallaudet children who had either 1 or 2 sets of deaf grandparents; (b) 1 of 4 New York children had college-educated parents, while 16 of 17 Gallaudet mothers and 14 of 17 Gallaudet fathers had some college; (c) none of the New York mothers breast-fed their children, while 4 of 7 Gallaudet mothers for whom we have data breast-fed their children. (New York data are found in Galenson et al., 1979, pp. 131–133.)

SUMMARY AND CONCLUSIONS

In summary, we can say that the 17 profoundly deaf children of 2 deaf parents included in this study exhibited attachment patterns following almost exactly those reported for hearing children of similar ages. Half of the children younger than age 3 showed signs of distress when separated from their parent in the laboratory setting; the majority sought proximity and were sociable with the parent upon reunion while 2 exhibited avoidance or resistance to the parent's overtures. Five of the 7 children age 3 or older had achieved the more advanced attachment pattern ("goal-corrected partnership" with the parent); the remaining 2 were classified as "secure" in their attachment while not yet achieving the more mature pattern.

These data were compared with others reported from clinical observations in different settings, and some reasons for differences in the results were suggested.

We conclude that deaf children of deaf parents may follow a variety of developmental patterns. These may depend even more heavily on parental characteristics, history, and environment than the developmental course of non-hearing-impaired children. The developmental complexities created by deafness should be of great interest to behavioral scientists and clinicians alike, and it is clear that many issues remain to be resolved.

REFERENCES

Ainsworth, M. D. S. (1973). The development of infant-mother attachment. In: *Review of Child Development Research, Vol. 3*, ed B. M. Caldwell & H. N. Ricciuti. Chicago: University of Chicago Press.
—— Blehar, M. C., Waters, E. & Wall, S. (1978). *Patterns of Attachment*. Hillsdale, N.J.: Lawrence Earlbaum Associates.

Altshuler, K. Z. (1974). The social and psychological development of the deaf child; problems and their treatment and prevention. *Amer. Ann. Deaf*, 119:365–376.

—— Deming, W. E., Vollenweider, J., Rainer, J. D. & Tendler, R. (1976). Impulsivity and profound early deafness; a cross cultural inquiry. *Amer. Ann. Deaf*, 121:331–345.

Bowlby, J. (1969). *Attachment and Loss; Vol. 1, Attachment.* New York: Basic Books.

Brasel, K. E. & Quigley, S. P. (1977). Influence of certain language and communication environments in early childhood on the development of language in deaf individuals. *J. Speech Hear. Res.*, 20:81–94.

Erting, C. (1978). Language policy and deaf ethnicity in the United States. *Sign Language Studies*, 19:139–152.

Galenson, E., Miller, R., Kaplan, E. & Rothstein, A. (1979). Assessment of development in the deaf child. *This Journal*, 18:128–142.

Greenberg, M. T. & Marvin, R. S. (1979). Patterns of attachment in profoundly deaf preschool children. *Merrill-Palmer Quart.*, 25:265–279.

Grinker, R. R. (1969). *Psychiatric Diagnosis, Therapy and Research on the Psychotic Deaf.* Washington D.C.: Social Rehabilitation Service, Department of Health, Education and Welfare.

Harris, R. I. (1978). Impulse control in deaf children; research and clinical issues. In: *Deaf Children: Developmental Perspectives*, ed. L. Liben. New York: Academic Press, pp. 137–156.

Heider, F. & Heider, G. M. (1941). Studies in psychology of the deaf. *Psychol. Monogr.*, 53(No. 242).

Levine, E. S. (1956). *Youth in a Soundless World, a Search for Personality.* New York: New York University Press.

Maccoby, E. E. & Feldman, S. S. (1972). Mother-attachment and stranger-reactions in the third year of life. *Monogr. Soc. Res. Child Developm.*, 37 (3, Serial No. 148).

Marvin, R. S. (1972). Attachment-, exploratory- and communicative behavior in 2-, 3-, and 4-year-old children. Unpublished doctoral dissertation, University of Chicago.

—— (1977). An ethological-cognitive model of the attenuation of mother-child attachment. In: *Advances in the Study of Communication; Vol. 3. Development of Social Attachments*, ed. T. M. Alloway & L. Krames, New York: Plenum Press.

Meadow, K. P. (1967). The effect of early manual communication and family climate on the deaf child's development. Unpublished Ph.D. dissertation, University of California, Berkeley.

—— (1968a). Early manual communication in relation to the deaf child's intellectual, social, and communicative functioning. *Amer. Ann. Deaf*, 113:29–41.

—— (1968b). Parental responses to the medical ambiguities of deafness. *J. Hlth. Soc. Behav.*, 9:299–309.

—— (1969). Self-image, family climate, and deafness. *Soc. Forces*, 47:428–438.

—— (1980). *Deafness and Child Development.* Berkeley, Calif.: University of California Press.

—— Greenberg, M. T., Erting, C. & Carmichael, H. (1981). Interactions of deaf mothers and deaf preschool children; comparisons with three other groups of deaf and hearing dyads. *Amer. Ann. Deaf*, 126:454–468.

Mindel, E. D. & Vernon, M. (1971). *They Grow in Silence—The Deaf Child and Family.* Silver Spring, Md.: National Association of the Deaf.

Moores, D. F. (1978). *Educating the Deaf.* Boston: Houghton Mifflin.

Rainer, J. D., Altshuler, K. Z. & Kallmann, F. J. (1969). *Family and Mental Health Problems in a Deaf Population*, ed. 2. Springfield, Ill.: Charles C Thomas.

Rawlings, B. W. & Jensema, C. J. (1977). *Two Studies of the Families of Hearing Impaired Children*. Washington, D.C.: Office of Demographic Studies, Gallaudet College.

Schein, J. D. (1979). Society and culture of hearing-impaired people. In: *Hearing and Hearing Impairment*, ed. L. J. Bradford & W. G. Hardy. New York: Grune & Stratton, pp. 479–487.

Schlesinger, H. S. (1978). The acquisition of bimodal language. In: *Sign Language for the Deaf*, ed. I. M. Schlesinger & L. Namir. New York: Academic Press.

—— (1979a). The deaf child. In: *Basic Handbook of Child Psychiatry, Vol. 1*, ed. J. D. Call, J. D. Noshpitz, R. L. Cohen & I. N. Berlin. New York: Basic Books, pp. 421–426.

—— (1979b). From object to subject. *J. Rehabil. Deaf*, 12:viii-xii.

—— & Meadow, K. P. (1972). *Sound and Sign: Childhood Deafness and Mental Health*. Berkeley, Calif.: University of California Press.

Spradley, T. S. & Spradley, J. P. (1978). *Deaf Like Me*. New York: Random House.

Stokoe, W. C. & Battison, R. (1981). Sign language, mental health, and satisfactory interaction. In: *Deafness and Mental Health*, ed. L. K. Stein, E. D. Mindel & T. Jabaley. New York: Grune & Stratton, pp. 179–194.

Stuckless, E. R. & Birch, J. W. (1966). The influence of early manual communication on the linguistic development of deaf children. *Amer. Ann. Deaf*, 111:452–460; 499–504.

Vernon, M. & Koh, S. D. (1970). Early manual communication and deaf children's achievement. *Amer. Ann. Deaf*, 115:527–536.

Waters, E. (1978). The reliability and stability of individual differences in infant-mother attachment. *Child Developm.*, 49:483–494.

Weinraub, M. & Lewis, M. (1977). The determinants of children's responses to separation. *Monogr. Soc. Res. Child Developm.*, 42 (4, Serial No. 172).

Winefield, R. M. (1981). Bell, Gallaudet, and the sign language debate; a historical analysis of the communication controversy in education of the deaf. Unpublished doctoral dissertation, Graduate School of Education, Harvard University.

Part IV

TEMPERAMENT STUDIES

The significance of temperamental individuality as an influential variable in a wide variety of situations of both normal and deviant psychological development continues to be emphasized in the research literature. The practical as well as the theoretical implications of the new data that have emerged from the most recent studies are evident in the papers of this year's section on temperament studies.

Previous studies from our own research unit as well as from other centers have provided evidence that as a group temperamentally easy children differ significantly in their developmental course from temperamentally difficult children. Wachs and Gandour explore the early beginnings of such differences and their developmental implications in a study of 100 six-month-old infants. They find specific differences in the reactions of the temperamentally easy infants to environmental parameters from the difficult babies. The authors emphasize that the differences found appear to be a genuine case of individual differences mediating the response to the environment rather than differences in the environment mediating development. They offer several alternative explanations for their findings and suggest the value of studying the question of what other individual difference parameters, besides sex or temperament, may also mediate the impact of the early environment, and indicate the implications of such studies for elucidating the specific dynamics of genetic-early environmental interactional patterns.

The paper by Wilson and Matheny, from the Louisville Twin Study Center, takes up a number of questions of theoretical and methodological interest. Extensive data were gathered through structured laboratory assessment and parental reports, using the Toddler Temperament Scale. Three principal dimensions were revealed by factor analysis. Of special interest, in view of some of the questions raised in the field as to the validity of parental reports, is the finding of convergent reliability between the staff laboratory ratings and the parental reports. This may well reflect the care taken in this study to structure the laboratory pro-

189

cedures into a set of prescribed activities. These were designed to present each infant with specific opportunities for interaction with the caretakers and engagement in play, as a means of detecting the infant's predominant behavioral style. This provided observational ratings based on a wide range of situations and stimuli. These more closely approximated the range of behaviors in the home setting which provided the basis for the parents' reports than have other observational strategies.

The concept of temperament is relatively complex, and its measurement presents a number of problems, as it is based on the evaluation of the child's typical behavioral response to a wide range of stimuli and situations. Inevitably, there is the temptation to short-circuit some of these methodological issues to reformulate theoretical concepts so as to simplify research strategies. William Carey, a leading worker in the field of temperament studies, identifies some of the outstanding pitfalls in infant temperament research and suggests how they might be remedied. He takes up the issues of definition, origins of temperament differences, temperament stability, measurement, and clinical applications. His comments and suggestions offer useful guides to future research efforts to deal with the challenging issues he raises.

In our own temperament studies we have, from the beginning, emphasized that the functional significance of temperament does not lie in the temperamental characteristics themselves, but in their active role in helping to shape the nature of the organism-environment interaction. In analyzing the dynamics of this interactional process we have found the "goodness of fit" concept to be most useful in categorizing those relationships between the child's characteristics and capacities and the demands of the environment which promote healthy development (goodness of fit) versus those relationships which are suboptimal or even pathogenic (poorness of fit). Lerner reports an ingenious study in which this goodness of fit model is tested in the adaptation of a group of adolescents to school in both social and academic contexts, with positive findings, and suggests possibilities for further tests of this model.

12

Temperament, Environment, and Six-Month Cognitive-Intellectual Development: A Test of the Organismic Specificity Hypothesis

Theodore D. Wachs and Mary Jane Gandour

Purdue University, USA

The major question asked in the present study was whether temperamental differences mediated the infants' response to the early environment (organismic specificity). A corollary question involved the nature of the relationship between temperament and cognitive-intellectual development. Subjects were 100 six-month-old infants who were observed in their homes three times over a three-week period. Home observations were coded into social and physical environmental parameters. During this time period infant temperament and level of sensorimotor development were independently assessed. Canonical and univariate analyses revealed the following relationships: (1) Infants classified as temperamentally "easy" were more sensitive to environmental parameters than temperamentally "difficult" babies; when environmental influences were relevant for "difficult" infants, they tended to have a negative impact upon development. (2) Tempera-

Reprinted with permission from the *International Journal of Behavioral Development*, 1983, Vol. 6, 135–152. Copyright 1983 by North-Holland.

The authors wish to acknowledge the help of Jane Doherty, Grete Wachob, Mark Reinecke and Marlene Baldizon for their aid in observation of babies, and Grete Wachob, Deanne Defibaugh and Jolanda Torres in assisting us in the preparation of data for analysis. Special thanks goes to Nancy Hubert for her work in testing infants on the IPDS. Our appreciation to all those parents who let us do observation and testing with their infants goes without saying.

mental characteristics associated with difficultness were also associated with an inability to coordinate specific sensorimotor schemes. Implications of the above for our understanding of early environmental action were discussed.

Historically early experience has been viewed as a global phenomenon in terms of its impact upon the individual (Hunt, 1977; Wachs and Gruen, 1982). That is, "positive" early experiences have been viewed as uniformly facilitating development for all individuals, whereas "negative" early experiences have been viewed as having uniformly depressing effects upon development. In reviewing the available evidence on early cognitive-intellectual development, we (Haywood and Wachs, 1981; Wachs and Gruen, 1982) have suggested that the data more closely support an "organismic specificity" hypothesis than they do a global model of early environmental action. The organismic specificity hypothesis predicts differential reactivity by different individuals to similar early environmental stimulation, thereby making individual differences a central consideration in early experience research.

Most of the available evidence on individual differences in reactivity to the early environment has dealt with sex differences (Honzik, 1967; Moore, 1968; Miller and Dyer, 1975). A major problem with the above findings is that it is unclear whether the results are due to genuine differential reactivity of males and females to similar environmental circumstances, or to different environments being provided for each of the sexes. The only published data which consider this potential confounding of individual and environmental characteristics are two studies by Wachs (1978, 1979) and one by Pedersen (Pedersen et al., 1979). These data suggest that sex differences in reactivity to the environment are a function of differential reactivity to similar environments, rather than different environments being provided to male and female babies.

The present study was designed as a further test of the organismic specificity hypothesis. Based on recent theorizing from the New York Longitudinal Study (Thomas et al. 1963, 1968; Thomas and Chess, 1977), we chose to investigate infant temperament as an individual difference likely to be associated with differential reactivity to the early environment. We asked the following *major question*: Are there differences in patterns of reactivity to the early environment between babies who are classified as temperamentally easy (i.e., positive in mood, low in intensity, adaptable) versus those who are classified as difficult?

In addition to this major question, we also addressed a *corollary* question: What is the nature of the relationship between temperament and cognitive-intellectual development per se? Both Sostek and Anders (1977) and Field (Field et al., 1978) have reported significant relationships between measures of infant temperament and later Bayley performance. These reports are limited in their generalizability, however, due to small sample sizes (Sostek and Anders, 1977) and the use of high-risk populations (Field et al., 1978). The present paper looked at possible relationships between temperament and cognitive-intellectual development using a large sample of normal babies.

METHOD

Subjects

Subjects were 100 normal six-month-old infants (50 males, 50 females); the overwhelming majority (93) were Caucasian. Parental SES level ranged from lower class through upper middle class. Infant names were obtained through use of birth listings in the local daily newspaper. Acceptance rate among those contacted was 62%, with no dropouts among parents who agreed to let their infants be in the study.

Instruments

Four measurement instruments were used. Cognitive-intellectual development was measured on the Infant Psychological Development Scale (IPDS; Uzgiris and Hunt, 1975). the IPDS is a Piaget-based measure of sensorimotor intelligence which assesses development in eight specific areas including object permanence, development of schemes and development of an understanding of causality. Each of the eight subscales consists of a series of separate ordinal steps which delineate the stages of development within a subscale. Available evidence indicates significant reliability, ordinality, and predictive and construct validity for the IPDS (Uzgiris, 1976).

The infant's physical environment was measured using Sections 1–3 of the Purdue Home Stimulation Inventory (PHSI; Wachs et al., 1979). The PHSI provides a description of the infant's physical environment through interview and direct observation of the home environment. The inventory consists of 33 items measuring the infant's daily schedule, physical stimuli characteristics of the home, and physical stimuli at the child's disposal. Previous data indicate a median interobserver agreement on PHSI items of 0.85, with a median retest reliability over twelve months of 0.69 (Wachs, 1979). Previous research has also yielded relationships between specific PHSI items and early cognitive development (Wachs, 1978, 1979). Factor analytic data on the PHSI (Wachs et al., 1979) indicate that the 33 PHSI items reduce down to 12 factors, nine of which clearly seem to be tapping physical dimensions of the infant's environment.

The infant's social environment was measured through direct observation, utilizing an adaptation of the Yarrow et al. (1975) "Manual for Observation of the Home Environment and Mother-Infant Interaction" (referred to here as the Yarrow scale). The Yarrow scale includes 16 observational categories which focus on social stimulation of the infant and parental mediation of inanimate objects for the infant. Data from these observational categories are used to compute 11 summary scores which describe the infant's social environment. In previous research (Yarrow et al., 1975), interobserver reliability for observational categories ranged from 0.85 to 0.99; specific summary scores have been related to various aspects of cognitive development (Yarrow et al., 1975).

Infant temperament was measured utilizing the Revised Infant Temperament Questionnaire (RITQ; Carey and McDevitt, 1978a). The RITQ consists of ninety-five statements describing behaviors of young infants which the parents rate on a 6-point scale from "almost never" to "almost always." Available evidence on the RITQ indicates median retest reliability of 0.75 with a range from 0.66 to 0.81 (Carey and McDevitt, 1978a). A weighted averaging procedure is employed to obtain scores on each of the nine New York Longitudinal Study temperament categories. Six of the nine category scores (rhythmicity, approach, activity, adaptability, intensity and mood) are used to divide infants into temperamental clusters (easy, intermediate low, slow-to-warm-up, intermediate high, difficult) (Carey and McDevitt, 1978a). All clusters were derived using a computer scoring program for the RITQ developed by Gandour and Gandour (1980).

Although other instruments were available for assessing temperament at six months (see Hubert et al., 1982, for a review), we chose the Revised Infant Temperament Questionnaire (RITQ) for several reasons. First, practical considerations required that we use a parent questionnaire to obtain our temperament data, rather than interview (e.g., Thomas and Chess, 1977) or physiological measures (e.g., Rothbart and Derryberry, 1981). Second, our interest in the NYLS conceptualization of temperament required that we use an instrument which reflected this theoretical framework. The Carey questionnaires are considered "the instruments of choice for parental ratings of the NYLS dimensions" (Plomin, 1982a) because of their adequate psychometric properties, relatively diverse item pools, appeal to parents, and wide usage. Third, our hypothesis of organismic specificity required that we measure temperament as an organismic characteristic of the infant to the fullest extent possible. Although there is current debate about the validity of temperament questionnaires as measures of the infant's organismic characteristics (Bates, 1980, in press; Thomas et al., 1982; Sameroff et al., 1982; Kagan, 1982; Rothbart, 1982), there seems to be little question that parent reports do, to some extent, represent "real" characteristics of the infant as indicated by replicated correlations among mother, father, and/or observer reports (Dunn and Kendrick, 1981; Kagan, 1982; Olson et al., in press; Rothbart, 1980; Billman and McDevitt, 1980; Field and Greenberg, 1982; Lyon and Plomin, 1981; Bates et al., 1979). The emphasis of the RITQ on ratings of very specific infant behaviors rather than global perceptions or general information would also seem to reduce the possibility of parental bias (Carey and McDevitt, 1978a; McDevitt and Carey, 1981).

For the purpose of the present study, "easy" babies were those in the easy and intermediate low diagnostic clusters; "difficult" babies were those falling into the difficult, intermediate high and slow-to-warm-up clusters. The rationale for these groupings is rooted in past temperament research. By definition, intermediate high and difficult infants cluster together as do intermediate low and easy (Carey, 1970; Carey and McDevitt, 1978a). Historically slow-to-warm-up babies have been treated as a distinct group. However, recent evidence (Carey and McDevitt, 1978b; Berry and Weizmann, 1978) indicates that they more closely resemble difficult infants than they do easy babies. Thus, an argument can be made for including slow-to-warm-up infants in our "difficult" grouping. For the present study we analyzed our results for the "difficult" grouping both with and without the slow-to-warm-up infants included. When exclusion of the slow-to-warm-up babies did make a difference in our results, we used only the difficult and intermediate high babies.

Given the current controversy surrounding the term "difficult" infant (Bates, 1980, in press; Thomas et al., 1982; Kagan, 1982; Rothbart, 1982; Plomin, 1982a, 1982b), it is important to note that the terms "easy" and "difficult" are hereafter used to refer to the *groupings* described above, rather than the pure diagnostic clusters. It is also important to point out that infants classified as difficult based upon RITQ results, may not necessarily be seen as difficult by their parents.

Procedure

Data collection consisted of four home visits, within a three week period, starting when the infant reached six months of age. During visit 1 the mother signed the informed consent form and filled out the RITQ. In addition, the observer completed Sections 1 and 2 of the PHSI based on interview and direct observation. Visit 1 also served to familiarize mother and infant with the procedure of being observed.

Visits 2 and 3 involved 90 minutes of observation each, using the Yarrow scale. During this procedure the observer watched for 30 seconds and recorded for 60 seconds. Timing signals were provided by an auditory signal played through a prerecorded cassette tape audible only to the observer. In addition, during the last 45 minutes of visits 2 and 3 the observer also completed the Section 3 PHSI ratings. Visit 4 consisted of administration of the IPDS.

All observers were graduate students or upper-level undergraduate students at Purdue University. Prior to actual field observation, each observer had obtained at least a 0.90 level of interobserver reliability on both the PHSI and Yarrow scales over several practice observations. Periodic reliability checks during the course of the study indicated that this level of interobserver reliability was being maintained. The observer for visit 1 was not the one doing visit 2 and 3, though for any given infant the same observer completed visits 2 and 3. IPDS testers were the first author or an advanced graduate student, neither of whom had seen the babies before and who were thus blind to the infants' scores on the temperament and environmental measures. Prior to actual testing, both testers had obtained essentially perfect interscorer reliability on IPDS administration and scoring.

STATISTICAL ANALYSIS

The major focus of our data analyses was to determine the relationships between our predictor measures of temperament, physical environment, and social environment, and our criterion variable, cognitive-intellectual development, both for the total group and the easy and difficult temperament groups. More specifically our predictor variables were the infant's temperament (the nine category scores from the RITQ for the total group or the grouping of easy or difficult), the infant's social environment (11 summary scores from the Yarrow scale), and the infant's physical environment (33 items from the PHSI). In all cases the criterion variable was the level of the infant's performance on each of the eight IPDS subscales. The major analytic procedure was canonical correlation between each set of predictors and the criterion (Harris, 1975). For each significant canonical root, items with weights of ±0.40 or greater were retained for data interpretation [1].

In addition to this multivariate approach, univariate correlations were also run between predictor and criterion variables. The purpose of this analysis was to assess the support or lack of support for our multivariate findings using an alternative approach to data analysis. A basic problem with univariate correlations involving a large number of variables is the generation of large-scale correlation matrices, and the possibility of chance significant correlations. In order to minimize consideration of such random correlations, all univariate matrices were subjected to cutting-score analysis (Wachs et al., 1971; Wachs, 1979). Basically, the cutting-score procedure is a logical approach to identifying those environmental predictors that are most consistently related to development, in terms of their frequency and consistency of direction (see Wachs, 1979, for a more detailed description of this procedure).

The last step in univariate analysis was to compare univariate correlations meeting cutting-score criteria with their comparable opposite matrix correlations, by means of z transformation technique. The purpose of this analysis was to determine if correlations from the temperament groups were actually significantly different from each other. Finally, we computed the Hotelling T^2 (Harris, 1975) statistic to determine whether subjects differed from each other on environment and development variables.

RESULTS

Total Sample

For the total sample of 100 infants, 3 canonical correlations were computed relating temperament, physical environment and social en-

---

[1] Given the small number of slow-to-warm-up babies in our sample ($N = 10$) it was impossible to compute multivariate correlations for this group. Univariate correlations were computed. Given the small sample on which these correlations are based they will be briefly summarized in the results section rather than reported in detail. A complete description of the univariate results for the slow-to-warm-up babies is available from the first author.

vironment to IPDS level [2]. Results for the total sample indicated that there was a significant canonical correlation only between temperament category scores and IPDS performance ($R = 0.57, X^2 = 99.75, p < 0.05$). The canonical weights indicate that a combination of high infant activity (0.40), withdrawal (0.43) and intensity (0.65) predicted an advanced level of gestural imitation (0.74) but a lower level of uses of objects as means (−0.46).

In addition to these canonical correlations, univariate correlations were also computed for the total sample, relating temperament categories to IPDS level. After cutting-score procedures, four temperament categories were found to have consistent significant correlations with IPDS performance. These items are shown in Table 1. These data suggest that both high intensity and high activity are positively related to schemes and gestural imitation. Intensity, rhythmicity, and withdrawal, however, are all negatively related to object permanence.

Easy Versus Difficult Infants

For both the social and physical environment canonical analyses, exclusion of the slow-to-warm-up infants from the difficult grouping made no difference in the results. Thus, these analyses were conducted with

Table 1
RITQ categories meeting cutting score criteria for predicting IPDS subscale scores for the total sample. Correlations between temperament and cognitive-intellectual development at 6 months.

Item	r (RITQ: IPDS)	
Intensity	Object permanence	−0.17 [a]
	Schemes	0.26 [b]
	Gestural imitation	0.38 [b]
Activity	Schemes	0.29 [b]
	Gestural imitation	0.38 [b]
Rhythm	Object permanence	−0.23 [b]
	Schemes	−0.19 [a]
Approach/withdrawal	Object permanence	−0.17 [a]
	Means	−0.19 [a]

[a] $p < 0.05$
[b] $p < 0.01$

[2] The same analyses were also run for male and female infants. Results for males mirrored the results for the total sample. Results for females were generally non-significant. Readers wishing the results for males and females can obtain these data by writing to the first author.

the slow-to-warm-up infants included as part of the difficult grouping ($N = 46$). For the univariate cutting-score analysis, exclusion of the slow-to-warm-up infants did lead to some differences in results; therefore, for this latter analysis the difficult grouping was based on only the difficult and intermediate high babies ($N = 36$).

For the babies falling in the easy grouping ($N = 54$) canonical analyses revealed significant canonical correlations between IPDS performance and both Yarrow scale scores ($R = 0.80$, $X^2 = 111.89$, $p < 0.05$) and PHSI scores ($R = 0.94$, $X^2 = 286.28$, $p < 0.05$). Items having weights of ± 0.40 or greater for each of the significant canonical roots are shown in Table 2.

Results shown in Table 2 indicate that a social environment characterized as low in auditory stimulation (contingent vocalization), but high in kinesthetic and emotional (broad smile) stimulation, predicts a cognitive-intellectual pattern characterized by advanced levels of object permanence but lower levels of foresight and schemes in relation to objects. Results shown in Table 2 also describe a physical setting where the child

Table 2

Temperament, environment and 6-month cognitive development for easy babies: significant canonical correlation and retained weights.

	Weights
I. Yarrow Scale and IPDS ($R = 0.80$, $X^2 = 118.89$, $p < 0.05$)	
Set I	
Auditory stimulation	-0.53
Contingent responding–vocalization	-0.49
Kinesthetic stimulation	0.44
Broad smile	0.40
Set II	
Object permanence	0.40
Foresight	-0.60
Schemes	-0.43
II. PHSI and IPDS ($R = 0.94$, $X^2 = 286.28$, $p < 0.05$)	
Set I	
Child has exclusive toys	0.52
Access to papers/magazines	0.40
Access to household objects	0.46
Mobile over crib	-0.46
Child's room decorated	0.44
Floor freedom	0.56
Set II	
Schemes	0.73
Vocal imitation	0.67
Gestural imitation	-0.76

has exploratory freedom (floor freedom) in a stimulus rich environment (exclusive toys, access, room decorations). This type of physical environment is related to a cognitive pattern characterized by advanced levels of vocal imitation and schemes for relating to objects but low levels of gestural imitation.

In sharp contrast to the above, for the difficult grouping neither the IPDS-Yarrow or the IPDS-PHSI canonical correlations reached an acceptable level of statistical significance.

The above pattern of results suggest a greater sensitivity to the social and physical environment by infants who tend to be characterized as temperamentally easy. However, given the non-significant results for more difficult babies, these data do not address the question of whether infants characterized as temperamentally difficult react to the same environmental factors as infants characterized as temperamentally easy. To test this question our univariate cutting-score analysis seemed most appropriate. Significant differences in environment-development relationships for the two groups would suggest the possibility of differential reactivity, as well as the differential sensitivity suggested by our canonical analysis. For the easy grouping 6 Yarrow scale and 10 PHSI items met our cutting-score criterion of 2 or more significant correlations with the IPDS. For the difficult grouping 6 Yarrow scale and 4 PHSI items met this criterion.

Those items meeting the cutting-score criterion for each group were compared to their corresponding correlations by means of z test analysis. The results of the z test analysis are shown in Table 3. Our results indicated significant differences in environment-development relationships between easy and difficult groups on four of the Yarrow scales (reactivity to contingent vocalization, personal-social play, reinforcement and visual stimulation) and on 8 PHSI items (in-neighborhood visits, stimulus training, number of children's books, physical restrictions on exploration, number of persons and number of strangers visiting home, regularity of naptime, and number of stimulus sources in the home). The most consistent differences were seen for *contingent responses to vocalizations*, with the relationships being positive for easy infants and negative for difficult infants, *number of strangers in the home*, with the relationships being positive for difficult infants and negative for easy infants, and *number of stimulus sources*, with the relationship being negative for difficult infants and zero order for the easy group [3].

---

[3] For slow-to-warm-up babies little differential reactivity to the social environment was shown. With regard to the physical environment they appeared to be more influenced by the presence of objects and the presence of familiar persons and situations than either the easy or difficult groups. -

Table 3
"Difficult" and "easy" univariate correlations that met cutting score criteria and were also significantly different from the corresponding correlations for opposite temperament babies.

	r Easy	r Difficult	z
Yarrow – IPDS			
Contingent response to vocalization –			
Foresight	0.27	−0.29 [a]	2.88 [b]
Causality	0.31 [b]	−0.11	2.15 [a]
Means	0.19	−0.28 [a]	2.40 [a]
Personal-social play –			
Foresight	0.38 [b]	−0.02	2.10 [a]
Schemes	−0.04	0.35 [a]	2.02 [a]
Social mediation with reinforcement – Foresight	0.24 [a]	−0.20	2.24 [a]
Visual stimulation – Verbal imitation	−0.15	0.35 [a]	2.58 [b]
PHSI – IPDS			
In neighborhood visits – Causality	0.44 [b]	0.05	2.11 [a]
Skill training – Foresight	0.46 [b]	−0.52 [b]	5.36 [b]
Number childrens books – Schemes	0.34 [b]	−0.06	2.07 [a]
Physical restrictions on exploration – Means	−0.28 [a]	0.12	2.04 [a]
Number people visiting home – Verbal imitation	−0.25 [a]	0.25	2.55 [a]
Number strangers visiting home –			
Causality	0.01	0.44 [b]	2.31 [a]
Verbal imitation	−0.38 [b]	0.30 [a]	3.55 [b]
Regularity of Naptime – Gestural imitation	−0.15	0.35 [a]	2.58 [b]
Number of stimulus sources in home –			
Causality	0.12	−0.29 [a]	2.10 [a]
Verbal imitation	0.18	−0.42 [b]	3.15 [b]

[a] $p < 0.05$
[b] $p < 0.01$

Alternative Explanations

Given the above data indicating different environment-development patterns for easy versus difficult groupings of babies, alternative explanations for these findings had to be considered prior to claiming evidence for organismic specificity. One suggested explanation (Clarke-Stewart et al., 1979), which has been offered for early experience research in general, is the possibility that highly specific relationships between environment and development are simply random. To test this possibility all subjects were randomly assigned to one of two groups. For each of these random split groups we then reran our canonical analysis between environment and development. If the Clarke-Stewart et al. explanation is correct, for our data we would expect to find a significant canonical correlation between IPDS scores and the Yarrow and/or PHSI scales for one random subgroup but not the other, which would thus resemble our present results using an easy-difficult split. Our analysis indicated that none of the environment development canonical correlations reached statistical significance for either random subgroup.

A second alternative explanation is that our results are not due to differential reactivity per se but rather different *concurrent* environments for the easy and difficult groups. To test this possibility, differences between the 6-month physical and social environments of the easy and difficult groupings were compared using the Hotelling T^2 procedure (Harris, 1975). For the social environment the overall T^2 and all post hoc univariate t tests were non-significant. A similar pattern of findings also occurred for the PHSI. The overall T^2 was non-significant while only 2 out of the 33 post hoc PHSI comparisons were statistically significant (difficult babies tend to have more small objects available ($t = 2.14$, $p < 0.05$) and more people visiting in the home ($t = 2.10$, $p < 0.05$)). These results suggest minimal differences, at best, in the 6-month social and physical environments of the easy and difficult groups.

A third possible explanation is that, even though the environments of easy and difficult infants are highly similar, their levels of cognitive-intellectual development are highly discrepant from each other. To test this possibility, differences between the 8 IPDS subscales for the easy and difficult groups were compared using the Hotelling T^2 procedure. The overall T^2 was non-significant. Only the post hoc comparison for object permanence was significant ($t = 2.39$, $p < 0.05$), indicating that the characteristic level of performance for easy infants was a complete visible displacement (the infants could find an object they had seen being completely covered) while for difficult infants, it was only a partial visible displacement (the object could be found only when a portion of it was showing after being covered).

DISCUSSION

Minor Question: Temperament and Development

As described in the introduction, previous research (Sostek and Anders, 1977; Field et al., 1978) has reported a significant relationship between temperament and early development. However, the generalizability of this research is limited by small sample sizes and the use of high risk populations.

The present results from our sample of 100 normal infants indicates that several temperament dimensions associated with the difficult child are related to cognitive development. First, our canonical analysis for the total sample revealed that a temperament component comprised of withdrawal, intensity and high activity predicts a developmental pattern characterized by a negative weighting of means' end behavior and a positive weighting of gestural imitation. Intensity and withdrawal characterize the difficult child by definition (Thomas et al., 1963, 1968; Thomas and Chess, 1977) while high activity has been associated with continued difficulty into early childhood (Carey and McDevitt, 1978b). The cognitive pattern described above suggests an infant who, at 6 months, is reactive to the environment but has not yet reached the stage of differentiated actions (Uzgiris, 1976) wherein specific schemes are intercoordinated.

The inability of the difficult infant to coordinate specific schemes may be mediated by delayed object permanence for this group. Our cutting score results for the total sample indicated a negative relationship with object permanence for three out of five characteristics of the difficult infant (high intensity, arythmicity, and withdrawal). Along the same lines our T^2 analyses of the IPDS for the easy and difficult groupings, while showing no overall difference between the groups, did reveal a significant post hoc univariate relationship indicating that the difficult group was significantly more delayed in object permanence than the easy group. Previous developmental data have emphasized the critical nature of object permanence as a developmental precursor for other sensorimotor abilities (Uzgiris, 1973; Wachs, 1975). The delay in the development of object permanence for infants categorized as difficult may thus underlie the previously reported relationship between difficult temperament and cognitive risk status (Field et al., 1978).

Major Question: The Organismic Specificity Hypothesis

The observed pattern of results are contrary to predictions that would be derived from a global model of environmental action, wherein all infants should be equally sensitive to all aspects of the environment. Rather, by illustrating the mediation of the environment by individual differences the results of the present research lend support to the organismic specificity hypothesis. Specifically, present findings indicate a significant canonical relationship between cognitive development and the social and physical environments for those infants categorized as temperamentally easy but not for those categorized as temperamentally difficult. These data suggest a greater reactivity to the environment by easier babies. It is important to note here that those specific environmental parameters to which easy infants appear more reactive (i.e., kinesthetic stimulation, exploratory freedom) are those which have been demonstrated in previous research (Wachs and Gruen, 1982) to be particularly salient for intellectual development in the first 12 months of life.

Our univariate analysis also indicates that when difficult babies do react to the environment they tend to react to different environmental parameters than do easy babies. For those infants categorized as easy in temperament the impact of social interactions upon development is a positive one. In contrast, particularly for proximal environmental parameters involving social contingencies, the impact of the social environment appears to be negative for more difficult infants. Difficult infants do not appear to react negatively to the presence of people per se but rather to interactions from people. Also of theoretical interest is evidence suggesting that difficult infants may be more sensitive to negative physical characteristics in the environment such as noise-confusion. This pattern is congruent with previous research which also illustrates the role of individual differences (sex of infant) in mediating the impact of noise-confusion upon development (Wachs, 1979).

It must be further emphasized that the differences between our easy and difficult groups appear to be a genuine case of individual differences mediating the response to the environment (i.e., organismic specificity) rather than differences in the environment mediating development. Both our T^2 procedure and the post hoc t tests yield little evidence for easy and difficult babies living in significantly different social or physical environments at 6 months. This is not an isolated finding. A similar lack of relationship between infant temperament and mother-infant interaction at 6 months has also been reported in two other studies, using different measures of temperament (Vaughan et al., 1981; Bates et al., 1982). These findings seem to challenge, at least at six months, the prediction from transactional models (e.g., Sameroff and Chandler, 1976) that infants of differing temperaments elicit different types of maternal responses, which in turn would lead to differences in the infants' environments.

Although the present results support the possibility of differential reactivity to the environment by easy versus difficult babies, what is not clear is why this differential reactivity should be occurring. Two possible explanations exist, each having to do with the nature of difficult infants. Interestingly, the pattern described for our difficult group of babies (less sensitive to positive social stimulation; more sensitive to negative physical experience) bears a striking resemblance to the arousal model recently proposed by Field (1981). Specifically, Field hypothesizes that certain high-risk infants have a higher threshold for attentive/orienting responses and a lower threshold for aversive/defensive reactions (i.e., a narrower arousal range). Our difficult group of babies seemed to have this same narrow range in terms of being less sensitive to social interactions (attention) and more sensitive to physical environment overstimulation (aversion).

A second, alternative explanation [4], is that difficult infants are so tuned in to their own internal discomforts (caused perhaps by their high intensity responses to new situations and people—Thomas and Chess, 1976, or their heightened sensitivity to negative aspects of the physical environment—our own data) that they simply tune out social interactions as such. Thus, social interactions may not form an "effective environment" (Thomas and Chess, 1976) for difficult infants. Clearly, further research needs to be done to compare the validity of these alternative hypotheses.

Given the available evidence for the potential validity of the organismic specificity hypothesis, the next logical step would seem to be the question of what other individual difference parameters, besides sex or temperament, may also mediate the impact of the early environment. A taxonomy describing those individual difference parameters which mediate the effects of the early environment may provide hypotheses about the nature and rationale of differential reactivity. Further, the study of individual differences in reaction to the environment offers the possibility of an interface between those interested in nurture (i.e., early-experience researchers) and those interested in nature (i.e., genetically oriented researchers). Although it is now obvious that development is a function of both nature and nurture, there is still little interface between the disciplines in terms of describing how this interaction occurs. Focusing on individual differences as mediators of environmental influence may offer one approach to this question.

REFERENCES

Bates, J. E. (1980). The concept of difficult temperament. *Merrill-Palmer Quarterly,* 26: 299–319.
Bates, J.E. (in press). Issues in the definition and assessment of difficult temperament. *Merrill-Palmer Quarterly.*

[4] The authors are indebted to both Gerald Gratch and Ina Uzgiris who, independently, came up with the same hypothesis on the second rationale for differential reactivity.

Bates, J.E., Freeland, C.B. and Lounsbury, M.L. (1979). Measurement of infant difficultness. *Child Development,* 50: 794–803.

Bates, J.E., Olson, S.L., Pettit, G.S. and Bayles, K. (1982). Dimensions of individuality in the mother-infant relationship at six months of age. *Child Development,* 53: 446–461.

Berry, D. and Weizmann, F. (1978). Temperament and patterns of attachment. Unpublished manuscript. York University.

Billman, J. and McDevitt, S.C. (1980). Convergence of parent and observer ratings with observations of peer interaction in nursery school. *Child Development,* 51: 395–400.

Carey, W.B. (1970). A simplified method for measuring infant temperament. *Journal of Pediatrics,* 77: 188–194.

Carey, W.B. and McDevitt, S.C. (1978a). Revision of the Infant Temperament Questionnaire. *Pediatrics,* 61: 735–739.

Carey, W.B. and McDevitt, S.C. (1978b). Stability and change in individual temperament diagnoses from infancy to early childhood. *American Academy of Child Psychiatry,* 17: 331–337.

Clarke-Stewart, K.A., Vanderstoep, L. and Killian, G. (1979). Analysis and replication of mother-infant relations of 1 year of age. *Child Development,* 50: 777–793.

Dunn, J. and Kendrick, C. (1981). Interaction between young siblings: Association with the interaction between mother and firstborn. *Developmental Psychology,* 17: 336–343.

Field, T. (1981). Infant arousal, attention and affect during early interaction. In: L. Lipsitt (Ed.), *Advances in infant behavior and development.* Norwood, NJ: Ablex.

Field, T. and Greenberg, R. (1982). Temperament ratings by parents and teachers of infants, toddlers, and preschool children. *Child Development,* 53: 160–163.

Field, T., Hallock, N., Ting, G., Dempsey, J., Dabira, C. and Shuman, H. (1978). A first year followup of high risk infants: Formulating a cumulative risk index. *Child Development,* 49: 119–131.

Gandour, J. and Gandour, M.J. (1980). A computer program for scoring the Infant Temperament Questionnaire (revised). *JSAS: Catalogue of Selected Documents in Psychology,* 10, 62 (Ms. No. 2073).

Harris, R. (1975). *A primer of multivariate statistics.* New York: Academic Press.

Haywood, H.C. and Wachs, T.D. (1981). Intelligence, cognition and individual differences. In: M. Begab, H.C. Haywood, and H. Garber, (Eds.), *Psychosocial influences in retarded performances.* Baltimore, MD: University Park Press.

Honzik, M. (1967). Prediction of differential abilities at age 18 from the early family environment. *APA Proceedings,* 2: 151–152.

Hubert, N.C., Wachs, T.D., Peters-Martin, P. and Gandour, M.J. (1982). The study of early temperament: Methodological and conceptual issues. *Child Development,* 53: 571–600.

Hunt, J. McV. (1977). Specificity in early development and experience. O'Neal invited lecture. Meyer Childrens Rehabilitation Institute, University of Nebraska Medical Center, Omaha, NE.

Kagan, J. (1982). The construct of difficult temperament: A reply to Thomas, Chess & Korn. *Merrill-Palmer Quarterly,* 28: 21–24.

Lyon, M. and Plomin, R. (1981). The measurement of temperament using parent ratings. *Journal of Child Psychology and Psychiatry,* 22: 47–54.

McDebitt, S.C. and Carey, W.B. (1981). Stability of ratings vs. perceptions of temperament from early infancy to 1–3 years. *American Journal of Orthopsychiatry,* 51: 342–345.

Miller, L. and Dyer, J. (1975). Four preschool programs: Their dimensions and effects. *Monographs of the Society for Research in Child Development,* 40.

Moore, T. (1968). Language and intelligence: A longitudinal study of the first eight years. *Human Development*, 11: 1–24.

Olson, S.L., Bates, J.E. and Bayles, K. (in press). Maternal perceptions of infant and toddler behavior: A longitudinal, construct validation study. *Infant Behavior and Development*.

Pedersen, F., Rubenstein, J. and Yarrow, L. (1979). Infant development in Father Absent Families. *Journal of Genetic Psychology*, 135: 51–61.

Plomin, R. (1982a). Childhood temperament. In: B. Lakey and A. Kazdin (Eds.), *Advances in clinical child psychology*. New York: Plenum.

Plomin, R. (1982b). The difficult concept of temperament: A response to Thomas, Chess & Korn. *Merrill-Palmer Quarterly*, 28: 25–33.

Rothbart, M.K. (1980). Longitudinal home observation of infant temperament. Paper presented at the International Conference on Infant Studies, New Haven, April.

Rothbart, M.K. (1982). The concept of difficult temperament: A critical analysis of Thomas, Chess & Korn. *Merrill-Palmer Quarterly*, 28: 35–40.

Rothbart, M.K. and Derryberry, D. (1981). Development of individual differences in temperament. In: M.L. Lamb and A.L. Brown (Eds.), *Advances in developmental psychology*, Vol. 1. Hillsdale, NJ: Erlbaum.

Samcroff, A. and Chandlcr, M. (1976). Reproductive risk and the continuum of caretaking casualty. In: F. Horowitz (Ed.), *Review of child development research, IV*. Chicago, IL: University of Chicago Press.

Sameroff, A.J., Seifer, R. and Elias, P.K. (1982). Sociocultural variability in infant temperament ratings. *Child Development*, 53: 164–173.

Sostek, A.M. and Anders, T.F. (1977). Relationships among the Brazelton Neonatal Scale and the Bayley infant scale, and early temperament. *Child Development*, 48: 320–323.

Thomas, A. and Chess, S. (1976). Behavioral individuality in childhood. In: L. Aronson, E. Tobach, D. Lehrman and R. Rosenblatt (Eds.), *Development and evolution of behavior*. San Francisco, CA: Freeman.

Thomas, A. and Chess, S. (1977). *Temperament and development*. New York: Bruner/Mazel.

Thomas, A., Chess, S. and Birch, H. (1968). *Temperament and behavior disorders in children*. New York: New York University Press.

Thomas, A., Chess, S. and Korn, S. (1982). The reality of difficult temperament. *Merrill-Palmer Quarterly*, 28: 1–20.

Thomas, A., Chess, S., Birch, H., Hetzig, M. and Korn, S. (1963). *Behavioral individuality in early childhood*. New York: New York University Press.

Uzgiris, I. (1973). Patterns of cognitive development in infancy. *Merrill-Palmer Quarterly*, 19: 181–204.

Uzgiris, I. (1976). Organization of sensorimotor intelligence. In: M. Lewis, *Origins of intelligence*. New York: Plenum.

Uzgiris, I. and Hunt, J. McV. (1975). *Assessment in infancy*. Urbana, IL: University of Illinois Press.

Vaughn, B., Taraldson, B., Crichton, L. and Egeland, B. (1981). The assessment of infant temperament: A critique of the Carey Infant Temperament Questionnaire. *Infant Behavior and Development*, 4: 1–18.

Wachs, T.D. (1975). Relation of infants performance on Piaget scales between twelve and twenty-four months and their Stanford-Binet performance at thirty-one months. *Child Development*, 46: 929–935.

Wachs, T.D. (1978). The relationship of infants physical environment to their Binet performance at 2½ years. *International Journal of Behavioral Development*, 1: 51–65.

Wachs, T.D. (1979). Proximal experience and early cognitive-intellectual development:

The physical environment. *Merrill-Palmer Quarterly*, 25: 3–42.

Wachs, T.D. and Gruen, G.E. (1982). *Early experience and human development*. New York: Plenum.

Wachs, T.D., Francis, J. and McQuiston, S. (1979). Psychological dimensions of the infants physical environment. *Infant Behavior and Development*, 2: 155–161.

Wachs, T.D., Uzgiris, I. and Hunt, J.McV. (1971). Cognitive development in infants of different age levels and from different environmental backgrounds: An exploratory investigation. *Merrill-Palmer Quarterly*, 17: 283–317.

Yarrow, L., Rubenstein, J. and Pedersen, F. (1975). *Infant and environment*. New York: Wiley.

13

Assessment of Temperament in Infant Twins

Ronald S. Wilson and Adam P. Matheny, Jr.
University of Louisville School of Medicine

A structured laboratory assessment of temperament is described, and the results are presented for 84 infant twins at 12 months of age. Ratings were made of emotional tone, attention span, activity, co-operation, and orientation to staff during a standardized sequence of interactions between the twins and the staff. The twins' behavior was videotaped and then rated for successive 2-minute periods from the videotape, after which the ratings were condensed into a composite temperament profile. A factor analysis revealed three principal dimensions in the ratings, the primary one involving positive emotional tone, sustained attention, and receptiveness to staff. The Toddler Temperament Scale (Fullard, McDevitt, & Carey, Note 1) was also filled out by the parents for each twin, and it revealed a strong first factor anchored on four categories of temperament: adaptability, approach, attention and persistence, and positive mood. A canonical analysis performed on the factor scores from the two data sets showed significant continuity in the expression of temperament between home and lab. The strongest linkage was between the core variables of each set, as represented in the Factor 1 scores. The results demonstrated

Reprinted with permission from *Developmental Psychology*, 1983, Vol. 19, No. 2, 172–183. Copyright 1983 by the American Psychological Association, Inc.

This research was supported in part by Research Grant 90–C–922 from the Office of Child Development, Grant BNS 76–17315 from the National Science Foundation, and a grant from the John D. and Catherine T. MacArthur Foundation. We are indebted to the many co-workers who have contributed so much to this program, including A. Dolan, S. Nuss, M. Hinkle, J. Krantz, M. Riedesel, R. Arbegust, P. Gefert, and K. Adkins.

that the infant's temperament profile could be reliably detected and rated; the results also demonstrated convergent validity between the lab ratings and parents' report.

The Louisville Twin Study has for some years been engaged in longitudinal research with young twins, principally in the areas of mental development and physical growth (e.g., Wilson, 1978, 1979). Beginning in 1976, however, the principal focus of the research program turned to the assessment of temperament in infant twins.

The transition was founded on three major factors: (a) a resurgence of interest in the intrinsic response style of the infant and how it influences the caretaker (Bell, 1974; Escalona, 1968; Lewis & Rosenblum, 1974); (b) an appreciation, in the twin sample, of the central role played by the infants' temperament in shaping the parents' reactions to the twins, especially where differences in temperament were evident; and (c) a detailed and provocative body of research on temperament from the New York Longitudinal Study (Thomas & Chess, 1977; Thomas, Chess, Birch, Hertzig, & Korn, 1963). The focus of the latter program was upon distinctive patterns of reaction found among infants in the early months of life and the extent to which these initial patterns were both persistent and influential in shaping later behavioral development.

In the New York Longitudinal Study, parents were asked to describe precisely how their infants behaved during specific routines of daily living such as sleeping, bathing, feeding, and responding to people. These descriptions, submitted to contrast analyses, were cast into nine categories of temperament that provided the framework for the rating scales and all additional analyses. Thomas et al. (1963) anticipated that the categories were not fully independent, and they (Thomas, Chess, & Birch, 1968) and others (Bates, Freeland, & Lounsbury, 1979; Garside, et. al., 1975; Scholom, Zucker, & Stollak, 1979) have indicated that three or four factors account for most of the individual differences found among the ratings.

In the main, the results from the New York Longitudinal Study have been focused on the extension and elaboration of the categories of temperament, often as applied within a clinical context. A substantial body of clinical research has also emerged that has employed the parent-report questionnaires developed by Carey and his colleagues to assess the nine New York Longitudinal Study categories of temperament (Carey & McDevitt, 1978; McDevitt & Carey, 1978; Fullard, McDevitt & Carey, Note 1).

Unfortunately, the significance of the clinical research has somewhat overshadowed systematic efforts to sharpen the definitions and measures of temperament within the context of normal infant development. In this regard, several discussions of temperament research (Carey, 1981; Rothbart & Derryberry, 1981; Wilson & Matheny, 1980) have recommended the use of multivariate, multimethod approaches for specifying the nature and number of temperament variables, and for providing empirical links between the various sources of data. In addition, heavy emphasis has been placed on directly observable behaviors rated by trained observers, as a crucial adjunct to parental reports.

RELATED BACKGROUND STUDIES AT LOUISVILLE

Research in this area began with interviews of mothers in which they reported whether their twins were concordant or discordant for various aspects of behavior (Wilson, Brown, & Matheny, 1971). Many pairs were discordant for a cluster of behaviors relating to temperament (i.e., temper frequency and intensity, crying, irritability, and demanding attention), and the mothers were often sharply aware of these differences in the first 6 months of life. When one twin displayed these behaviors in greater degree, the cotwin would typically be described as being more tractable, having a longer attention span, and remaining absorbed in an activity longer.

This temperament cluster was particularly evident in the first 2 years, after which it was supplemented by a cluster of behaviors related to sociability and seeking affection. A recent follow-up of data obtained since 1971 replicated the two basic clusters and further demonstrated that individual differences in temperament remained reasonably stable across ages (Matheny, Wilson, Dolan, & Krantz, 1981).

The maternal interview data were augmented by direct observations made by the staff during the testing sessions with the infants. Behavioral ratings were made by the examiners on Bayley's (1969) Infant Behavior Record, which had been used extensively as part of the mental testing program and for which ample normative data were available (Dolan, Matheny, & Wilson, 1974).

Prior results from the Infant Behavior Record had shown that monozygotic twins were more concordant than dizygotic twins (Matheny, Dolan, & Wilson, 1976); and a recent factor analysis of these temperament-related behaviors for 400 twins revealed three principal factors pertaining to emotionality, activity, and attentiveness and task persistence (Matheny, 1980). These prominent features of infant behavior, as rated by trained observers in a test setting, were notably congruent with the features of infant temperament reported in the mothers' interviews, and also as described in other investigations of infant twins (Freedman, 1965; Goldsmith & Gottesman, 1981).

Further, as part of the previous mental testing program, one twin had been kept in the playroom with the staff while the cotwin was being tested with the mother. This had furnished extensive experience with the specific caretaking problems and aspects of temperament that arose at each age, and the effective diversionary techniques to deal with them. In fact, a battery of soothing techniques and play activities was developed to cope with any distress and to keep the infant contented.

Therefore, as the research program turned to temperament, we drew from the collective experiences of dealing with these infants and began to formalize a detailed set of interactions between the staff and infant. In essence, the infant would be confronted with a succession of typical age-related challenges—the most notable being separation from the mother—and the staff would employ a graded series of soothing techniques and diversionary play activities, as required. The predominant behavioral style would then be reflected in how the infant responded to these challenges, and in how responsive or resistant the infant was to efforts at soothing and engagement in play.

In effect, the lab setting would become a microcosm of many experiences typically encountered by the infant, and the distinctive features of temperament would be inferred from the observable behaviors elicited in this standardized setting. The sessions would be videotaped, and the staff would subsequently rate the infant's behavior from the videotapes. The ratings would then serve to define each infant's temperament profile as displayed in the lab.

METHOD

Subjects

The twins were recruited as part of an ongoing longitudinal study described in more detail elsewhere (Wilson, 1978). Recruits were drawn from the entire twin birth registry in the Louisville, Kentucky area, with a special effort made to enroll and retain families of low socioeconomic status (SES). The full SES distribution was represented in the sample, with 27% of the families in the lowest two deciles of the occupational rating scales (Reiss, 1961), and the remaining families distributed in roughly equal proportions through the other eight deciles.

Recruited twins made quarterly visits to the research center during the first year, but it was not until the 12-month visit that the full range of laboratory procedures could be employed. The data to be reported were obtained from 84 infants who had completed the 12-month visit, with full data for all programmed episodes. The 84 infants were drawn from 18 male-male pairs, 16 female-female pairs, and 8 opposite-sex pairs. For technical and psychological reasons, the twins are not blood-typed until they are 3 years old, so zygosity was not definitely established for any of the same-sex pairs.

Outline For Each Visit

From pretesting, a basic outline evolved for the temperament assessment at each age, as follows: After the twins arrived there was a brief warm-up period including both twins, the mother, and the two staff members serving as interactionists. The mother subsequently left for an interview and the twins remained together with the interactionists, who engaged in specific activities vis-à-vis the twins. The mother returned briefly and then left with one twin for testing. The second twin remained alone with the staff members until the mother came back for a brief reunion; then the second twin went with the mother for testing and the first twin remained alone with the staff. In these solo episodes, the staff engaged each twin in a prescribed set of activities, or vignettes, for a fixed period of time, so that there would be uniformity of treatment across all participants. The vignettes were designed to confront each infant with specific opportunities for interaction with the caretakers and engagement in play, as a means of detecting the infant's predominant behavioral style. The schedule was carefully organized to yield 1 hour of videotaping for each pair, and in a format that was exactly duplicated for all twins.

For illustration, two of the vignettes employed at 12 months are described below. A full description of all vignettes and the associated rating scales may be found in Matheny and Wilson (1981).

Cuddling. The infant is picked up and held by the interactionist in an upright position with the infant's head resting on the interactionist's shoulder. The interactionist's free arm provides support for the infant's back. After the infant is placed in this position, the degree to which the infant's body stiffens, pushes away or yields to cuddling is noted. As the infant is held, the interactionist turns around slowly so that the infant's postural adjustment can be videotaped from several angles. The routine is carried out with the infant held at least once in the left arm and at least once in the right. (Time allotted, 2 minutes.)

Visible barrier. This vignette is based on a test item from the Cattell Infant Intelligence Scale (Cattell, 1947). The infant is seated in a feeding table that has a large tray in front and is given an attractive small toy. When the infant holds the toy and proceeds to play with it, the toy is taken from the infant and moved away, but within reach. As the infant reaches for the toy, a transparent plexiglass screen is placed upright between the infant and the toy. If the infant does not attempt to obtain the toy, the screen is removed and the same or another toy is given to the infant. If the toy evokes interest, the procedure is repeated. (Time allotted, 2 minutes.)

Behavioral Rating Scales

Several behavior rating categories were developed in conjunction with the standardized vignettes described above. The behavioral categories were drawn initially from Bayley's (1969) Infant Behavior Record, then progressively refined and anchored in observable behaviors through extensive pretesting. The rating categories and representative descriptors for the four scales most directly related to temperament are illustrated below.

Emotional tone. This refers to the principal emotional state manifested during the rating period: 1 = extremely upset, crying vigorously; 3 = upset, but can be soothed; 5 = bland, no apparent reaction; 7 = contented, happy; 9 = excited or animated.

Attention. This category refers to the degree to which an infant alerts to and maintains attention to objects and events: 1 = unoccupied, non-focused, vacant staring; 3 = minimal or fleeting attention, easily distractable; 5 = moderate attention—generally attentive but may shift; 7 = focused and sustained attention; 9 = continued and persistent attention to the point of being "glued" to object or event.

Activity. This refers to body motion with or without locomotion; it may involve whole or part body movements: 1 = stays quietly in one place, with practically no self-initiated movement; 3 = usually quiet and inactive, but responds appropriately in situations calling for some activity; 5 = moderate activity; 7 = in action for much of period; 9 = hyperactive; cannot be quieted for sedentary tasks.

Orientation to staff. This refers to the positive or negative aspects of social interaction: 1 = Actively negativistic, struggling, strongly avoidant; 3 = wary, hesitant, passively resistant; 5 = indifferent or ignoring; 7 = positive, friendly, approachful; 9 = very strongly oriented, demanding, possessive of interaction.

Scoring

After the visit was completed, the raters worked individually from the videotape and made the appropriate scale ratings for each successive 2-minute period. No rater scored the episode for which she was the principal interactionist with the twin.

Rater training is necessarily an intensive and demanding task, because all raters must apply the scales in a systematic manner according to a single standard. As a reliability check, the videotape for every seventh infant was rated independently by a second set of raters, permitting an assessment of interrater reliability. The reliabilities were computed in two ways: (a) as the percent of agreement (within one point) for the scale ratings made throughout the entire visit; and (b) as an intraclass correlation expressing the degree of concordance between raters. The results are presented in Table 1 for 25 cases that were scored by two raters.

The values indicate a high degree of consensus among raters in applying the scales to the observed behavior of the infants. The scale with the lowest interrater correlation (orientation to staff) had a restricted range of scores among these 25 cases, which attenuated the reliability estimate.[1]

Condensed scoring program. With ratings made for each 2-minute segment of the videotape, it should be apparent that a large matrix of ratings was generated by this procedure. Consequently, a scoring program was developed that would condense the ratings into two summary

Table 1
*Interrater Reliabilities for Behavior
Rating Scales*

| Rating scale | %
agreement | Correlation
between raters |
|---|---|---|
| Emotional tone | 92 | .92 |
| Attention | 86 | .81 |
| Activity | 87 | .90 |
| Orientation to staff | 81 | .65 |

Note. N = 25.

---

[1] Parenthetically, it should be emphasized that the use of structured vignettes, rather than nondirected free play, was a crucial feature of these assessments, and it contributed to high interrater reliability. The vignettes not only confronted each infant with a set of standardized challenges, but also gave a sharper focus to the actual behaviors elicited. Individual differences were thus more dependably detected, and raters were better able to make consensual judgments about the behaviors.

scores for each scale, one score reflecting the average value, and the other score reflecting the extent of variation or change over periods. The scoring program was applied to the ratings obtained for the twins together (mother absent) and then for each twin alone with the staff, since these were the principal episodes during which the vignettes were employed. The summary scores thus became the primary data for constructing each infant's temperament profile, as revealed under the successive challenges of the lab assessment.

Physical measures. When the laboratory assessment was completed, the twins were taken to an adjacent room for physical measurements, which included weight, length, and head circumference. The infants were undressed for the measurements—a procedure that is upsetting for some infants—and the measurement of length required that the infant be stretched out in a supine position and held stationary while a footboard was brought into contact with the heels. The necessary restraint often provoked outbursts of temper, and ratings were made by observers of the infant's emotional tone, cooperativeness, and activity during each measurement. Interrater agreement on these scales was 87%, 75%, and 65%, respectively. The temperament ratings made during physical measurements were combined with the summary scores from the videotaped assessment, and together they furnished a composite behavioral profile for each infant.

RESULTS

The first analysis was directed towards the internal consistency of the summary scores—how effectively did these scores represent the recurrent features of temperament displayed by each infant throughout the visit? Measures of response consistency and the range of individual differences are presented in Table 2.

Table 2
Measures of Rating Consistency and Range of Individual Differences at 12 Months

Rating	Overall M	SD	Range of individual means	Stability coefficient[a]
Videotaped assessment variables				
Emotional tone	4.5	1.63	1.8–6.3	.91
Attention	4.3	1.48	2.3–5.7	.83
Activity	4.7	1.22	2.7–6.0	.80
Orientation to staff	5.6	1.32	2.6–7.1	.81
Physical measures				
Emotional tone	4.7	2.35	1.0–7.5	.77
Activity	4.8	1.91	1.5–7.5	.56
Cooperation	4.3	1.81	1.5–6.8	.63

Note. N = 84.
[a] Based on 14 ratings for videotaped assessment variables; 4 ratings for physical measurements.

The stability coefficient in the final column of Table 2 is the same as the alpha coefficient for k combined observations, as often employed for internal consistency estimates (Cronbach, 1970, p. 161). It reflects the accurancy of the composite score in representing all ratings made for the infant throughout the observation periods. Emotional tone in particular was consistently displayed, ranging from the infant who was chronically upset and resistant to soothing ($M = 1.8$), to the infant who was relatively content in the face of all challenges ($M = 6.3$). These summary scores may be said to furnish a reliable picture of the infant's temperament profile as manifested in the lab assessment.[2]

Relationship Among Scales

With the ratings condensed into summary scores, intercorrelations were computed among the scales; the results are shown in Table 3. For two scales, the variability scores were included as well as mean scores, since there was a sufficient range of individual differences in the variability scores to justify inclusion.

The results from the videotaped assessment showed a strong association between positive emotional tone and sustained attention span, or conversely, between very distressed emotional tone and fleeting atten-

Table 3
Intercorrelations Between Behavioral Ratings at 12 Months

Rating variable	1	2	3	4	5	6	7	8	9
1. Emotional tone	—	−.35*	.63*	−.26*	.81*	.62*	.29*	.03	.27*
2. Emotional tone (Var)		—	−.17	.35*	−.31*	−.19	−.12	−.12	−.05
3. Activity			—	−.23	.55*	.21	.15	.10	.08
4. Activity (Var)				—	−.29*	−.30*	−.14	.02	−.21
5. Attention					—	.48*	.29*	−.03	.24*
6. Orientation to staff						—	.20	−.05	.21
7. Emotional tone (PM)							—	−.48*	.78*
8. Activity (PM)								—	−.67*
9. Cooperation (PM)									—

Note. Var = variability score. PM = physical measure. $N = 84$.
* $p \leq .05$.

---

[2] It is worth noting that the composite score for each scale benefited from repeated observations that progressively sharpened the picture of the infant's typical response and markedly enhanced the detection of a consistent pattern of reaction. The alpha coefficient for a single rating period ranged from .24 to .38 and reflected the nominal low-order predictive power for a single observation. However, when the infant's response was aggregated over multiple observations, the central value was sharpened. Epstein (1980) has recently presented a compelling argument for estimating behavioral stability from aggregate responses rather than a single observation, and the present data certainly reinforce Epstein's conclusions.

tion. Emotional tone was also significantly related to activity (the distressed child tended to be immobile) and to staff orientation (the distressed child was avoidant and withdrawn). By contrast, the child with positive emotional tone was more active, eager, and responsive with the staff.[3]

The variability scores showed a modest negative relationship with the mean ratings; the infant with considerable change over periods tended to be less positive in mood and less attentive. During physical measurements, positive emotional tone and cooperation were strongly related, and both were negatively correlated with activity, which became something of a struggle index against the restraints necessary for measurement. The modest correlations between the ratings for videotaped episodes and physical measurements showed that there was some influence of setting upon the expression of temperament. Evidently, the physical measurements provoked upset and distress in some infants who had handled the preceding experiences in the playroom with equanimity. In addition, the restraints incited an active struggle in some infants who were not otherwise disposed to high activity in the playroom.

Factor Analysis

With these results as background, a principal-components factor analysis (Harman, 1968) was performed to identify the major dimensions in the temperament ratings. Three factors were extracted with eigenvalues greater than 1.00, and a varimax rotation was also performed. However, the factor structure was not clarified by the rotation, so the original structure was retained. The factor loadings for each variable are shown in Table 4, with loadings smaller than .30 deleted.

The three factors accounted for 72.0% of the variance in the ratings, and the first factor was loaded heavily with the ratings of emotional tone, attention, and orientation to/cooperation with staff. This factor became the composite representation of the main temperament cluster described above, as revealed under the successive challenges of the playroom assessment.

---

[3] These strong relationships between scales were specifically induced by the challenges of the lab procedure and did not appear as strongly in a preliminary warm-up phase before the assessment started. During warm-up, emotional tone correlated with attention ($r = .19$), with activity ($r = .38$), and with orientation to staff ($r = .65$). Attention correlated with activity ($r = .05$) and with orientation to staff ($r = .07$). The clustering of temperament variables was thus not a byproduct of built-in overlap between the scales, nor would the cluster automatically appear in a nonchallenging situation, where all efforts of mother and staff were bent on soothing the infant.

Table 4

Factor Loadings for Behavioral Ratings at 12 Months

Rating variables	Factor 1	Factor 2	Factor 3
Emotional tone	.86	.32	
Attention	.84		
Orientation to staff	.65		
Emotional tone (PM)	.62	−.60	
Cooperation (PM)	.59	−.73	
Activity	.56	.43	.38
Activity (Var)	−.48		.66
Emotional tone (Var)	−.45	−.35	.56
Activity (PM)		.81	
Eigenvalue	3.42	2.05	1.01
Total variance accounted for (%)	38.0	22.8	11.2

Note. Var = variability score. PM = physical measure. Loadings smaller than .30 have been omitted.

The second factor was principally determined by the physical-measurement ratings—a high positive loading for activity and moderately negative loadings for emotional tone and cooperation. The distressed and uncooperative child tended to be actively resistant, rather than passively suffering through the routines measurement. This factor confirmed that the physical measurements yielded a perspective on the expression of temperament somewhat different from that obtained in the playroom.

The third factor was anchored almost entirely by the variability scores, and revealed that the degree of period-to-period change in emotional tone and activity was an independent aspect of temperament. This quality of changeableness showed an interesting association with rhythmicity of vegetative functioning, as will be described later.

Toddler Temperament Scale

As the direct assessment of temperament became fully developed, it seemed desirable to supplement the laboratory procedures with questionnaires that would draw on the cumulative observations of the parents at home. For this purpose, the questionnaires developed by Carey and his colleagues were selected because of their wide use, available norms, and extensive research and clinical applications. At 12 months, the appropriate questionnaire was the Toddler Temperament Scale (TTS; Fullard et al., Note 1). The questionnaire included 97 items rated on 6-point scales and combined into nine temperament categories. The categories are listed below, with brief descriptors for each and with illustrations of the extreme points on the scale. The authors report a median test-retest correlation of .81 for the nine scales.

1. Activity level—motor activity during daily routines as well as motility during the sleep-wake cycles. (Inactive . . . Very active)

2. Rhythmicity—regularity of vegetative functions. (Rhythmic . . . Very nonrhythmic)

3. Approach/withdrawal—initial positive or negative response to a new stimulus. (Approaches easily . . . Withdrawing, avoidant)

4. Adaptability—ease of transition to new or altered situations. (Adapts easily . . . Slow to adapt)

5. Intensity of reaction—degree of response. (Mild . . . Intense)

6. Quality of mood—amount of positive or negative affect. (Pleasant, happy . . . Negative, irritable)

7. Attention span and persistence—degree to which an interest is maintained or an activity is pursued in the face of obstacles. (Persistent, sticks to it . . . Nonpersistent, changes frequently)

8. Distractibility—effectiveness of extraneous stimuli to shift ongoing behavior. (Ignores distractions . . . Easily distracted)

9. Threshold of responsiveness—level of sensory stimulation required to evoke a response. (Indifferent to dirt, wetness, smells . . . Very sensitive)

The questionnaires, one for each twin, were taken home by the mother, who had instructions to complete and return the questionnaires within 2 weeks. It was apparent from written and spoken comments that the mothers had no difficulty in defining each twin's pattern of reaction and in preserving any differences in the ratings. This questionnaire became available only after several pairs had passed the 12-month visit, so the sample size was 48 for the questionnaire.

The infant's temperament profile on the TTS was represented by a vector of nine scaled scores, and these scores were intercorrelated for the available 12-month sample. The results are presented in Table 5.

From the mothers' perspective, there emerged a clear network of relations among the categories of temperament pertaining to approach, adaptability, mood, attention span, and resistance to distraction. With minor variations, all correlated moderately well with one another and seemed to sketch (at one extreme) the profile of an infant who was positive in mood, adapted easily, approached others readily, and main-

Table 5
Intercorrelations Between Toddler Temperament Categories at 12 Months

Categories	1	2	3	4	5	6	7	8	9
1. Activity	—	.02	−.06	−.13	.24	.19	.03	−.13	−.06
2. Rhythmicity		—	−.11	−.11	.11	.18	−.08	−.09	.01
3. Approach/withdrawal			—	.55*	.04	.50*	.57*	.25	.07
4. Adaptability				—	.20	.47*	.51*	.60*	.34*
5. Intensity					—	.28*	.18	.16	.10
6. Mood						—	.53*	.22	.24
7. Attention/persistence							—	.50*	−.10
8. Distractibility								—	.02
9. Threshold response									—

Note. N = 48.
* *p* ≤ .05.

tained attention in the face of superfluous distractions. The opposite extreme was of an infant predominantly negative in mood, avoidant of others, slow to adapt, short in attention span, and easily distracted.

A principal-components factor analysis was performed to help clarify this cluster and to identify other dimensions of temperament. Varimax rotation did not improve interpretability, however, so the original structure was retained. The results are presented in Table 6, with the factor loadings sorted according to size and with loadings smaller than .30 omitted.

Factor 1 was loaded heavily with the five categories of temperament

Table 6
Factor Loadings for the Toddler Temperament
Scale at 12 Months

Categories of temperament	Factor 1	Factor 2	Factor 3
4. Adaptability	.84		
7. Attention/persistence	.80		−.39
3. Approach/withdrawal	.74		
6. Mood	.73	.41	
8. Distractibility	.65		
5. Intensity	.33	.60	
1. Activity		.69	−.36
2. Rhythmicity		.52	
9. Threshold response			.87
Eigenvalue	3.02	1.43	1.17
Total variance accounted for (%)	33.5	15.9	13.0

Note. Factor loadings smaller than .30 have been omitted.

identified above, and this cluster represented the major constellation of behaviors that mothers perceived as expressive of temperament. Not unexpectedly, this factor represented the same characteristics noted as contributing largely to first or second factors in previous analyses; namely adaptability, approach/withdrawal, and mood (Scholom et al., 1979; Thomas et al., 1968).

Factor 2 picked up those aspects that, when combined with the negative extreme of Factor 1, could create a very trying temperament. An infant who responded intensely and who was highly active and nonrhythmic in vegetative functions would likely pose a special management problem when also avoidant, negative in mood, nonadaptable, and short in attention span. Prior studies have also isolated similar features relating to the kinetics of the infant's behavior (Garside et al., 1975; Scholom et al., 1979).

Factor 3 was defined almost exclusively by threshold of response, which captured the infant's sensitivity to tastes, smells, temperature, and cleanliness. In the vernacular, it signified a dimension ranging from picky and particular to unconcerned and indifferent. As an independent factor, it meant that one temperamental infant might be hypersensitive to such matters, whereas another temperamental infant might be indifferent.

Relationship Between Ratings

One of the pressing issues in the assessment of temperament is the relationship between direct observations and maternal reports. The latter are often criticized as being nonobjective and biased, whereas the former may suffer from having only a brief period of observation in an artificial setting. If there is a conjunction between the two views of infant temperament, however, it should emerge as a common bridge linking both sets of measurements.

As a first step, the correlations were computed between the TTS scores and the research ratings; results are shown in Table 7. In their original form, most of the TTS scales are scored in the opposite direction from the lab ratings, and consequently the TTS scores were inverted on Scales 3 through 9 before computing the correlations.

It is apparent that there were a number of significant relations between the direct observations and the maternal perceptions of the infants' temperament. As one might anticipate, the core variables within each set accounted for most of the relations, but there were some interesting exceptions.

Table 7
Intercorrelations Between Behavioral Ratings and Toddler Temperament Scale (TTS) at 12 Months

TTS categories	Videotaped assessment						Physical measures		
	Emot. tone	Emot. tone (var)	Activ.	Activ. (var)	Attn.	Orient. to staff	Emot. tone	Activ.	Cooper.
Activity	−.01	.00	−.06	.16	.02	−.11	.09	.22	−.16
Rhythmicity	.14	.38*	.12	.31*	.01	−.02	.07	.12	.10
Approach/ withdrawal	.57*	−.15	.46*	−.23	.47*	.47*	.33*	−.01	.34*
Adaptability	.32*	−.24	.31	−.26	.32*	.08	.26	−.08	.27
Intensity	−.03	.02	.21	−.15	−.01	−.13	.00	−.20	.05
Mood	.34*	−.15	.34*	−.18	.28*	.29*	.26	−.08	.26
Attention/ persistence	.33*	−.11	.44*	−.13	.34*	.14	.23	.16	.09
Distractibility	.29*	−.17	.19	−.10	.30*	.09	.02	.04	−.01
Threshold response	.19	.00	−.01	.13	.15	.09	.33*	−.18	.31*

Note. N = 48. Emot. = emotional; var = variability; Activ. = activity; Attn. = attention; Orient. = orientation; Cooper = cooperation.
* $p \leq .05$.

For example, rhythmicity of vegetative functioning correlated more highly with the two lab variability scores than with any other ratings. The infant perceived as nonrhythmic and erratic at home was the one seen as showing greater fluctuations in emotional tone and activity in the laboratory setting—perhaps reflecting some underlying aspect of lability in the organism.

Multivariate Analysis

Although the individual correlations in Table 7 are informative, each infant's temperament profile was represented by a multivariate vector of scores, and the preferred analysis would be to express the similarity in temperament profile between the two sets of scores.

The analysis was carried out in two stages. First, the factor analysis within each set had revealed a strong first factor that was heavily loaded by the core variables within each set. Therefore, factor scores were generated for all infants on Lab Factor 1 and TTS Factor 1. Each factor score represented a single weighted composite of the high-loading variables per set, and the linkage between the sets was assessed by a correlation between the factor scores. For Lab Factor 1 and TTS Factor 1, the correlation was .52 ($p < .001$).

Thus, when each infant's temperament profile was condensed into a single factor score, there was a highly significant relation between the factor scores based on direct observations and those based on maternal ratings. Despite the differences in observers, settings, rating instruments, and periods of observations, there was still considerable coherence between the two measures of temperament.

Canonical analysis. The second analysis expanded upon the preceding single-factor correlation by recognizing that other factors within each set might also be correlated. Since the factor analysis had reduced the original array of nine variables per set to a smaller array, the decision was made to select those factors in each set that would account for at least 80% of the variance in the original ratings. Under this proviso, four factors were extracted from the lab ratings; five factors were extracted from the TTS scores.

Nine factor scores were then computed for each infant, and a canonical correlation analysis was performed to determine the degree of similarity in the two sets of factor scores. A canonical analysis searches for the linear combination of scores in each set that will yield the largest correlation between the two sets, then for a second combination (orthogonal to the first) that yields the next largest correlation, and so on until the covariance between the two sets is exhausted (Cooley & Lohnes, 1971; Cohen & Cohen, 1975).

The results (shown in Table 8) revealed a canonical correlation of .60 between the first canonical variates, indicative of a substantial linkage between the two sets of factor scores. The pattern of loadings showed

Table 8
Canonical Correlations Between Lab Factor Scores and Toddler Temperament Scale (TTS) Factor Scores

Canonical variate	Canonical correlation	Factor variable	Canonical loadings	
			First variate	Second variate
First	.60*	Lab 1	.98	
Second	.46	Lab 2		−.48
		Lab 3		.76
		Lab 4		.42
		TTS 1	.88	
		TTS 2		.32
		TTS 3		
		TTS 4		.76
		TTS 5	−.47	−.47

Note. $N = 48$. Canonical loadings smaller than .30 have been omitted.
* $p < .01$.

that the first canonical variate was carried almost entirely by the first factor scores in each set. Recalling the earlier correlation of .52 for the first factor scores alone, the first canonical variate slightly enhanced this basal relationship, mainly through the contribution of TTS Factor 5. However, the strongest linkage was clearly through the core variables entering into Factor 1 of each set, as previously described.

The remaining canonical variates had smaller correlations and accounted for considerably less variance in the matrix; collectively, they added about 7% additional systematic variance to the cross linkage established by the first canonical variate. The pattern of loadings, however, was informative about what were associated as bridging factors. For the second variate, high loadings were obtained for Lab Factor 3 and TTS Factor 4, and these factors were based, respectively, on fluctuations in emotional tone and activity and on nonrhythmicity of vegetative functions. The canonical analysis thus isolated a bridging factor related to biobehavioral lability, as had been previously inferred from the cross correlations in Table 7.

DISCUSSION

The major aim of this study was to employ a multimethod battery for collecting temperament data from 12-month-old infants. The results indicated that behaviors rated in a standardized laboratory assessment and behaviors reported by the mother via questionnaire shared a substantial common link. The core variables from the laboratory—emotional tone, attentiveness, and social orientation to staff—loaded on a factor that was significantly related to the principal factor extracted from the maternal ratings.

The latter factor, made up of adaptability, attention/persistence, approach, mood, and distractability, might have been expected to correlate with the laboratory ratings on a priori grounds. However, the correlation between factor scores demonstrated a substantial degree of convergent validity not readily apparent from the individual correlations in Table 7 alone. In view of the differences in setting, in observers, and in rating instruments, the presence of a consistent within-the-individual component of temperament can be affirmed (Bates, 1980). Moreover, the results supported the argument that aggregate, rather than single, measures are more likely to yield a coherent picture of stable individual differences (Epstein, 1980).

The data also indicated that there are some aspects of temperament unique to each setting and confirmed Lytton's (1974) observation that each source of data has its own relative utility. Thomas and Chess (1980) had anticipated such results in their use of the concept of developmental interaction between the infant and the socializing environment. If that concept has any meaning, then variations in settings should elicit some degree of variation in infant behaviors.

For example, in a recent study some temperamental characteristics were more closely related to the child's behavior in nursery school than to his or her behavior at home with the mother (Hinde, Easton, Meller, & Tamplin, 1982). From another perspective, temperamental differences between firstborn children affected the degree of anxious and unhappy behavior displayed following the birth of a sibling; but the vulnerability of the anxious firstborns to prolonged disturbance was markedly influenced by their relationship with the mother (Dunn, 1982). These results make it evident that the child's behavior is a joint function of temperamental predispositions and the home/school environment in which these predispositions are expressed.

Turning to the issue of identifying dimensions of temperament, it is clear that both laboratory and maternal observations yielded a primary factor incorporating an emotional and social aspect. Therefore, it seemed that the essential pattern of temperament in the 12-month-old concerned the degree to which the infant was positive in mood, approachful to persons and events, adaptive to situational demands, and task oriented.

Comparable data from other observational studies are sparse; however, Plomin and Rowe (1978) conducted home observations for twins aged 13–37 months and found pronounced individual differences in social responsiveness, which included vocalizing, smiling, approach, playfulness, and separation distress. Reaction to a stranger was more discriminating of monozygotic/dizygotic differences (and presumed genetic effects) than reaction to the mother.

Results from temperament questionnaires have shown that mood, approach/withdrawal, adaptability, and intensity defined the first factor for ratings of infants' behaviors displayed preponderantly during the first 12 months (Thomas et al., 1968); and somewhat similar results were obtained from 6-month-old infants (Scholom et al., 1979). A factor analysis of items from a different questionnaire suggested that descriptions pertaining to mood defined the primary dimension of temperament (Bates et al., 1979). A recent questionnaire developed by Rothbart (1981) put forward six conceptually distinct attributes of temperament: activity, smiling and laughter, soothability, fear, duration of orienting, and distress to limitations. Whereas these titles differ somewhat from the category names employed by Thomas et al. (1968), there is considerable overlap between the reference behaviors—Rothbart intentionally chose titles that were more neutral and more easily operationalized than, say, adaptability.

Although there are some variations in the perceived essential characteristics of infant temperament, there is a surprising degree of consensus among the findings, particularly when one is mindful that the present study, and two previous studies (Bates et al., 1979; Rothbart, Note 2), demonstrated some convergence between direct observations and parental ratings. In an area where the measuring devices are still fairly primitive, the emergence of coherent relationships attests to the potency of these characteristics.

From a longitudinal perspective, the temperament profile becomes the prime vehicle for assessing stability over ages and addressing the question: Does the infant's profile reveal itself at an early age and appear recurrently at later ages, or are there major shifts in the profile over successive ages? If intrinsic factors play an influential role, one might expect a high degree of stability. However, as Carey (1981) pointed out, a number of factors may confound efforts to demonstrate stability, not the least of which are varying rates of maturation for the underlying central nervous system structures, and the appearance of age-linked behavioral competencies that may alter the mode of expression for a particular temperamental style.

The problem and the challenge is one of determining when a nominal change in profile represents an intrinsic developmental transformation, or instead, a modification arising from purely environmental causes. The present program is collecting temperament data at successive ages and a detailed assessment of the home environment in order to address this question.

REFERENCE NOTES

1. Fullard, W., McDevitt, S. C. and Carey, W. B. (1980). *Toddler Temperament Scale*. Unpublished manuscript, Temple University.
2. Rothbart, M. K. (1980). *Longitudinal home observations of infant temperament*. Paper presented at the International Conference on Infant Studies, New Haven, CT.

REFERENCES

Bates, J. E. (1980). The concept of difficult temperament. *Merrill-Palmer Quarterly*, 26: 299–319.
Bates, J. E., Freeland, C. A. B., and Lounsbury, M. L. (1979). Measurement of infant difficultness. *Child Development*, 50: 794–803.

Bayley, N. (1969). *Bayley scales of infant development.* New York: Psychological Corporation.

Bell, R. Q. (1974). Contributions of human infants to caregiving and social interaction. In M. Lewis and L. A. Rosenblum (Eds.), *The effect of the infant on its caregiver.* New York: Wiley.

Carey, W. B. (1981). The importance of temperament-environment interaction for child health and development. In M. Lewis and L. A. Rosenblum (Eds.), *The uncommon child.* New York: Plenum Press.

Carey, W. B., and McDevitt, S. C. (1978). Revision of the Infant Temperament Questionnaire. *Pediatrics*, 61: 735–739.

Cattell, P. (1947). *Cattell Infant Intelligence Scale.* New York: Psychological Corporation.

Cohen, J., and Cohen, P. (1975). *Applied multiple regression/correlation analysis for the behavioral sciences.* Hillsdale, NJ: Erlbaum.

Cooley, W. W., and Lohnes, P. R. (1971). *Multivariate procedures for the behavioral sciences* (2nd ed.). New York: Wiley.

Cronbach, L. J. (1970). *Essentials of psychological testing* (3rd ed.). New York: Harper & Row.

Dolan, A. B., Matheny, A. P., and Wilson, R. S. (1974). Bayley's Infant Behavior Record: Age trends, sex differences and behavioral correlates. *JSAS Catalog of Selected Documents in Psychology*, 4: 9–10. (Ms. No. 551)

Dunn, J. (1982). Temperamental differences, family relationships, and young children's responses to change within the family. In *Temperamental differences in infants and young children* (Ciba Foundation Symposium 89). London: Pitman.

Epstein, S. (1980). The stability of behavior: II. Implications for psychological research. *American Psychologist*, 35: 790–806.

Escalona, S. K. (1968). *Roots of individuality.* Chicago: Aldine.

Freedman, D. G. (1965). An ethological approach to the genetic study of human behavior. In S. G. Vandenberg (Ed.), *Methods and goals in human behavior genetics.* New York: Academic Press.

Garside, R. F., et al. (1975). Dimensions of temperament in infant school children. *Journal of Child Psychology and Psychiatry*, 16: 219–231.

Goldsmith, H. H., and Gottesman, I. I. (1981). Origins of variation in behavioral style: A longitudinal study of temperament in young twins. *Child Development*, 52: 91–103.

Harman, H. H. (1968). Factor analysis. In D. K. Whitla (Ed.), *Handbook of measurement and assessment in behavioral sciences.* Reading, MA: Addison-Wesley.

Hinde, R. A., Easton, D. F., Meller, R. E., and Tamplin, A. M. (1982). Temperament and behaviour. In *Temperamental differences in infants and young children* (Ciba Foundation Symposium 89). London: Pitman.

Lewis, M., and Rosenblum, L. A. (Eds.) (1974). *The effect of the infant on its caregiver.* New York: Wiley.

Lytton, H. (1974). Comparative yield of three data sources in the study of parent-child interaction. *Merrill-Palmer Quarterly*, 20: 53–64.

Matheny, A. P. (1980). Bayley's Infant Behavior Record: Behavioral components and twin analyses. *Child Development*, 51: 1157–1167.

Matheny, A. P., Dolan, A. B., and Wilson, R. S. (1976). Twins: Within-pair similarity on Bayley's Infant Behavior Record. *Journal of Genetic Psychology*, 28: 263–270.

Matheny, A. P., and Wilson, R. S. (1981). Developmental tasks and rating scales for the laboratory assessment of infant temperament. *JSAS Catalog of Selected Documents in Psychology*, 11: 81–82. (Ms. No. 2367)

Matheny, A. P., Wilson, R. S., Dolan, A. M., and Krantz, J. Z. (1981). Behavioral contrasts in twinships: Stability and patterns of differences in childhood. *Child Development*, 52: 579–588.

McDevitt, S. C., and Carey, W. B. (1978). The measurement of temperament in 3–7 year old children. *Journal of Child Psychology and Psychiatry*, 19: 245–253.

Plomin, R., and Rowe, D. C. (1978). Genes, environment, and development of temperament in young human twins. In G. M. Burghardt and M. Bekoff (Eds.), *The development of behavior*. New York: Garland Press.

Reiss, A. J. (1961). Occupations and social status. New York: Free Press of Glencoe.

Rothbart, M. K. (1981). Measurement of temperament in infancy. *Child Development*, 52: 569–578.

Rothbart, M. K., and Derryberry, D. (1981). Development of individual differences in temperament. In M. Lamb and A. Brown (Eds.), *Advances in developmental psychology* (Vol. 1). Hillsdale, NJ: Erlbaum.

Scholom, A., Zucker, R. A., and Stollak, G. E. (1979). Relating early child adjustment to infant and parent temperament. *Journal of Abnormal Child Psychology*, 7: 297–308.

Thomas, A., and Chess, S. (1977). *Temperament and development*. New York: Brunner/Mazel.

Thomas, A., and Chess, S. (1980). *The dynamics of psychological development*. New York: Brunner/Mazel.

Thomas, A., Chess, S., and Birch, H. G. (1968). *Temperament and behavior disorders in children*. New York: New York University Press.

Thomas, A., Chess, S., Birch, H. G., Hertzig, M. E., and Korn, S. (1963). *Behavioral individuality in early childhood*. New York: New York University Press.

Wilson, R. S. (1978). Synchronies in mental development: An epigenetic perspective. *Science*, 202: 939–948.

Wilson, R. S. (1979). Twin growth: Initial deficit, recovery, and trends in concordance from birth to nine years. *Annals of Human Biology*, 6: 205–220.

Wilson, R. S., Brown, A. M., and Matheny, A. P. (1971). Emergence and persistence of behavioral differences in twins. *Child Development*, 42: 1381–1398.

Wilson, R. S., and Matheny, A. P. (1980). Conference on temperament research: Abstracts of presentations. *JSAS Catalog of Selected Documents in Psychology*, 10: 10. (Ms. No. 1978)

14

Some Pitfalls in Infant Temperament Research

William B. Carey

University of Pennsylvania Medical School

After 27 years of daily contact with mothers and infants in pediatric settings, and more than half of that time in infant temperament research, I have become increasingly cognizant of the perils as well as the excitement associated with investigation in this area. Since the publication of the original version of the Infant Temperament Questionnaire (ITQ) (Carey, 1970) and its revision (Carey & McDevitt, 1978a), a number of other infant temperament scales have been introduced (Bates, Freeland, & Lounsbury, 1979; Bohlin, Hagekull, & Lindhagen, 1981; Persson-Blennow & McNeil, 1979; Rothbart, 1981). The varying uses to which the scales have been put, and the interpretations of the data derived from them, are the source of my concern and the subject of this commentary.

My plan is to identify some of the outstanding pitfalls in each of several aspects of temperament research and to suggest how these might be remedied.

DEFINITION: INDIVIDUAL DIFFERENCES VERSUS "MATERNAL PERCEPTIONS"

Temperament has been defined as behavioral style, or the "how" of behavior, rather than as the content of behavior, or capacities, or motivations (Thomas & Chess, 1977; see also Buss & Plomin, 1975; Rothbart, 1981). This view regards the difficult infant as one who is irregular,

---

Reprinted with permission from *Infant Behavior and Development*, 1983, Vol. 6, 247–254.

low in initial approach and adaptability, and intense and predominantly negative in mood (Thomas & Chess, 1977). Evidence abounds from parental and professional experience that these individual differences are real (Rutter, 1982), although the way they are reported depends on the observer's duration of exposure, sampling technique, and perspective. This inconsistency of observations should not distress us since even in the "hard" science of physics, events cannot be described with complete certainty and uniformity (Bronowski, 1973).

The chief pitfall here is the "Maternal Perceptions Fallacy" (Carey, 1981) that temperament differences (and especially difficult temperament) are all in the mind of the mother. A similar view maintains that temperamental traits may be real but that parents can report only their "perceptions" about them—a highly imperfect mixture of fantasy and reality (Bates, 1980). Moreover, some investigators have referred to ITQ ratings of difficult temperament as "maternal perceptions of difficult temperament" without regard for the fact that many mothers who rate their infants as difficult do not perceive them as such (Carey, 1970).

The confusion over what temperament differences are and where they "reside" can be reduced by several steps. First, a more precise definition is needed to clarify the phenomenon and to differentiate between it and other aspects of personality. Some further criteria as to hereditability and stability would be useful (Plomin, 1982). Rothbart and Derryberry (1981) have offered some valuable suggestions.

Second, the ability of parents to describe their children's individuality should be acknowledged. Although some studies (Sameroff, Seifer, & Elias, 1982; Vaughn, Taraldson, Crichton, & Egeland, 1981) have demonstrated modest correlations between parental attitudes and their ratings of their infants on the unrevised ITQ, there are possible explanations other than the one embraced by these authors, i.e., that mothers are merely projecting themselves onto their infants' behavior. Lyon and Plomin (1981) and Thomas, Chess, and Korn (1982) have shown that this projection is negligible when assessment methods are sufficiently sensitive. It is my view that research would be gravely impoverished and clinical practice impossible, if parental reports are discarded as worthless.

Finally, the present terminology of "perceptions" by parents and "observations" by professionals should be revised. Both parents and professionals can make observations (e.g., ratings) which are detailed descriptions of exactly what the infant does, and they both can have perceptions, which may be defined as hastily or partially formed general impressions. Perceptions by either may be as valid as ratings but are more likely to be influenced by the observer and the observer's situation. Both are useful clinically (Carey, 1982a,b).

ORIGINS OF TEMPERAMENT DIFFERENCES: GENETIC AND ENVIRONMENTAL FACTORS INTERTWINED OR SEPARABLE?

Temperament differences in infants and children are presently presumed to be partly genetic and influenced by both prenatal and postnatal environment (Carey, 1981; Thomas & Chess, 1977). Interaction with the environment seems to be constant with mutual modification. The genetic component of temperament, apparently, is not entirely expressed at birth, but becomes fully evident only later (Torgersen, 1982; Torgersen & Kringlen, 1978), as is the case with eye color and body size. Since it is difficult, if not impossible, to separate clearly the genetic and environmental components of infant temperament at any time, one is compelled to regard an infant's temperament as the behavioral style displayed at the time, acknowledging that there are always innate and experiential factors.

The two pitfalls most evident here are the assumption that behavior at birth provides a clear view of the genetic component or "congenital temperament" (Crockenberg & Acredolo, 1983) and that all further developments in it after birth reflect environmental influences. Newborn behavior is already affected by pre- and perinatal environments (Sameroff, 1978), and genetic dispositions may not emerge until later.

As new behavioral style characteristics, such as reactions to strangers or persistence at play, evolve during the months after birth, these are likely to be affected both by genetic and environmental factors. The relative amount of influence of these two factors cannot be measured easily at present. Therefore, it seems hazardous to interpret correlations between maternal attitudes and infant temperament as a unidirectional effect from the mother to infant (cf. Crockenberg & Acredolo, 1983). It is equally possible that predominantly genetically determined characteristics are molding maternal attitudes, feelings, and handling, or that mutual modifications are occurring.

Much needs to be learned about the origins of temperament traits. Two principal lines of inquiry are possible. The study of the genetic component, by investigating twins, as in the work of Plomin (1982), Torgersen (1982), and Wilson and Matheny (1982), should continue to illuminate the questions as to which traits are genetically determined and to provide estimates as to how strong the influence may be. It is not a technically perfect method, but it is the best we have currently available.

Assessing how the environment modifies the genetic components of the infant's temperament will be no less difficult or important. Neither prenatal nor postnatal environments are easily standardized. For example, toxemic or abusive mothers are not all alike. Correlational studies between environmental factors and temperament are inconclusive since they do not reveal the direction of effects or rule out some common prior cause for both. Detailed interactional studies seem at present to be the most promising way to increase our understanding.

TEMPERAMENT STABILITY: SUBSTANTIAL OR NEGLIGIBLE?

Research to date has demonstrated some evidence for stability and some for change in temperament (Carey & McDebitt, 1978b; Thomas & Chess, 1977). No current researcher has claimed to have shown temperament to be fixed at any point, nor has any project established that the environment can induce in temperament any change at all, or that stability of temperament is nothing more than persistence of "maternal perceptions." From relatively unstable patterns at birth (Sameroff, 1978), behavioral style seems to become more consistent as children get older (Hegvik, McDevitt, & Carey, 1982). Clinicians may regard stability as a relatively unimportant issue since what matters to them are the present interaction problems rather than future trends. However, behavioral scientists may be more concerned, since a viable definition of temperament requires that it be "relatively stable, at least within major developmental areas" (Plomin, 1982).

A common pitfall in studies of the stability of temperamental traits has been the failure to compare similar measures at the two points. The rapid development of infants and young children makes difficult the measurement of precisely the same behaviors at two points in time, but does not relieve the investigator of the responsibility of trying. Birns, Barten, and Bridger (1969) found evidence of consistency in the measures of irritability, sensitivity, tension, and soothability between birth and 4 months. By contrast, Crockenberg and Acredolo (1983) found little relationship between the newborn period and 3 months. However, the items and item clusters derived from the Neonatal Behavioral Assessment Scale (NBAS) (Brazelton, 1973) and the category ratings on the Infant Behavior Questionnaire (IBQ) of Rothbart (1981) used at 3 months differed in content and dimension. For example, NBAS irritability (Item 19) is scored 1–9 on the basis of *how many* of eight aversive stimuli (pinprick, Moro reflex, etc.) cause crying. The NBAS irritability cluster they used also includes Items 17 and 18, which are measures of the *degree* and *rapidity* of arousal by the stimuli. On the other hand, the IBQ distress category, against which the newborn measures were compared, rates *how often* the infant has shown distress in the last week under certain different circumstances: limitations and intense or novel stimuli. There is no evidence that these professionally and maternally rated behaviors correlate with each other at the same time, let alone over the course of a 3-month interval characterized by marked developmental change.

A second major pitfall is an environmentalist bias in the interpretation of data on the stability of temperamental traits. If the environment is responsible for all changes in temperament, then any change would be possible with appropriate manipulation of the child's setting. In his foreword to the book by Thomas and Chess (1977), Sameroff proposes "a new environmentalism," which acknowledges the existence of the child's contribution to the parent-child interaction, "but at the same time places the major responsibility for the child's outcome on the environment." This view overlooks the facts that we do not now know how to change children's temperaments other than, possibly, pharmacologically (Carey, 1982a) and that some traits and some individuals may be more modifiable than others. An important outcome of the work of Thomas and Chess (1977) has been to relieve parents of unjustified guilt as to the behavior of their children; this sort of environmentalist bias gives it back to them.

Better estimates of the stability of temperament have been obtained as behaviors at the two points have been matched and as more psychometrically sophisticated instruments have been used (Carey & McDevitt, 1978b). Also to be remembered in subsequent studies of stability should be the advice of Epstein (1980) on the importance of "aggregating behavior over situations and/or occasions, thereby cancelling out incidental uncontrollable factors relative to experimental factors."

MEASUREMENT: SEVERAL VALID SOURCES
VERSUS BRIEF PROFESSIONAL RATINGS

In recent years three methods have evolved for the measurement of temperament: parental interviews, parental questionnaires, and professional observations. The adequate internal consistency and retest reliability of the four questionnaires developed by our group (Carey, 1981) and others have been described elsewhere (Bohlin et al., 1981; Persson-Blennow & McNeil, 1979; Rothbart, 1981). A recent review of these and other temperament measurement techniques by Hubert, Wachs, Peters-Martin and Gandour (1982) judged their psychometric properties more harshly, but the value of that report is somewhat diminished by the authors' acceptance at face value of the results of a group of studies that is highly varied as to pertinence and sophistication.

The process of demonstrating the external validity of these questionnaires has been difficult because no standardized comprehensive professional rating scheme exists against which they can be compared. Although clinicians rely heavily on parental reports of their children, they know that behavioral descriptions are least likely to be verifiable if they are general impressions or retrospective ones, or if the parent reporting is of lower class status or emotionally disturbed. Yet, all the adequately designed studies reported so far have shown at least moderate validity (Carey, 1982b).

In the newborn period, when there is the NBAS for validity comparisons, Field, Dempsey, Hallock and Shuman (1978) demonstrated that mothers rated their infants with a high degree of accuracy on a questionnaire adapted from the NBAS (the MABI scale).

The chief pitfall in validation of temperament questionnaires has been the unjustified reliance on brief unmatched professional observations for comparison with maternal reports (Crockenberg & Acredolo, 1983; Sameroff et al., 1982; Vaughn et al., 1981). Lacking an adequate standardized professional observation rating technique, researchers have rated a child's temperament after just a few hours, or even minutes, with the child, and discrepancies with what the mother has reported have been taken as evidence that the mother was wrong. (This is equivalent to maintaining that a 2-week tour of China makes a person more of an expert on the country than someone who has lived there all his life, or that careful measurements of the weather for an hour in Boston are more informative than a detailed description by a long term inhabitant.) Where is the evidence that brief professional ratings of temperament are themselves valid? In view of this problem, one would expect that considerable effort would be expended to match maternally and professionally rated behaviors as to content and dimension. The three studies cited above failed to do this. "As to matching content and dimensions from observational to rating data, I would agree that we made no attempt to match. I would also argue that such matching should not be necessary." (Vaughn, B. E., Personal communication, Aug. 5, 1981).

The development of a comprehensive, standardized professional rating technique for infant temperament should help solve these problems. Observations will have to be sufficiently long and representative to sample adequately the full range of the infant's behavior and must match exactly what the mother is reporting if used for validation. Then the existing questionnaires (and brief professional rating techniques) can be adequately tested and improved where necessary. To be helpful to clinicians, researchers should not just be critical of parental reports but should try to find ways of making them better.

Physicians have traditionally relied on information from several sources in the process of diagnosis and management: the history, the physical exam, and laboratory tests. Progress in clinical and research determination of infants' temperament undoubtedly will come from similar "eclectic, multimethod strategies" (Plomin, 1982) using parental interview, questionnaire, and professional observations to obtain a well rounded picture of the child's behavioral style.

CLINICAL APPLICATIONS: PROGRESS THROUGH COLLABORATION VERSUS INDEPENDENT STRUGGLING

Infant temperament and its interaction with environmental factors have already been demonstrated to be related to a variety of clinical problems such as behavior disorders (Thomas, Chess, & Birch, 1968), accidents, and colic and are likely to be shown to have an even greater sphere of influence (Carey, 1981). The ultimate social value of temperament research lies in contributions to the management of these problems.

The chief pitfall here is the assumption by both clinicians and behavioral scientists that they can progress adequately without interdisciplinary collaboration. A host of methodological problems awaits the medical clinician who assumes he knows all about measuring behavior; the same is true for the behavioral scientist who presumes detailed knowledge of physical and neurological problems.

Our differing skills and points of view can be a strength rather than a source of friction. Pediatricians and psychiatrists can learn a great deal from psychologists, especially about theory and statistical method. Also, pediatricians and psychiatrists can offer psychologists a broader perspective on the clinically relevant issues in child development, improved techniques for obtaining valid information, and advice on specific matters such as sample selection. Furthermore, our pediatric practices can supply researchers with the relatively stable populations indispensible for the longitudinal studies necessary to resolve most clinical issues. Together we can work toward building theoretically sound and practically useful ways of understanding and dealing with the important phenomenon of infant temperament and other issues that concern us all.

REFERENCES

Bates, J. E. (1980). The concept of difficult temperament. *Merrill-Palmer Quarterly*, 26: 299–319.

Bates, J. E., Freeland, C. A. B., and Lounsburg, M. L. (1979). Measurement of infant difficultness. *Child Development*, 50: 794–803.

Birns, B., Barten, S., and Bridger, W. H. (1969). Individual differences in temperamental characteristics of infants. *Transactions of the New York Academy of Sciences*, 31: 1071–1082.

Bohlin, G., Hagekull, B., and Lindhagen, K. (1981). Dimensions of infant behavior. *Infant Behavior and Development*, 4: 83–96.

Brazelton, T. B. (1973). *Neonatal Behavioral Assessment Scale*. Philadelphia, PA: J. B. Lippincott Co.

Bronowski, J. (1973). *The ascent of man*. Boston, MA: Little, Brown and Company.

Buss, A. H., and Plomin, R. (1975). *A temperament theory of personality development*. New York: Wiley.

Carey, W. B. (1970). A simplified method for measuring infant temperament. *Journal of Pediatrics*, 77: 188–194.

Carey, W. B. (1981). The importance of temperament-environment interaction for child health and development. In M. Lewis and L. Rosenblum (Eds.), *The uncommon child*. New York: Plenum.

Carey, W. B. (1982). Clinical use of temperament data in pediatric practice. In R. Porter and G. Collins (Eds.), *Temperamental differences in infants and young children*. London: Pittman Books. (a)

Carey, W. B. (1982). Validity of parental assessments of development and behavior. *American Journal of Diseases of Children*, 136: 97–99. (b)

Carey, W. B., and McDevitt, S. C. (1978). Revision of the infant temperament questionnaire. *Pediatrics*, 61: 735–739. (a)

Carey, W. B., and McDevitt, S. C. (1978). Stability and change in individual temperament diagnoses from infancy to early childhood. *Journal of the American Academy of Child Psychiatry*, 17: 331–337. (b)

Crockenberg, S., and Acredolo, C. (1983). Infant temperament ratings: A function of infants, of mothers, or both? *Infant Behavior and Development*, 6: 61–72.

Epstein, S. (1980). The stability of behavior. II. Implication for psychological research. *American Psychologist*, 35: 790–806.

Field, T. M., Dempsey, J. R., Hallock, N. H., and Shuman, H. H. (1978). The mother's assessment of the behavior of her infant. *Infant Behavior and Development*. 1: 156–167.

Hegvik, R., McDevitt, S. C., and Carey, W. B. (1982). The middle childhood temperament questionnaire. *Journal of Developmental and Behavioral Pediatrics*, 3: 197–200.

Hubert, N. C., Wachs, T. D., Peters-Martin, P., and Gandour, M. J. (1982). The study of early temperament: Measurement and conceptual issues. *Child Development*, 53: 571–600.

Lyon, M. E., and Plomin, R. (1981). The measurement of temperament using parental ratings. *Journal of Child Psychology and Psychiatry*, 22: 47–53.

Persson-Blennow, I., and McNeil, T. F. (1979). A questionnaire for measurement of temperament in six-month-old infants: Development and standardization. *Journal of Child Psychology and Psychiatry*, 20: 1–13.

Plomin, R. (1982). Childhood temperament. In B. Lahey and A. Kazdin (Eds.), *Advances in clinical child psychology* (Vol. 6). 1–80.

Rothbart, M. K. (1981). Measurement of temperament in infancy. *Child Development*, 52: 569–578.

Rothbart, M. K., and Derryberry, D. (1981). Development of individual differences in temperament. In M. L. Lamb and A. L. Brown (Eds.), *Advances in developmental psychology* (Vol. 1). Hillsdale, NJ: Lawrence Erlbaum Associates.

Rutter, M. L. (1982). Temperament: Concepts, issues, and problems. In R. Porter and G. Collins (Eds.), *Temperamental differences in infants and young children*. London: Pitman Books.

Sameroff, A. J. (1978). Organization and stability of newborn behavior: A commentary on the Brazelton neonatal behavioral assessment scale. *Monographs of the Society for Research in Child Development*, 43 (5–6, Serial No. 177).

Sameroff, A. J., Seifer, R., and Elias, P. K. (1982). Sociocultural variability in infant temperament ratings. *Child Development*, 53: 164–173.

Thomas, A., and Chess, S. (1977). *Temperament and development*. New York: Brunner/Mazel.

Thomas, A., Chess, S., and Birch, H. (1968). *Temperament and behavior disorders in children*. New York: New York University Press.

Thomas, A., Chess, S., and Korn, S. (1982). The reality of difficult temperament. *Merrill-Palmer Quarterly*, 28: 1–20.

Torgersen, A. M. (1982). Influence of genetic factors on temperament development in early childhood. In R. Porter and G. Collins (Eds.), *Temperamental differences in infants and young children*. London: Pitman Books.

Torgersen, A. M., and Kringlen, E. (1978). Genetic aspects of temperamental differences in infants: A study of same-sexed twins. *Journal of the American Academy of Child Psychiatry*, 17: 433–444.

Vaughn, B. E., Taraldson, B. J., Crichton, L., and Egeland, B. (1981). The assessment of infant temperament: A critique of the Carey infant temperament questionnaire. *Infant Behavior and Development*, 4: 1–17.

Wilson, R. S., and Matheny, A. P. (1983). Assessment of temperament in infant twins. *Developmental Psychology*, 19: 172–183.

15

The Role of Temperament in Psychosocial Adaptation in Early Adolescents: A Test of a "Goodness of Fit" Model

Jacqueline V. Lerner

Stanford University

This study assessed the role of temperament in adolescents' adaptation to school social and academic contexts, and whether temperament when matched with contextual demands provides better adaptation than when not matched. Temperamental attributes of 48 male and 51 female junior high school students and both actual and perceived demands of the two school contexts were assessed. As predicted, Ss whose attributes fit best (were least discrepant) with the demands of the two contexts were more likely to have better scores on teacher-, peer-, and self-rated measures of adaptation than Ss whose attributes fit less well. Fit scores for the perceived contexts were better predictors than were fit scores for the actual contexts. Methodological issues are discussed, and future tests of the present "goodness of fit" model of person-context relations are suggested.

Reprinted with permission from the *Journal of Genetic Psychology*, 1983, Vol. 143, 149–157. Copyright 1983 by The Journal Press.

This article is based on a dissertation submitted to the Department of Educational Psychology, The Pennsylvania State University, in partial fulfillment of the requirements for the degree of doctor of philosophy. The author thanks Francis J. Di Vesta, Committee Chair, and David S. Palermo, Juris G. Draguns, and Paul A. Games, Committee Members, for their support and guidance in this research. The author also thanks Richard M. Lerner for a critical reading of the current version of the manuscript.

INTRODUCTION

The contextual paradigm of human development, unlike the more traditional organismic and mechanistic models, emphasizes the relation between the developing person and his or her changing social and psychological world (10). Derived from this view is the notion that a person's developing behavioral (e.g., temperamental) and/or physical (e.g., constitutional) characteristics evoke differential reactions in significant others, and that these reactions feed back to affect further development (5). Through the establishment of such "circular functions" in ontogeny (13), a child's own characteristics may provide a significant source of stimulation for his own development (6). Considerable data support the use of this idea (1,8). An exemplary case is the research of Thomas and Chess (14, 15) on the role of temperamental individuality in such circular functions. This research leads also to a stress on the relation between person and context as central in such circular functions.

Temperament is defined by Thomas and Chess (14) as behavioral style or individuality—that is, how a person goes about doing whatever he does (e.g., fast or slow or with much or a little intensity)—and consists of nine attributes: rhythmicity, activity level, adaptability, approach/ withdrawal, mood, threshold of responsiveness, intensity of reaction, distractibility, and attention-span. Thomas and Chess (14, 15) suggest the impact of temperament for psychosocial adaptation lies in whether a person's characteristics of individuality provide a "goodness of fit" with the demands present in the physical and social context. A person's individuality, in meeting these demands, will provide a basis of the feedback he receives; thus, people whose temperamental characteristics fit their setting should show evidence of more adaptive behavioral functioning than should mismatched people.

Because goodness of fit has not been directly measured in the New York Longitudinal Study [NYLS (14)], data from the study provide only an indirect test of the model. In order to provide a more direct test, the present study assessed the temperamental attributes of adolescents in two junior high school contexts: academic (involving the teacher) and social (involving peers). The peer and teacher contexts were selected on the basis of their constituting two of the three most salient contexts (the family being the other) to adolescents (9). Teacher and peer demands/expectations regarding the temperamental attributes were assessed. Indices of personal and social adaptation were grade-point average, teacher's judgments of pupil academic and social competence, positive and negative peer relations, and self-esteem. It was predicted that temperamental differences should relate to both personal and social adaptation scores, and that better fit would be positively related to better adaptation scores.

METHOD

Subjects

Ss were enrolled in four eighth-grade classes of a junior high school located in a large suburb of New York City. All classes were taught by the same teacher. Of the 110 students in these classes 48 males and 51 females (mean age = 13.5 years, SD = .29) agreed to participate. Most Ss (75%) were white, 21% were black, and 4% were of another racial background. The largest proportion (64%) of students were Catholic, 28% were Protestants, 5% Jews, and 3% followed other religions.

Measures and Scoring

a. *Temperament*. The temperamental attributes of the Ss were assessed by having them respond in a group testing situation to the Dimensions of Temperament Survey (DOTS) developed by Lerner, Palermo, Spiro and Nesselroade (11). The version of the DOTS used consisted of 89 questions, each having a dichotomous ("more false than true," "more true than false") response format. Each item pertains to one of the nine categories of temperament associated with the Thomas and Chess (14) definition of temperament. The range of raw scores for each DOTS dimension is as follows: Activity Level, 0–12; Rhythmicity, 0–23; Adaptability, 0–10; Threshold, 0–10; Intensity of Reaction, 0–8; Mood, 0–6; Attention Span and Persistence, 0–6; Distractibility, 0–5; and Approach/Withdrawal, 0–9. High scores corresponded directly to the strength or degree of the respective dimensions. Since each attribute has different ranges of scores, all raw attribute scores are standardized by conversion Z scores. Reliability and validity data for this version of the DOTS are presented in Lerner et al. (11).

b. *Demands/expectations about temperament*. Demands/expectations were assessed for the school-social and the school-academic situation. For each situation actual and perceived demands were obtained. For each set of demands nine items were presented, one for each of the nine DOTS temperament dimensions. Actual demands were assessed by use of two questionnaires. The social (peer) demands questionnaire asked an S to indicate the actual demands regarding behavioral style held in regard to his peers. The second questionnaire asked the teacher to indicate behavioral style demands held in regard to his students. For the peer demands context, questions were phrased according to the following frame: "I *think* children should usually. . . ." For the teacher context the frames were, "I *expect* my students to be. . . ." Three response alternatives were available per item, and, since within a class the actual demands for both situations were the same for all Ss, 2 was used as the mean and a set of deviations was derived for each situation by subtracting the deviations of each actual demand from 2.[1]

Perceived demands were assessed by use of two questionnaires asking Ss to indicate the behavioral style demands they *perceived* imposed on them. For the peer context, questions were framed as, "My friends at school *want me* to usually. . . ." For the teacher context, questions were framed as, "My teacher *wants* me to usually. . . ." Perceived demands scores were standardized by conversion to Z scores.

c. Discrepancy scores. To assess goodness of fit, all Ss received four sets of discrepancy scores, one for each context: perceived peer, perceived teacher, actual peer, and actual teacher. Within each context there were nine different discrepancy scores, one for each temperamental attribute. The absolute value of the difference between an S's Z score for each attribute and the deviation score of the demand that pertained to that attribute were used to make up the set of discrepancy scores for all Ss over all contexts. For example, a Z score of +2.00 for the attribute Activity Level coupled with a Z score of −1.00 on the perceived demand for the peer situation would yield a discrepancy score of +3.00 for Activity Level. In addition, discrepancy scores were summed over the attributes for each context to obtain a total discrepancy score for each of the four situations. These scores indicated the total amount of discrepancy between attributes and demands for each situation, with high scores indicating a maximum amount of mismatch between attributes and demands, and low scores indicating a maximum amount of match between attributes and demands.

d. Self-esteem. Several outcome measures were obtained for each S. First, a measure of self-esteem was obtained. Twenty-five items from Coopersmith's Self-Esteem Inventory [SEI (4)] were used. Response alternatives were dichotomous ("like me" *vs* "unlike me") and scores ranged from zero to 25.

e. Positive and negative peer relations. An index of positive and negative peer relations, used by Lerner Lerner (8) and Lerner and Korn (7), was

---

[1] Copies of all demands questionnaires can be obtained from the author on request.

derived for each S by use of a list of positive and negative bipolar phrases describing nine positive social and personal attributes (other boys and girls like him/her, most want as a friend, happy, doesn't fight, has many friends, will be picked leader, picks the games to play, kind, and neat) and nine negative personal and social attributes (least want as a friend, gets teased, is left out of games, mean, sloppy, fights, sad, has few friends, and will not be picked leader). Ss respond by naming a boy (girl) in their class who best fits each item. An S's positive and negative peer relations score was derived by summing the favorable or unfavorable mentions, respectively, received from peers.

f. Teacher judgments of pupil academic and social competence. The teacher judged how competent he thought each S was academically and socially (irrespective of academic performance), by rating each one on a seven-point Likert-type scale with response alternatives ranging from "1" = "competence is extremely below average" to "7" = "competence is extremely above average."

g. Achievement. Current grades were gathered for all Ss, and were converted to a nine-point scale in order to obtain a grade-point average. The scale used was as follows: A+ (95–100) = 8; A (90–94) = 7; B+ (85–89) = 6; B (80–84) = 5; C+ (75–79) = 4; C (70–74) = 3; D+ (65–69) = 2; D (60–64) = 1; and F (0–59) = 0.

Procedure

In all classes testing was done on a group (classroom) basis during two 45-minute classes on successive days. During the first day Ss responded to the DOTS, and the teacher completed the actual demands questionnaire and rated the Ss' academic competence. During the second day the Ss responded to the SEI, the peer relations questionnaire, and the perceived and actual demands questionnaires, and the teacher gave his appraisal of the Ss' social competence.

RESULTS

Multiple Regressions

Preliminary analyses indicated no significant sex or classroom differences. Data were collapsed across these dimensions for further analysis. Multiple regression analyses were used to address the question of how well the temperamental attributes and the degree of match between attributes and demands predicted the outcome measures. The temperamental attributes and discrepancy scores were used as the predictors, and grade point average (GPA), teacher judgments of pupil academic competence (PAC) and pupil social competence (PSC), positive peer relations (PPR), negative peer relations (NPR), and self-esteem (SE) were used successively as the criterion measures.

Consistent with the work of Thomas and Chess (14) and the first prediction of this study, when the temperamental attributes are used as the predictors, all of the outcome measures were predicted (see Table 1). Data in the table also provide some support for the second prediction; that is, in most cases discrepancy (goodness of fit) scores also predict psychosocial adaptation. Specifically, for the two perceived contexts, the discrepancy scores predicted all outcome measures in regard to the perceived peer context, and in regard to the perceived teacher context all measures were predicted except PPR. For the actual contexts, the discrepancy scores from the actual peer context predicted all of the outcome measures except PPR, and the actual teacher context predicted four of the measures—GPA, PAC, PSC, and PPR.

In addition, the perceived discrepancy scores were related to more of the outcome measures than the actual discrepancy scores, indicating that it may be a person's perception of how his temperament fits the demands of his context that has most import for psychosocial adaptation. Furthermore, it seems that the peer contexts, both actual and perceived, are

TABLE 1
SUMMARY OF MULTIPLE REGRESSION ANALYSES: TOTAL R^2 ASSOCIATED
WITH SET OF PREDICTORS

	Predictors					
Outcome measure	TS	PSS	PSA	ASS	ASA	Total
Grade-point average	.322	.272	.205	.181	.135	.222
Perceived academic competence	.311	.281	.263	.148	.133	.238
Perceived social competence	.269	.258	.260	.178	.230	.128
Positive peer relations	.104	.156	—	—	.102	—
Negative peer relations	.240	.129	.114	.182	—	—
Self-esteem	.187	.152	.169	.104	—	—

Note: Predictors: TS = Temperament attribute scores alone; PSS = Perceived school-social context (nine discrepancy scores); PSA = Perceived school-academic context (nine discrepancy scores); ASS = Actual school-social context (nine discrepancy scores); ASA = Actual school-academic context (nine discrepancy scores); Total = Four total within-context discrepancy scores. Only R^2 values greater than .10 are reported.

more sensitive in the prediction of the outcome measures.[2] Finally, the fact that there is not perfect covariation between temperament scores and discrepancy scores in the prediction of the adaptational outcome measures of this study may be due to the differential limits of reliability of the measures derived from the different number of items used to obtain the discrepancy scores (nine items) and the temperament scores (89 items).

Analyses of Variance

In order to address further whether Ss assessed as having good fit were better adapted than those assessed as having poor fit, analyses of variance were performed. In these analyses the independent variable was the degree of fit (high vs low) for each situation. The 33 Ss with the lowest and highest total discrepancy scores were selected for each analysis ($X = 66$). There were significant differences for the high and low groups in two of the four situations, the perceived teacher and the perceived peer situations. For the perceived teacher context, the groups differed significantly on only one of the dependent measures, PSC, $F(1, 64) = 8.7$, $p < .005$. For the perceived teacher context, the congruent and incongruent groups differed significantly on the following: GPA, $F(1, 64) = 9.4$, $p < .003$; PSC, $F(1, 64) = 10.0$, $p < .003$; and PAC, $F < 1, 64) = 7.4$, $p < .009$. These findings provide some additional, moderate support for the second prediction—that Ss with the lowest discrepancy (best fit) scores would have higher adaptation scores than would Ss with the highest discrepancy scores. In addition, these findings again highlight the greater role of Ss' perception of their fit than of their actual fit.

DISCUSSION

The results indicate that temperament was implicated in the psychosocial adaptation to two features of the school context among the present sample of adolescents. These data are thus consistent with those existing for younger age levels (14), and provide some support for the view that

---

[2] Not all temperament dimensions, with respect to either temperament scores alone or the discrepancy scores, were equally implicated in the prediction of each of the six outcome measures. A table presenting the amount of variance accounted for by each temperamental dimension in each multiple regression analysis may be obtained from the author on request.

the link between temperament and adaptation may lie in whether temperament provides a goodness of fit with the demands of one's context. That is, those adolescents with the lowest discrepancy scores were better adapted than those with the highest discrepancy scores. This pattern was especially marked in the case of the perceived situations. That the perceived situations were more involved in the prediction of adaptation than were the actual situations suggests the importance of the role of cognitive processes in mediating between a person and his/her context. Such a phenomenon has been noted by others. Combs and Snygg (3), for example, maintain that a major factor governing the behavior of individuals is their unique perception of themselves and the world in which they live and the meanings things have for them. They also maintain that behavior is a reasonable and necessary result not of the physical situation or the objective situation but the perceived situation as it appears to the behaver. Similar views are also forwarded by Bronfenbrenner (2) and Sameroff (12).

The present results are limited by some of the methodological features of this research. That the discrepancy scores for the actual situations did not predict the outcome measures and the discrepancy scores from the perceived situations and, in particular, from the perceived peer situation, may be due to the fact that the demands for the actual situations were the same for all Ss, thus limiting the variability of the actual discrepancy scores. Similarly, although the DOTS' scores have adequate reliabilities for Ss of the age level assessed in this study (11), the demands questionnaires, comprised of only nine items each, may have both attenuated reliability and variability. Thus, discrepancy scores obtained from differences between attributes and demands may not have been as accurate as might have been the case had a set of demands questionnaires having more items been used. This could account for why there was not complete correspondence between discrepancy scores and the temperament scores alone in the prediction of the outcome measures.

In sum, because of the methodological issues raised here, the results of the present study must be interpreted with caution. Nevertheless, the fact that the data lend some support to the Thomas and Chess (14, 15) contextual goodness of fit model, even with these limitations, provides an encouraging basis for future research. Such research should expand on the present research design to include several contexts and longitudinal assessments. In addition, recasting the DOTS into a demands questionnaire could be done to obtain a reliable measure that can then be compared to attribute scores in order to derive more reliable discrepancy scores. Finally, a wide age range should be investigated in order to evaluate the generalizability of the model to all developmental periods, as well as the period of adolescence.

REFERENCES

1. Berscheid, E., and Walster, E. (1974). Physical attractiveness. In L. Berkowitz (Ed.), *Advances in experimental social psychology.* New York: Academic Press.
2. Bronfenbrenner, U. (1979). *The ecology of human development: Experiments by nature and design.* Cambridge, MA.: Harvard University Press.
3. Combs, A. W., and Snygg, D. (1959). *Individual behavior: A perceptual approach to behavior.* New York: Harper.
4. Coopersmith, S. (1967). *The antecedents of self-esteem.* San Francisco, CA: Freeman.
5. Lerner, R. M. (1976). *Concepts and theories of human development.* Reading, MA: Addison-Wesley.
6. Lerner, R. M., and Busch-Rossnagel, N. (1981). Individuals as producers of their development: Conceptual and empirical bases. In R. M. Lerner and N. Busch-Rossnagel (Eds.), *Individuals as producers of their development: A life-span perspective.* New *as producers of their development: A life-span perspective.* New York: Academic Press.
7. Lerner, R. M., and Korn, S. J. (1972). The development of body build stereotypes in males. *Child Development,* 43: 908–920.
8. Lerner, R. M., and Lerner, J. V. (1977). The effects of age, sex, and physical attractiveness on child-peer relations, academic performance, and elementary school adjustment. *Developmental Psychology,* 13: 585–590.
9. Lerner, R. M., and Spanier, G. B. (1980). *Adolescent development: A life-span perspective.* New York: McGraw-Hill.
10. Lerner, R. M., Hultsch, D. R., and Dixon, R. A. (in press). Contextualism and the character of developmental psychology in the 1970s. *Annals of the New York Academy of Science.*
11. Lerner, R. M., Palermo, M., Spiro, A., III, and Nesselroade, J. R. (1982). Assessing the dimensions of temperamental individuality across the life span: The Dimensions of Temperament Survey (DOTS). *Child Development,* 53: 149–159.
12. Sameroff, A. J. (1975). Transactional models in early social relations. *Human Development,* 18: 65–79.
13. Schneirla, T. C. (1957). The concept of development in comparative psychology. In D. B. Harris (Ed.), *The concept of development.* Minneapolis: University of Minnesota Press.
14. Thomas, A., and Chess, S. (1977). *Temperament and development.* New York: Brunner/Mazel.
15. ———. The role of temperament in the contributions of individuals to their development. In R. M. Lerner and N. A. Busch-Rossnagel (Eds.), *Individuals as producers of their own development: A life-span perspective.* New York: Academic Press.

Part V

SPECIAL STRESS AND COPING

In our own New York Longitudinal Study we have been deeply impressed by the human capacity for flexibility, adaptability, and mastery in the face of all kinds of adverse and stressful life situations. As we have said, "The emotionally traumatized child is not doomed, the parents' early mistakes are not irrevocable, and our preventative and therapeutic intervention can make a difference at all age-periods."

However, this does not mean that children or adults can be invulnerable to long-continued special stresses with which they cannot cope successfully. This we have seen in those of our subjects who developed persistent behavior disorders, and is also evident over and over again in clinical practice. The papers in this section examine different types of stress to which specific groups of children have been subjected, their coping mechanisms, and the short- and long-term effects.

Eiduson reports on the impact of conflict and stress on children in nontraditional families and compares the findings from studies of traditional family types. She finds that different life styles resonate differently to stressful events, and details a number of these differences. But she finds that as far as the children are concerned, alternative life styles offer no panaceas that will protect them from conflict or stress.

Wallerstein contributes a related report on her long-term study of the impact of divorce on the child. She emphasizes that this special stress poses long-term continuing demands for major psychological, social, and often economic reorganization, which may stretch over the years of childhood and adolescence. She formulates a series of six closely interrelated coping tasks which follow a temporal, hierarchical sequence beginning at the time of parental rupture and extending through adolescence. She emphasizes the positive psychological consequences for the child who copes successfully with these sequential tasks, though she also feels there may even then be some emotional residues which may or may not have negative consequences. She also indicates the influence of factors within the family following the divorce.

Our own report from the New York Longitudinal Study focuses on the relationship of early parental attitudes and divorce to young adult outcome. As such, it serves to complement Wallerstein's detailed account of the sequential coping demands on the children of divorce through the adolescent years. Our findings suggest that youngsters can usually cope more successfully with a single stress, even one as traumatic as parental divorce, than they can with one that is long-continued and persistent, such as parental conflict.

Kaffman and Elizur take up the issue of the early effects on and long-term consequences for preadolescent children of the death of their fathers in the Israeli-Egyptian war of October 1973. Of special interest is the difference in the responses of the kibbutz children and those living in urban settings. Clearly, it was not the single event of the father's death alone which was responsible for the child's ability to deal with this sudden bereavement experience. Rather, it was the nature of the family and community structure and support system, as well as the additional stressful changes that resulted from the father's death, which affected the child's ability to cope with this traumatic event.

Finally, Terr reports a four-year follow-up of the psychological consequences of the Chowchilla school-bus kidnapping on the children involved in this most terrifying experience. Her first report concerned the acute psychological disturbances after the event, which in many cases were ubiquitous, varied in their manifestations, and severe. In this four-year follow-up she reports the persistence of a number of symptoms such as anxiety and repetitive nightmares. Her findings indicate, however, that for most of the children the symptoms were diminishing, and the children were functioning adequately, academically and socially. Denial and conscious repression were frequent and effective coping devices. It was also evident that for a number of the children, the kidnapping did not represent a single, time-limited trauma. Recognized by strangers, they were frequently reminded by others of the event, and asked to describe what had happened. This they found embarrassing and disturbing, perhaps because this interfered with the success of their denial coping strategies. Thus, this follow-up report indicates that a severe unique traumatic event can have psychological consequences which are not short-lived, but that children can find coping mechanisms which over time can ameliorate and resolve the effects of such a terrifying experience.

16

Conflict and Stress in Nontraditional Families: Impact on Children

Bernice T. Eiduson

School of Medicine, University of California at Los Angeles

Particular stresses and certain kinds of conflict appear to be associated with each of the different family styles under study. Responses to stressful events also differ distinctly by family style. Aspects of children's intellectual performance and social-emotional behavior are negatively affected by stress, but in some types of families children are found to be more buffered than in others.

If the current divorce rate in the United States is any indication, being married is a hazardous enterprise. It is hazardous for the adults directly involved, and for the children of divorce who are put at emotional risk for potentially long-standing, in some cases irreversible, effects.[12,16] This paper will consider the extent to which alternative family styles differ from traditional two-parent nuclear families with respect to interpersonal strife and conflict. In particular, it will focus on whether the nontraditional family provides ways of living that are less stressful for children.

Some of the participants in our study of alternative life styles had become cognizant as children of the unhappiness of their own parents with each other, and of the emptiness of their families during their

Reprinted with permission from the *American Journal of Orthopsychiatry*, 1983, Vol. 53, No. 3, 126–435. Copyright 1983 by the American Orthopsychiatric Association, Inc.

Presented at the 1982 annual meeting of the American Orthopsychiatric Association in San Francisco. Research was supported in part by grants from the Carnegie Corporation of New York (B4198–09); U.S. Public Health Service; National Institute of Mental Health (5R01, MH24947–09); and by a Research Scientist Award (NIMH 70541–10).

childhood.[9] Although generally successful and affluent, their parents had been troubled by alcoholism, ulcers, and neuroses. The nontraditional family was not seen by our participants as an environment in which conflict was absent; in fact, the early dissolution of many of the "new families" attested to their strife and divisiveness.[2] Conflict-free utopias have historically been elusive, frustrating, and disappointing. Yet, the study participants hoped that countervailing forces in their alternative family styles might mitigate relationship difficulties, and protect children from the scars of unhappy homes.

Our consideration of the kinds of conflicts and stresses faced by non-traditional families will be based on a number of data sources:

1. The nature of conflicts specific to each of the four family styles represented in our study, as derived from interview and questionnaire data, will be reported.

2. A second source is a quantitative study that identified and compared the kind and extent of stress found in each family style.[7] In this study, 45 stressful events likely to have a negative effect on the young child were derived from data collected in the project. These were assigned weights for their likely deleterious effect on the child by six clinicians, and total stress scores for each year of the child's life were developed. Scores for four subcategories of stressors were also obtained: a) scores for life-style change events, such as moves, separations, and divorces; b) scores for parent psychological status events, such as depression or emotional disturbance; c) scores for parent-child relationship problems, such as neglect or rejection; and d) scores for stresses directly impinging upon the child, such as development of a physical impairment.

3. A third data source is a composite or summary score developed to reflect conflict or tension between mates.

The impact on the child in terms of cognitive and intellectual findings and social and emotional behavior, including the development of symptoms and problems during the first four years of the child's life, will also be considered.

COMMUNAL LIVING GROUPS

Parkinson's Law states that the level of conflict in a family rises exponentially with the number of persons in the family. In the communal living group there are two-and-one-half times as many people, on the average, as in a two-parent nuclear family: twice as many adults and twice as many children.[18] Almost all of our communal families share public space as well as having private quarters. Participants report that conflict arises from reality difficulties that accompany sharing space, tasks, and assignments. Consulting everyone to make decisions and pursue activities can be trying and tedious and lead to the feeling that nothing is ever easily done. Rivalries and resistances lead to dissension and open quarrels.[15]

Participants feel they have limited control over their interpersonal lives. Because much relevant decision-making about roles and relationships is taken over by the family group, roles and relationships are frequently rehashed and reclarified, with group members seeming in constant negotiation with each other.[14] Power coalitions develop and change, and these affect what is happening in dyadic relationships —between men and women, and between adults and children.

It is often difficult to resolve interpersonal problems in the fishbowl atmosphere of a communal group. Everyone knows when partners quarrel, when a mother is depressed, when marriages are under strain. The group inevitably seems to intrude on personal difficulties,[13] and a self-consciousness in relationships results. Adults report the need to maintain the image of being a good parent or contented wife, a burdensome and guilt-producing responsibility. When a small family unit that is nested within the larger communal group has troubles, there are forces that impede their problem-solving, and that make it easier for them to give up. Each partner in a troubled couple is continually in contact with other people who may be seen as potential replacements in the relationship. At the same time, group roles, the individual's tasks and assignments, are primarily delegated on an individual basis; one can remain part of the communal group even if the dyadic relationship is dissolved.[3]

Parents in a communal group feel the pressure of the judgmental eyes of the others.[14] Differences in parenting styles and preferences are rampant; even in highly structured groups, there may be some general perspectives on handling life situations but few specific guidelines.[18] In many situations, parents feel themselves to be on shaky ground, and the advice of others is sometimes given too freely. At times, however, other families in the communal group may provide needed assistance to parents in their relationships with their children. For example, an adolescent may live temporarily with another family group until the intensity of a problem with his or her parents diminishes.

By and large, communal living groups present problems for the children. They can have too many adults to listen to. While there are many mammas, children often have the feeling that no single one will protect and stand up specifically for them. Children who see their own parents treating all children equally may feel insecure about "who's for me."

This is especially true in group families having many children, where there is competition, intense activity, and many "battles" to settle. Non-biological "brothers and sisters" do, however, act as allies, companions, and teachers who care very deeply for each other.[2]

Among our four family types, the communal living group is characterized by the highest number of parent-child separations of more than a two-week period during the child's first three years.[8] In the communal family, children also seem to be more unscheduled (data usually noted in home observations). Another stress unique to this type of family is the relative absence of stimulating toys and playthings. There is also a greater likelihood that the young child will be exposed to adult sexuality. In the domestic living groups, the families in which social, artistic, and political commonalities act as bonds of friendship, mothers report having a harder time with children. This type of family group also experiences severe financial stresses. By the time the child is between three and four years old, the same stresses experienced in the first three years continue to impinge on these families. In addition, in some families, there is parental neglect of the child, with the home environment being reported by observers as having more potential dangers.

Despite these kinds of stresses, the communal group also has the lowest total stress levels of all our alternative families. In line with this finding, when we look at the extent of tension between mates or living partners, we find that communal families receive the lowest scores at all time periods in the first six years, as compared to the other family styles. The only point at which stress scores were more elevated than in the other groups (and this to a statistically significant degree) was in the first year, when we found stressful events associated with parent-child relationships particularly high for creedal living groups. This is a consistent finding in every one of the first four years, although there are no significant differences among alternative families in years two and four.[8]

THE SINGLE-MOTHER FAMILY

By contrast, the stresses that are idiosyncratic to our smallest family unit, the single-mother family, derive not from having a lot of people around but from being isolated and missing consistent and satisfying interpersonal interactions with others.[4] Our single mothers report loneliness, a need for companionship, and dissatisfaction with their status, once the blush of being a "pioneering" single woman wears off. By the time the child is a year old the realities of the single life—economic, occupational, and parental—are unmistakable, and problems of overload and unhappiness mitigate the satisfactions the infant provides. Single mothers miss having someone with whom to share the financial, work, and domestic burdens and joys that come with having a child. As is the case in the general population, our single-parent families are financially handicapped, having lower vocational skills than other alternative women, and considerably lower than our traditionally married mothers.[10]

The single mother lives in a household beset by frequent changes.[6] There are more changes in roommates (male or female) than in any other type of family, and more marriages during the first three years of the child's life. Family members are more often observed or reported as rejecting of the child than in other family groups.[8] There is also a higher incidence of single parents than others reported by our interviewers and observers as being emotionally troubled. Of the three children given up for adoption by age four, two are children of single mothers. In addition, the highest incidence of overprotection of the child is reported in this sample.

Our findings point to the first year of the child's life as being most stressful for the single-parent household. Total stress scores are significantly higher than for communal group or traditional families. In the child's second year, the total stress scores remain high but are not significantly different from those of other types of families. An overall summary of the incidence of weighted stressful events during the child's first through third years finds the single mothers at the top of the list. By the time the child is three or four, single-mother families continue to show high stress scores, second only to those of social-contract families.

The difficulties to which single-mother families are most prone are in the area of parental psychological stress. Contributing to high scores in this area are such discrete events as the mother's being unemployed against her will, suffering extreme financial hardships, or being reported as emotionally disturbed, even hospitalized for emotional reasons. It is with respect to parents' psychological status that significant differences are found among our family groups. Although the differences among groups did not rest primarily in the differences between single mothers and all other women, invariably the single mother tended to receive high stress scores. While there is some conflict with roommates or persons sharing quarters, this is far lower than in other groups simply because more than 50% of this sample of women remain single during the child's early life.

THE SOCIAL-CONTRACT FAMILY

The social-contract family is particularly interesting in regard to conflict, since it depends on maintaining strong emotional involvement and positive interpersonal relationships.[17] No formal ties exist. A partner can break up the family at any moment by walking out. Intimacy and directness are strong features of this relationship. Families do everything together, and enjoy each other's closeness. Children in social-contract families generally do not perceive their families as being any different than those of traditional, married parents. The children have close contacts with their father, who is likely to do more caretaking than other fathers, since he is often committed to egalitarian sharing of parental roles.[11] Because they spend more time with their parents, children are expected to adjust to adult activities and interests.[9] They go almost everyplace with parents and often spend less time with baby-sitters or grandparents than do children in other families.[10] The demand is made on children to grow up rapidly, to be sensitive to any shifts in the home, and to get their satisfactions from the small, intimate, close family unit, as their parents do.[3]

There are fewer economic resources in this family than in other families where fathers are present.[10] As a result, the children are less frequently sent to nursery school in the preschool years or to caretakers outside the home, at least until age four.[10] Because of this family's resistance to dependence on existing societal institutions and on professional experts, the children are also least likely to have had experiences that prepare them for conventional schools or involvement with other traditional community institutions.[6]

In the social-contract family, which was formed without legal bonds between parents, we find the highest number of marriages in the first three years of the child's life and the highest number of divorces between ages three and four.[8] Relations have some permanency; 68% of the social-contract partners are with their original partners through the child's fourth year, with half having married and the others still living together. The parents in this family group are involved with the highest number of social problem events—unemployment, occasional short periods in jail, drug abuse, etc.[8] When the child is three years old, there are significantly more social-contract women working at night than in other families. This family also had fewer births following that of the child being studied.

In the first two years of the child's life, social-contract families have the second highest total stress scores, exceeded only by the single-mother family.[7] In the third year the total stress scores are the highest of any group, a statistically significant finding. The stressful events notable in the social-contract family are parental psychological stresses—the same group affecting single-parent families. In the first year of the child's life, and for the first three years taken together, parental psychological stress is higher in this family group than in any other. In the child's fourth year, the level of parental psychological stress is more than one-and-one-half times the average of the rest of the sample.

The level of tension between mates is higher in the social-contract family than in any other group. However, in subsequent years, the amount of tension steadily drops; by the time the child is six, tension with mate is the lowest in any family unit, a finding brought about by the separation of parents who could not get along.

THE TRADITIONAL MARRIED FAMILY

The traditional married sample has the most stable life style of any of our participants.[10] They have fewer marriages, fewer mate changes, fewer divorces, fewer residential changes, fewer changes in household membership, and less drug use. However, the number of mothers who have worked full-time since the project child was born is the highest in this group. Our traditional marrieds also have had more new babies in the family following the birth of the target child. In all the early years of childhood, scores reflecting parental psychological stress, parent-child difficulties, or events reflecting reality changes in the household tend to run in the low or middle ranges for this sample.

However, when we look at the extent of conflict or tension with mate, the traditional married families have the highest scores. This finding was first made when the child was one year old, again at three, and at six years, the points in time at which data were summarized. This is a consistent finding whether we look at families traditionally married at the time the sample was selected or at all the families who have become traditionally married in the subsequent years of the project. Thus, interpersonal problems that are expressed in the high divorce rate in the general population, and which our alternative subjects saw in their own parents at least two decades ago, characterize our traditional two-parent nuclear families. However, our traditional families have a lower divorce rate than is found in the general population during the first three years of the child's life. It appears that these traditional parents struggle and live with tensions that some in our other groups resolve by making family changes.

IMPACT ON COGNITIVE AND INTELLECTUAL DEVELOPMENT

Our studies of the cognitive development of children in alternative families show that, in general, the child who experiences elevated levels of stress in the family is likely to have lower scores on intelligence tests, such as the Stanford-Binet, by age three.[7] This holds for the entire sample as well as for each family style. Children exposed to frequent moves, family break-ups, or heavy drug or alcohol use have a greater likelihood of performing at a lower level than do children whose family stress levels have not been so elevated. This important relationship between infant development (Bayley) scores and stress scores is noted in the child's first year, and persists, though not as strongly, into the second and third years. The relationship holds more strongly for children of single mothers and children in traditional families, than for those in social-contract and communal families.[17] The latter are families in which change events and stress seem more "ego-syntonic"; thus, perhaps the impact on the child's intellectual development during the early years is mitigated.[7]

There also appears to be a difference between alternative and traditional families in the level of stress that triggers disruptions in a child's intellectual growth. In the traditional married group, which has low levels of stress (the lowest total stress score of all our groups), a child who experiences even minimal stress levels shows lowered intellectual functioning at three years. Apparently, in a generally stable and uneventful environment, the occurrence of relatively little stress affects the child's intellectual development; children may be unprepared to cope with it.

The events most likely to affect intellectual performance at three years are those that relate to the parent's personal sense of well-being, and those that refer to a troubled relationship between parent and child. While this is true for the sample as a whole, in the first three years, the child most susceptible to low cognitive scores if the mother herself has psychological problems is the child of a single parent. However, it is the communal group child whose intellectual scores are lowered when there are parent-child relationship stresses. Life-style changes taking place in the second year lower third-year functioning of the social-contract and communal group child.

When the communal group child is three, stressful events that directly impinge on the child—such as adoption, child hospitalization, accidents, physical deformities, or congenital problems—depress the child's intellectual functioning. For the social-contract child of three years, parental psychological events, those that also handicap the child of the single mother, seem critical. For the child in the traditional married family, however, such changes as moves, divorces, or separations in the family are the kinds of events that lower cognitive scores. Our data therefore suggest that the different kinds of stress which we have identified as more likely to be associated with the various family groups, differentially affect how a child functions intellectually.

IMPACT ON SOCIAL AND EMOTIONAL COMPETENCE

The social and emotional competence of the three-year-old was assessed using summary measures of behavior such as cooperativeness, compliance, aggression, hostility, anxiety, etc., each of which was separately measured on a variety of assessments such as the Ainsworth Strange Situation Test, tests of frustration tolerance, independence, fantasy play, etc.[5] In general, life-style events—mobility, changes in household membership, etc.—were the types of stress that negatively affected the social and emotional competence of the three-year-old child, and most severely so for the single-mother and social-contract families.

However, low social and emotional competence scores do not necessarily go hand in hand with elevated stress in the family. For example, children of single mothers seem most likely to have poor social and emotional competence scores under stress, even when family stress scores for this sample are lower than for other groups. As a group, children of single mothers fare well with respect to overall social and emotional competence summarized at age three. However, when family stress centers around parent-child relationships, the toll is expressed in lowered social and emotional competence. The child with one parent seems poorly equipped to cope with such relationship problems.

Whatever the life style, when the parent shows personal psychological problems, the social and emotional competence of the offspring tends to be lowered. If such problems occur as early as age one in social-contract families, or ages two and three in single-parent households, children's functioning is lowered.[1]

CHILD SYMPTOMATOLOGY

Mothers reported symptoms of children on a standard symptom checklist at ages four, five, and six. Prior to age four, functional difficulties or problems in eating, sleeping, toilet habits, and other developmental behavior were also recorded. Using these reports, we summarized the extent of problems for each child, and thus were able to identify children who might be vulnerable.

Our preliminary analyses of these data show that, for the sample as a whole, high stress scores are associated with parents' having negative perceptions of their children. (Four factors had been produced when parents periodically rated their child on 98 adjectives; the factors were shy, independent, confident, and difficult. Ratings done independently at each time period proved to be highly positively correlated over time.) Elevated family stress levels in the first year are associated with the child being called shy at 18 months, and associated with the child being called shy and difficult at 24 months. High stress at age two is associated with children being perceived by parents as difficult at that point. Families with high weighted stress scores over the first three years perceive children as difficult at 24 months. The parents' psychological status events and parent-child relationship events at age one and parent conflicts at age two are found positively related to parents' perception of children as difficult and not independent or confident at 18 and 24 months. Further, if a parent reports that a child has numerous problems in the early years, there is good likelihood that the parent will consider that child difficult at 24 months.

From our analyses of the summary scores reflecting children's problems from birth on, family life style does not seem to make a difference with respect to the number of problems. The average number of problems for the entire sample is low—between three and four out of a possible 36—and there are no life-style differences in the number or type of problems children develop at ages one, three, or six. There are also no statistically significant differences in terms of the number of symptoms identified by mothers at four, five, or six, as a function of life style. Thus, whether a child has grown up in an alternative or a traditional family does not seem to predispose the child to symptomatology, on the basis of parental reports.

CONCLUSIONS

None of the alternative life styles studied is free from conflict, tension, or stress. However, the traditional, married two-parent nuclear family, overall, experiences fewer of the kind of events considered likely to be stressful for the young child. Different types of stress seem to be present in different kinds of families. For the traditional family, two types of experience are particularly stressful: 1) moves and changes in the household, and other reality or external events; and 2) conflict or tension between mates, which is generally higher throughout the first six years than in any other family group. There are fewer divorces and separations than in other types of families, suggesting that the traditional couple is likely to stay together in spite of conflict. In the social-contract family and for the single-mother group, parents' psychological status events, such as maternal depression and emotional disturbance, are noteworthy. For the communal group, stresses in the parent-child relationship area stand out.

Different life styles resonate to stressful events differently. A relatively small amount of stress is likely to be extremely disruptive to the child in the traditional family. Family groups that are used to solving problems through effecting external changes, as do social-contract or communal families, can experience a great deal of stressful change of the kind normally considered disruptive, but these do not prove to be as stressful to their children; in these families, change is a common way of solving problems. The single-mother family, while not necessarily experiencing the greatest amount of stress, is most susceptible when it occurs.

Family style thus has a bearing on whether or not conflicts and stress affect the child. The child of a single mother seems the most poorly buffered against conflict and stress. Cognitive performance as early as one year is negatively affected, and this consistently holds at two years (maternal ratings) and at three (when Stanford-Binet scores are lowered). The social competence of the social-contract child is affected in a significant way by stresses during the first year. These remain high in subsequent years, although they are not associated in a statistically significant way at two and three years. Attachment to the mother, tested typically at one year, finds the social-contract child who has experienced stress to be more anxiously attached than are children in any other family group.

Child symptomatology at four, five, and six does not differ by life style. Nor is there any association between level of parental tension and symptom formation in the children. However, there are significant associations between children perceived as difficult or shy by parents at 18 and 24 months and the symptoms shown in early life.

So far as children are concerned, alternative life styles offer no panacea that will protect them from conflict or stress. There are plusses and minuses in being raised in each of the various family styles, and some potentially negative fallout for the child. Our later data should add more conclusive information to these trend data.[1] As yet, there is no family life style that can be recommended as free of conflict or stress for the developing child.

REFERENCES

1. Alexander, J. (1978). Marriages without weddings: Changes in the American family. Unpublished doctoral dissertation. Institute for Clinical Social Work: Los Angeles.
2. Cohen, J. and Eiduson, S. (1975). Changing patterns of childrearing in alternative life styles: Implications for development. In *Child Personality and psychopathology: Current topics*. A. David ed. John Wiley, New York.
3. Eiduson, B. (1978). Emergent families of the 1970's: Values, practices, and impact on children. In *The family: Dying or developing*. D. Reiss and H. Hoffman, eds. Plenum Press, New York.
4. Eiduson, B. (1980). Contemporary single mothers. In *Current topics in early childhood education* (Vol. 3). L. Katz, ed. Ablex, Norwood, N.J.
5. Eiduson, B. (1981). Parent-child relationships in alternative family styles. Presented to the Society for Research in Child Development, Boston.
6. Eiduson, B. (1982). Non-nuclear families: vulnerabilities, stresses and implications for policy. Presented to the American Orthopsychiatric Association, San Francisco.
7. Eiduson, B. and Forsythe, A. (1981). Life change events in alternative family styles. In *Life-span developmental psychology: Non-normative life events*. E. Callahan and K. McCluskey, eds. Academic Press, New York.
8. Eiduson, B. and Forsythe, A. (1982). Comparative study of parent-child stresses in non-traditional and traditional families. Presented to the International Conference for Infant Studies, Austin.
9. Eiduson, B., Cohen, J. and Alexander, J. (1973). Alternatives in child-rearing in the 1970s. *Amer. J. Orthopsychiat.* 43:721–731.
10. Eiduson, B. et al. (1981). Comparative socialization practices in alternative family settings. In *Nontraditional families*. M. Lamb, ed. Plenum Press, New York.
11. Eiduson, B. and Weisner, T. (1978). Alternative family styles: Effects on young children. In *Mother/child, father/child relationships*. J. Stevens and M. Mathews, eds. National Association for the Education of Young Children, Washington, D.C.
12. Hetherington, E., Cox, M. and Cox, R. (1977). The aftermath of divorce. In *Mother/child, father/child relationships*. J. Stevens and M. Mathews, eds. National Association for the Education of Young Children, Washington, D.C.
13. Kanter, R. (1972). 'Getting it all together': Some group issues in communes. *Amer. J. Orthopsychiat.* 42(4):632–643.
14. Kanter, R., Jaffe, D. and Weisberg, D. (1975). Coupling, parenting, and the presence of others: Intimate relationships in communal household. *Fam. Coord.* 24:433–452.
15. Slater, P. (1963). On social regression. *Amer. Sociol. Rev.* 28:339–364.
16. Wallerstein, J. and Kelly, J. (1980). *Surviving the breakup: How children and parents cope with divorce.* Basic Books, New York.
17. Weisner, T., Eiduson, B. and Forsythe, A. (1981). Cultural mediation of stress in conventional and nonconventional families. Presented to the Society for Research in Child Development, Boston.
18. Weisner, T. and Martin, J. (1979). Learning environments for infants: Communes and conventionally married families in California. *Alternative Lifestyles* 2:201–242.

17

Children of Divorce: The Psychological Tasks of the Child

Judith S. Wallerstein, Ph.D.

Center for the Family in Transition, Corte Madera, California

Long-range outcomes for the child of divorce are related to factors within the family following divorce, and to the child's mastery of specific threats to development, which are here conceptualized as six interrelated hierarchical coping tasks. Beginning at the separation and culminating in young adulthood, these tasks add substantially to the normal challenges of growing up.

Divorce represents a special kind of stressful experience for the child who has been reared within a two-parent family. The child's experience in divorce is comparable in several ways to the experience of the child who loses a parent through death or to the child who loses his or her community following a natural disaster. Each of these experiences strikes at and disrupts close family relationships. Each weakens the protection that the nuclear family provides, leaving in its wake a diminished, more vulnerable family structure. Each traces a pattern of time that begins with an acute, time-limited crisis, and is followed by an extended period of disequilibrium which may last several years—or even longer—past the central event. And each introduces a chain of long-lasting changes that are not predictable at the outset and that reach into multiple domains of family life.

Reprinted with permission from the *American Journal of Orthopsychiatry*, 1983, Vol. 53, No. 2, 230–243. Copyright 1983 by the American Orthopsychiatric Association, Inc.

Presented at the 1982 annual meeting of the American Orthopsychiatric Association, in San Francisco. Research was supported by the San Francisco Foundation and the Zellerbach Family Fund.

Thus, divorce, bereavement, and the loss of community pose powerful continuing demands for major psychological, social, and often economic reorganization. For the child, the readjustments that are required are likely, in our observations, to stretch over the years of childhood and adolescence. We have conceptualized these required readjustments as a series of tasks to be addressed immediately as well as over the many years that follow. In accord with Erikson's architectural conception of the tasks that attend the successive stages of the life cycle,[4] and in accord with the formulations of Lindemann[10] and Caplan[3] regarding the succession of tasks imposed by bereavement, elaborated later and more complexly within crisis theory, this paper will delineate a series of tasks that attend the child's experience in the divorcing family. These are the coping tasks that are shaped by the threats or perceived threats to psychic integrity and development which the divorce process poses to the child. They are conceptualized as hierarchical, as following a particular time sequence beginning with the critical events of parental separation and culminating at late adolescence and young adulthood.

The reorganization and readjustments that are required of the child of the divorcing family, namely the tasks that need to be addressed, represent a major addition to the expectable customary tasks of childhood and adolescence in our society. In this view, the child of divorce faces a special set of challenges and carries an added burden.

There is, as we have found from many years of observation, no necessary progression toward resolution or closure to the dissolution experience. Although many divorcing families make their way through the acute phase of the divorce experience and after several years of disequilibrium reach stability and closure in the postdivorce or remarried family, the family may remain fixated for many years at the acute phase of the divorce. Chronically litigating couples certainly fall within this category of conflict-fixated behavior; but others who never enter the court arena may also remain fixated at the acute, conflict-ridden phase. Or, the adults or one adult may remain for years fixated at the state of transition or disequilibrium of "trying out a range of coping strategies," as Hetherington[5] characterized this phase, or as a *chronically reconstituting family*, as described felicitously by Hunter and Schuman.[7] Children in these families are especially hindered in their own efforts to reach closure. And while they may sometimes succeed in addressing the tasks imposed by divorce, they are more likely under these difficult circumstances to falter or to fail at any point along the way. Oppositely, if the parents have resolved their conflicts following the divorce, and successfully made use of the second chance provided by the divorce to improve the quality of life for adults *and* children, then the children are more likely to emerge happy and well.

The child's resolution of the tasks of divorce is profoundly influenced by the family ambiance and by the extent to which the family has made progress in addressing the many issues to which divorce gives rise. We have earlier reported the various factors within the family that are significantly linked with good or poor outcome during the post-divorce years.[16] Certainly, the adjustment within the family is a major influence on the child's capacity to navigate successfully the divorce-engendered problem. The family's balance of unresolved conflict, of qualified support or nonsupport of the child's struggles, of continued deprivation or exploitation of the child all play a very formative role in helping the child's ultimate outcome. Yet, all of these factors notwithstanding, it is still the child who must carry the burden of mastery and resolution on the way to a successfully achieved adulthood. For there is no necessary *determining* relationship between the resolutions and the adjustments achieved by either of the adult parties to the divorce proceedings and the outcome for any particular child. And, in fact, within the same divorcing family there is considerable variation in the outcomes that are achieved by siblings, dependent on both their particular role in the strife-torn family constellation and their individual developmental position and psychological strengths and resourcefulness. Therefore, mastery or failure as outcomes require separate scrutiny and understanding of the child and of the child's efforts on his or her own behalf.

My colleagues and I have followed over many years the course of 60 divorcing families with children from the time of the decisive marital separation and the initial filing for dissolution through the first five years following divorce and, more recently, through the first ten-year period. The sample drawn in 1971 from a Northern California population of primarily, but not entirely, white, middle-class families consisted at the outset of 60 divorcing families with 131 children aged three to 18 at the time of the decisive separation. The families were seen again a year later, or approximately 18 months after separation. By that time most were legally divorced. They were seen again at the five-year mark by the same clinical team. At that time, 58 of the original 60 families were recontacted. Finally, during the year 1981–82, at the ten-year mark, we have renewed contact with the same families using three members of the original five-person clinical team, and we have been successful thus far in reaching 86%, or 51 families and 98 children. The methods of the project and its findings at the decisive separation, at 18 months and at five years have been previously reported.[8,9,11–18]

The children's initial response to the marital rupture as manifest in play, fantasy, verbal communication, and behavior in the various settings of clinic, home, and school were described in detail in the early publications of the project. By and large, the acute symptomatic responses such as separation phobias, anxiety reactions, ego regressions, sleep disturbances, and acute mourning reactions came to an end within the first year or year-and-a-half following the decisive separation. It was not uncommon for the symptomatic responses of the children to subside before the adults had reached a state of restored equilibrium. There was no significant relation between the intensity and pervasiveness of the child's initial symptomatic response and the child's overall adjustment at the five-year mark. But the feelings aroused by the separation, the anger at one or both parents, the profound and sometimes pervasive sorrows, the sense of vulnerability, the concern with being unloved and perhaps unlovable, the yearning for the departed parent, the intense worry over the parents, the loyalty conflict, the general sense of neediness and being overburdened, the nostalgia for the intact family—these were more likely to remain in place and endure long after the symptomatic responses and regressions had disappeared.

Indeed, it is strikingly clear that five and ten years after the marital rupture the divorce remains for many children and adolescents the central event of their growing-up years and casts a long shadow over these years. Its effects are difficult to observe and even more difficult to separate out precisely because early symptoms and initial regressions do not endure and because, in fact, many responses do not appear as symptoms at all. But the effects are incorporated within the character, the attitudes, the relationships, the self-concept, the expectations, and the world view of the child. Over the course of time they are profoundly modified by the enfolding developmental stages and by subsequent life experiences and life decisions related and unrelated to events within the family. Each of these experiences interweaves complexly within the overall functioning of the child and yet at time stands out sharply. We have been startled to find young adults at the ten-year follow-up who remain intensely preoccupied with a parent's infidelity ten years earlier or other youngsters, who were age two or three at the time of the marital separation, who wept uncontrollably and seemed unable to leave our office, where they cried for an intact family they had hardly known and for close contact with a father they had encountered over the years as a capricious or disinterested parent.

This paper is an attempt to integrate some of these findings into theoretical formulations that can shed light on the long-term impact of divorce on the child. The concept of *task* will be presented as a guide in threading our way through the many unresolved issues and complex questions that attend and perhaps bedevil current efforts to examine long-term relatedness. Since 1980 my colleagues and I in the newly established Center for the Family in Transition, in Northern California, have attempted to translate these formulations. The family-centered and group-centered programs that have grown out of this work, together with a comprehensive assessment of their effectiveness and their limitations, will be presented at a future time.

SIX PSYCHOLOGICAL TASKS

We turn now to the tasks themselves. As formulated here they are six in number. They fall into an enfolding sequence with varying time spans attached for the accomplishment of each. Several tasks, namely Task I, Acknowledging the Reality of the Marital Rupture, and Task II, Disengaging From Parental Conflict and Distress and Resuming Customary Pursuits, need to be addressed immediately at the time of the decisive separation and then optimally resolved within the first year. The child's successful mastery of the two immediate tasks is tied to the maintenance of his or her appropriate academic pace and overall developmental agenda after the initial dip at the time of crisis. But the child's successful mastery of the divorce engendered stress is only partially related to the early period following the marital rupture. Task III, which is conceptualized as the Resolution of Loss; Task IV, which involves Resolving Anger and Self-Blame; and Task V, which involves Accepting the Permanence of the Divorce, are unlikely to be resolved during the first year or two following the marital rupture. Rather, they extend over many years and, as we have described elsewhere,[16,18] are worked and reworked by the child over a long period of time until they become salient together with Task VI during adolescence. This last task, which we have called Achieving Realistic Hope Regarding Relationships, presents a set of issues that the young person confronts primarily during the adolescent years and perhaps at entry to young adulthood, as well.

Task I: Acknowledging the Reality of the Marital Rupture

The first and simplest task for the child is to acknowledge the reality of the marital rupture and to understand the family and household changes that ensue separate from the frightening fantasies which have been evoked in the child's mind.

Overall, the child's perceptions and understanding of the family events are filtered through a prism that has been cut and shaped by the child's chronological age and developmentally-related needs, conflicts, and wishes, as well as a great many factors, including individual differences. The major divorce-related obstacles to an accurate, age-appropriate acknowledgement are the child's vivid and terrifying fantasies of parental abandonment and disaster; these have been triggered by the parental conflict, by the troubled—sometimes wildly raging, bizarre, and unprecedented—behavior of one or both parents, and by the departure of one parent from the home. And as so often happens, the macabre conclusions to which the child's fantasy constructions lead far exceed the unhappy reality. Additionally, the hapless child's fear of being overwhelmed by the intense feelings of sorrow, anger, rejection, and yearning further block the acknowledgement of the family rupture. Therefore, the child's powerful need to deny, to defer, and to avoid the terrifying thoughts and feelings is greatly strengthened and is joined with the comfort derived from fantasy and denial. Sometimes the power of fantasy is called upon additionally to undo and reverse the distressing reality. Indeed, fantasy can undo the child's feelings of powerlessness and enable the child heroically to mend the rift and reunite the parents or reunite the child with the departed parent. All of the preschool children in our study who played house placed the mother and father dolls in bed together, hugging each other. The complex ego-syntonic interweaving of denial through fantasy with the child's enfolding developmental agenda was so well reflected in the response of little girls at the oedipal stage of development in their response to the father's departure:

> "My daddy sleeps in my bed every night," we were informed by a smiling child who had not seen her father for many weeks. "He will come back to me when *he* grows up," another bravely assured us and herself.

We have elsewhere described the diminished parenting, the lessened supports from the parents and other adults, and the failure of so many parents to explain the family events to the children or to prepare them for what lay ahead.[16] Given the powerful fears generated by the family events it is understandable that the falling away of parental support at this critical time would gravely burden the child, especially the young child, in this first task of coming to grips with reality.

Younger children are especially disadvantaged in grasping the meaning of divorce. This observation may shed light on the severity of the responses that we found in the preschool and early latency groups. Their limited grasp of time, of calendar, of space, of distance, of concepts such as marriage, separation, and divorce burdened their struggles to understand the course of events in the family:

> "Where is Oakland?" wailed one seven-year-old boy whose father had moved to Oakland. "Is Oakland in Mexico, and where is Mexico?" he asked us anxiously.

The lacunae in the young children's understanding fostered greater dependence on fantasy and further blocked understanding. Their age-appropriate difficulty in separating reality and fantasy rendered them especially vulnerable to intense, frightening fantasies. And the anxiety-driven ego regressions reinforced their vulnerability.

Yet, the older youngsters were not spared. Many of the older children, particularly a significant subgroup of preadolescents and young adolescents, responded to their parents' announcement of their decision to divorce as if to a cataclysm. Overcome by the fantasy of being in grave danger, several youngsters ran shrieking through the house or to a neighbor to ask for help. Others developed acute vomiting and other symptoms of acute distress verging on panic. They, too, suffered with ego regressions that further reduced their capacity to discern and understand the reality.

All of the children whom we studied mastered this first task by the end of the first year of separation. A significant number achieved this recognition earlier. Older children and adolescents were helped in their understanding of the divorce because of the high incidence of divorce in their community which, while it did not reassure or comfort them, did promote realistic understanding.

The acknowledgement of the reality of the marital rupture presents a separate task from the more difficult task of acknowledging its permanence. Children address the issue of permanence with great reluctance and over a several-year period. We shall discuss this separately as Task V.

Task II: Disengaging From Parental Conflict and Distress and Resuming Customary Pursuits

The second task of the child is to return to customary activities and relationships at school and at play, and to do so with the capacity for learning and for appropriate interests and pleasure unimpaired by the family crisis. This task poses a dual challenge. At a time of family disequilibrium, when one or both parents may be troubled, depressed, or very angry, when the household is likely to be in disarray,[5] the child needs to find, establish, and maintain some measure of psychological distance and separation from the adults. In order to achieve this distance the child needs actively and very painfully to disengage from the parental distress or conflict despite what may be profound worry over a parent and despite what may be the intense need of one or both parents for nurturance and support from the child. In effect, with little or no expectable parental help, the child needs to take appropriate steps to safeguard his or her individual identity and separate life course.

The second part of this task requires that the child remove the family crisis from its commanding position in his or her inner world. The achievement of this task rests in turn on the mastery, or at least the diminution of anxiety, depression, and the many conflicting feelings that attend the marital rupture in order to gain or regain the perspective and composure sufficient to enable the child's return. Only by mastery of both aspects of this task, namely that which faces outward toward the family and involves relative disengagement from the parental orbit, and that which faces inward, namely toward the child's inner thoughts and feelings and involves relative mastery of anxiety and depression, can the child maintain his or her development unimpaired by the family crisis and make his or her way back to the world of children or adolescents.

Following the marital rupture, youngsters at every age experience difficulties in maintaining their usual round of activities. They feel wretched, too worried or dispirited to find interest anywhere. A significant subgroup in our study stayed at home or close to home. It was not uncommon for a great many children, during the several months following the marital rupture, to state in response to the request for their three wishes they had nothing to wish for except the restoration of the family. The pervasive sense of desolation that we observed in a significant number of the children was such that it was difficult to evoke even a brief pleasurable response:

> Arthur, a nine-year-old lad, told us soberly, "I'm at a dead end in the middle of nowhere." Roberta, age seven, volunteered sadly, "No one likes me because I don't have a house."

Teachers described children at this time as unable to concentrate, daydreaming, preoccupied, bored, restless, inattentive in the classroom, and irritable, manipulative, aggressive, or withdrawn on the playground. A full half of the 57 children in our sample who were between the ages of seven and 11 at the time of the separation suffered a significant decline in their learning during the entire year following the marital rupture.[16] Other studies[2] have reported school difficulties in this population, including higher drop-out rates, greater absence and tardiness, and widespread difficulty in learning.

A significant number of the latency age and preadolescent youngsters whose parents were newly involved in sexual relationships with lovers reported that they had difficulty concentrating and that they were preoccupied with their parents' sexual activities. We have elsewhere[18] referred to Gwen, age ten:

> Gwen complained to us that she had lost interest in her school, in her friends, and in her piano lessons, "in everything since Dad left." She reported that she thought all day that he was "making out with his girlfriend." She also thought constantly about her mother together with her boyfriend. "How," asked the child, "can I concentrate at school thinking about Mom and Dad kissing and making love with other people?"

Unlike the first task, the mastery of this task of disengagement was not easier for the older children. It may, in fact, have been rendered more difficult by the fine shading between an all too realistic worry and phobic anxiety. How shall we assess the behavior of the many youngsters who paced the floor nervously when the parent was late in returning home? Or how shall we assess the behavior of the children who begged the custodial parent to quit smoking, asking, "What will happen to me if you get cancer?" Or how assess the despair of children to whom a parent had confided a suicidal preoccupation and who realized full well that their presence was needed by the parent in order to stave off the suicide attempt or the threat of ego disintegration?

Adolescent commitments to school and their usual round of extracurricular activities seemed particularly vulnerable to disruption at this time. Several adolescents became acutely depressed:

> One 14-year-old youngster who had distinguished herself at school and competitive sports was truant for the remainder of the school year following the parental separation and was found to be riding the local buses six hours daily, preoccupied with suicidal thoughts.

Some became newly involved at this time in sexual activity or delinquency, most notably stealing.

By the end of the first year or year-and-a-half following the separation most youngsters in our study were able to reestablish their earlier levels of learning and to reinvest in their other activities. They were able to regain relationships with friends whom they had driven away by their moodiness and their irritability during the period immediately following the marital separation. Children in families where the siblings formed a supportive subgroup appeared to have some advantage in addressing this difficult task. Nevertheless, it should be noted that a significant number of children at every age, but notably at adolescence, were not able to find their way back to an age-appropriate agenda after the derailment of the family crisis.

Task III: Resolution of Loss

Divorce brings multiple losses in its wake, of which the most central is the partial or total loss of one parent from the family. But the losses of divorce may include, as well, the loss of the familiar daily routines, the loss of the symbols, traditions, and continuity of the intact family, and the loss of the protective physical presence of two parents who can spell and buffer each other as needed. Often, as well, the losses of divorce include the loss of the family home, school, and neighborhood, and sometimes the loss of a more privileged way of life, including private school and a wide range of pleasurable, exciting activities. While the departure of a parent who has been physically or psychologically brutal or demeaning to the child or parent provides great relief, by and large children who have not been frightened on their own behalf or on behalf of a parent are likely to mourn the loss of one parent's departure even in the absence of a close relationship or frequent contact during the marriage.

This task of absorbing loss is perhaps the single most difficult task imposed by divorce. The child is required to mourn the multiple losses in order to come to terms with the constraints, limitations, and potentialities of the postdivorce or remarried family. At its core this task demands that the child overcome his or her profound sense of rejection, of humiliation, of unlovability, and of powerlessness which the one parent's departure so often engenders. Children at all ages are likely to feel rejected. "He left me," they say and are likely secretly to conclude, "He left because I was not lovable." Our beginning findings regarding children who remain in the custody of their father suggest that these feelings of unlovability, unworthiness, and rejection are even stronger where the mother has relinquished or abandoned the child or is an inconsistent visitor.

This task is greatly facilitated by the establishment of a reliable visiting pattern which can enable father and child to restore a sense of psychic wholeness and rightness in their respective new roles of part-time parent and part-time child. The building of a good enough parent-child relationship within the visiting structure, which is governed realistically by the opportunities and the constraints of the visit, rests upon the working through of the yearning for the father within the intact family and an openness to the new relationship. It is reasonable that only if the loss of the full-time presence of the departed parent is accepted by both parent and child does the visiting relationship and its potential become fully realizable.[17] There is also the strong possibility that the child's relationship to the stepparent requires some modicum of resolution of this mourning process.

The resolution of this task often lasts many years. The voluntariness of both the divorce and the parent's departure burdens the child's coping efforts and increases the child's suffering, making this loss more difficult to assimilate than the involuntary loss associated with bereavement. This task is, of course, most easily accomplished when the loss of the relationship with the father (or the mother) is partial, and the outside parent and child are able to establish and maintain a loving relationship within an ongoing, reliable visiting pattern or under conditions of a good joint-custody plan. Even under ideal conditions this is no small achievement.

Many children fail to negotiate this task. They remain disappointed year in and year out by unreliable, disinterested, or absent fathers or mothers. Youngsters are trapped for many years by their inability to renounce the vain hope that the absent parent will return while knowing full well that this is unlikely to occur. Placed equally between these two opposite expectamcies, they seem unable to achieve closure. Although we have described a subgroup of youngsters who were able at adolescence to break free of their ties to a disinterested or rejecting parent by a process of active identification spurred by anger, we lack long-term findings regarding the psychological and developmental implications of this counter-rejection.[16]

Unfortunately, many children who experienced rejection seemed unable to master their sense of unlovability and unworthiness. We did not find that either age at the time of the marital rupture or the sex of the child was related to the ability of the youngster to resolve the loss successfully.

Task IV: Resolving Anger and Self-Blame

In order to understand this task it is important to note the importance of the social context of marital dissolution. Unlike bereavement or natural disaster, divorce is entirely man- or woman-made and represents a voluntary decision for at least one of the marital partners. The children are aware that divorce is not inevitable, that the immediate cause is the decision of one or both parents to separate and that its true cause is the unwillingness or failure to maintain the marriage. Moreover, the children, like the community, will have different responses when the divorce is sought to remedy a brutal or an unhappy marriage, when the divorce is sought to pursue a postponed career, or when the divorce occurs because of one adult's impulsive decision to join a lover.

Our work indicates clearly that children and adolescents do not believe in no-fault divorce. They may blame one or both parents or they may blame themselves. Divorce characteristically gives rise to anger at the one parent who sought the divorce or both parents for their perceived self-centeredness or unresponsiveness to the wishes of the child to maintain the intact family. The anger that these children experience is likely sometimes to be intense and long-lasting, especially among older children and adolescents who disapprove of the conduct of one or both parents. We have earlier reported[16] the intense anger and sorrow expressed by one 14-year-old boy:

> In a school composition written five years after the marital rupture, he wrote, "My father picked up his suitcases one day and walked out because, as he said, he wanted his freedom. We thought we were a close-knit family, and it was an unexpected shock. It was the death of our family."

Our observations are that anger that has been generated within the context of divorce may well remain undiminished by the passage of time. Such anger not only keeps youngsters alienated from one parent but often, in our observation, correlates significantly with acting-out behavior at adolescence, including delinquency, school difficulty, and low achievement. Most of all, anger that does not subside seems to keep youngsters from achieving closure with regard to the divorce experience. The anger does seem to diminish within the context of greater understanding of the parents and their relationship with each other; this rests, in turn, on the achievement by the older child or the adolescent of some perspective regarding the reasons that prompted the divorce and a greater understanding of one or both parents.

Thus, the cooling of the anger and task of forgiveness go hand in hand with the growing emotional maturity of the child and the greater capacity to recognize the divergence of interests and directions among the different family members. As the anger gives way, the young person is able to obtain both closure and relief. Only in this way are the narcissistic injury of the divorce and the sense of powerlessness engendered in the child finally resolved. A significant aspect of forgiveness is a child's capacity to forgive himself or herself for having wished the divorce to happen or having failed to restore the intact marriage. And, indeed, it may well be that there is a profound connection between children's capacity to forgive themselves and the capacity to forgive one or both parents. Further, the close relationships and friendships between parents and children that Weiss[19] and others have described as emerging out of this crisis may have their roots in part in a triumph over anger.

Among the distinguishing attributes of some of the parent-child relationships at the ten-year mark is a growing closeness between youngster and parent which seems to have the hallmarks of a significant, long delayed reconciliation:

> Barbara reported at age 17, ten years after the marital rupture, "My mom and I are real close now. I stopped being angry at her when I was 15 when I suddenly realized that all of the kids who lived in tract houses with picket fences were not any happier than I was. It took me a long, long time to stop blaming her for not being in one of those houses."

Task V: Accepting the Permanence of the Divorce

Closely related to all of the foregoing tasks, and particularly to the task of successfully mastering the distress evoked by the father's departure, is the child's gradual acceptance that the divorce is permanent and will not be undone. Time and again we have been impressed with the tenacity of the fantasy that the divorced family will be reunited. We have observed children, adolescents, and adults decades after the divorce persisting in this expectation that the intact family will be restored, weeping for the father that they hardly knew, finding omens of reconciliation in a harmless handshake or a friendly nod. Even the remarriage of both parents sometimes did little to diminish the intensity of this persistent fantasy, wish, hope, or expectation. Our clinical experience includes a middle-aged woman patient who sought help from two therapists simultaneously, a man and a woman, and who finally confessed to each her central preoccupation: that she wished to bring both therapists together within the same room so that they could hold hands and restore the intact family that she had lost as a preschool child. It proved difficult to dissuade this functioning, nonpsychotic woman that the actualization of her enduring childhood fantasy with the participation of both therapists would not immediately cure her recurrent severe depressions.

We have concluded that the child of divorce faces a more difficult task in accepting permanence than does the bereaved child. The bereaved child, despite intense hopes to the contrary, knows full well that death can never be undone, whereas the living presence and availability of two parents gives continuing credence to the child's wish to restore the marriage. In effect, the reality that both parents are alive and that divorce is always possible, as is remarriage, fuels the fantsy and permits it, even encourages it to flourish. It is by now quite clear that the fantasy of restoration taps into deep wellsprings within the child's functioning and yields to reality only very gradually, perhaps only when the child finally makes and consolidates a clear psychological separation between self and parent during the adolescent years.

Developmental factors seem relevant to the resolution of this task. It may well be that the younger children encountered greater difficulty in relinquishing the restoration fantasy than their peers who were older at the time of the marital breakup. Another factor of importance was the extent to which one or both parents also continued to long for the restoration of the marriage. Such adult fantasies reinforced the fantasies of the children. We did not find, however, that the adult wishes to restore the marriage governed the widespread fantasies and hopes of the children.

Task VI: Achieving Realistic Hope Regarding Relationships

Finally we come to the task that is perhaps the most important both for the child and for society, namely the resolution of issues of relationship in such a way that the young person is able to reach and sustain a realistic vision regarding his or her capacity to love and be loved. This is the task that occupies the child of divorce during the adolescent years and lends its particular cast and additional burden to the many developmental tasks that the adolescent confronts. It is also the task that brings together and integrates the coping efforts of earlier years and provides in this way an opportunity for the full-dress reworking of the impact of the divorce experience.

In this task we come full circle in comparing the child of divorce with his or her counterpart in bereavement. In the same way that the child who loses a parent through death must learn to take a chance on loving with the full and reinforced knowledge that humans are mortal and that all relationships will indeed end, so too the child of divorce must learn to take a chance on a loving relationship that may fail but with the realistic hope that it will flourish and endure.

As the adolescent youngsters examined their parents and themselves and considered their future, many were frightened at the possible repetition of marital or sexual failure in their own lives:

> Pamela, at age 24, told us at the ten-year follow-up, "I'm afraid to use the word love. I tell my boyfriend that I love him, but I can't really think about it without fear."

A significant number of young people during late adolescence turned away from a parent's behavior in anger, having measured it and found it wanting. As expressed at the ten-year follow-up by one 26-year-old young man who had elected to follow an entirely different life style from that of his father:

> "Some day I will say to my dad, 'Are you proud of what you have done with your life?' But," he said bitterly, "what can he answer me?"

We have reported earlier[18] the pointed and poignant comments of the youngsters during the adolescent years and their sober efforts to evolve strategies that might safeguard them from failure and help consolidate a separateness from the parents' experience:

> "My parents cheated and lied, but I decided never to do that." "I will live with a guy for a long time. I won't rush in." "They should both have been more considerate. My mother is selfish, and my father should never have married." "The trouble with my parents is that they each gave too little and asked too much."

Nevertheless, it seems evident that youngsters whose adjustment was otherwise adequate foundered on this last task. Sometimes the cynicism expressed was startling:

> Jay, at age 14, told us, "Dad left because Mom bored him. I do that all the time."

Others insisted that they would never marry because they were convinced that their marriages would fail. Still others were caught in a web of promiscuity and low self-esteem and spoke cynically and hopelessly of ever achieving a loving relationship or other goals. And, we have noted, we have been concerned at the emergence of acute depression during adolescence, especially what appears to be a delayed depression among adolescent girls many years following the marital rupture.[18]

Unfortunately we lack the long-term findings that would enable us to gauge success or failure of the efforts of these young people to select a different or a better direction for their lives. Our own findings from the ten-year follow-up are still in the preliminary phase. And it might well be argued that even tentative conclusions would need to await the time when the child of divorce becomes, in turn, a parent as well as a marital partner.

Bearing in mind that the resolution of life's tasks is always relative and probably never complete, it nevertheless appears that this last task is built on the successful negotiation of those that went before. For in order to trust in the reliability of relationships and maintain the capacity to love and be loved, the child of divorce will need to have acquired confidence in his or her lovability and self-worth. He or she will have had to consolidate separateness from the parental orbit and conflicts and establish an independent direction; will have had to master the depression, the anxiety, and the conflicts stirred by the divorce that have remained residually over the years; will have had to complete the mourning over the loss of the intact family or the departed parent; will have had to resolve early issues of intense anger and guilt stirred by the marital rupture and arrive at some forgiveness, understanding, and compassion for the parents and for self; and will have had to come to terms with the permanence of the parental divorce and relinquish longings for the restoration of the childhood family. All of the tasks come together for reworking within the context of the many tasks of adolescence. And it is this last task, in the "second chance" that Blos[1] has proposed adolescence beneficently provides, that enables the child of divorce to reach or restore a sense of wholeness and integrity by rescuing a realistic vision of love and constancy in human relationships to which the developing youngster can aspire in adulthood and, in turn, transmit to children.

CONCLUSION

The child's long-range adjustment following marital disruption is significantly related to many factors within the family that reflect the quality of family life following divorce as compared with that within the failing marriage. Nevertheless, the child's own capacity and efforts at mastery are of significance in the ultimate outcome. Efforts at mastery and readjustment that are required of the child in order to maintain psychic integrity and development have been conceptualized and presented here as a series of six coping tasks which are closely interrelated, hierarchical, and fall into a temporal sequence that begins at the time of the marital rupture and culminates with the close of adolescence. These tasks represent a substantive addition to the usual tasks of growing up. Successful resolution would enable the child to achieve closure to the divorce experience, a well-earned sense of independence and pride, and an intact capacity to trust and to love. It is likely, however, that even where these tasks are successfully resolved there will remain for the child of divorce some residue of sadness, of anger, and of anxiety about the potential unreliability of relationships which may reappear at critical times during the adult years.

One important goal in the formulation of the tasks which the child of divorce confronts during his or her developmental years is to construct the conceptual building blocks that are needed for the formulation of preventive interventions designed specifically for this population.

REFERENCES

1. Blos, P. (1962). On Adolescence: A Psychoanalytic Interpretation. Free Press, New York.
2. Brown, B. (1980). A study of the school needs of children in one-parent families. Phi Delta Kappan (April):537–540.
3. Caplan, G., ed. (1955). Emotional Problems of Early Childhood. Basic Books, New York.
4. Erikson, E. (1950). Childhood and Society. Norton, New York.
5. Hetherington, E., Cox, M. and Cox, R. (1978). The aftermath of divorce. In Mother-Child Relations, H. Stevens and M. Mathews, eds. National Association for the Education of Young Children, Washington, D.C.
6. Hetherington, E. (1979). Divorce: a child's perspective. Amer. Psychol. 34:851–858.
7. Hunter, J. and Schuman, N. (1980). Chronic reconstitution of a family style. Soc. Wk 25:446–451.
8. Kelly, J. and Wallerstein, J. (1976). The effects of parental divorce: experiences of the child in early latency. Amer. J. Orthopsychiat. 46:20–32.
9. Kelly, J. and Wallerstein, J. (1977). Part-time parent, part-time child: visiting after divorce. J. Clin. Child Psychol. 6:51–54.
10. Lindemann, E. (1944). Symptomatology and management of acute grief. Amer. J. Psychiat. 101:141–148.
11. Wallerstein, J. and Kelly, J. (1974). The effects of parental divorce: the adolescent experience. In The Child in His Family, E. Anthony and C. Koupernik, eds. John Wiley, New York.

12. Wallerstein, J. and Kelly, J. (1975). The effects of parental divorce: the experiences of the preschool child. J. Amer. Acad. Child Psychiat. 14:600–616.
13. Wallerstein, J. and Kelly, J. (1976). The effects of parental divorce: experiences of the child in later latency. Amer. J. Orthopsychiat. 46:256–269.
14. Wallerstein, J. (1977). Some observations regarding the effects of divorce on the psychological development of the pre-school girl. *In* Sexual and Gender Development of Young Children, J. Oremland and E. Oremland, eds. Ballinger, Cambridge, Mass.
15. Wallerstein, J. (1977). Responses of the preschool child to divorce: those who cope. *In* Child Psychiatry: Treatment and Research, M. McMillan and S. Henao, eds. Brunner/Mazel, New York.
16. Wallerstein, J. and Kelly, J. (1980). Surviving the Breakup: How Children and Parents Cope With Divorce. Basic Books, New York.
17. Wallerstein, J. and Kelly, J. (1980). Effects of divorce on the visiting father-child relationship. Amer. J. Psychiat. 137(12):1534–1539.
18. Wallerstein, J. (in press). Children of divorce: stress and developmental tasks. *In* Stress, Coping and Development, N. Garmezy and M. Rutter, eds. McGraw-Hill, New York.
19. Weiss, R. (1979). Going it Alone. Basic Books, New York.

18

Early Parental Attitudes, Divorce and Separation, and Young Adult Outcome: Findings of a Longitudinal Study

Stella Chess, Alexander Thomas, and Mary Mittelman
New York University Medical Center
Sam Korn
Hunter College, New York
Jacob Cohen
New York University

Effects of early parental attitudes, divorce and separation on adult adaptation are reported in 132 young adults followed anterospectively and longitudinally from early infancy (the New York Longitudinal Study). Ratings of child adjustment at home at age 3 and 5 and at school at age 5 derived from repeated interviews. A separate parent interview at age 3 provided 8 clusters of parental attitudes and environmental features. Early adult adaptation ratings were derived from direct subject interviews. Parent conflict, especially regarding child management but including other issues, predicted poor adult adaptation, but separation-divorce without this conflict did not.

Reprinted with permission from the *Journal of the American Academy of Child Psychiatry*, 1983, Vol. 22, No. 1, 47–51. Copyright 1983 by the American Academy of Child Psychiatry.

This research was supported by NIMH Grant MH 31333. A revised version of this paper was presented at the Annual Meeting of the American Academy of Child Psychiatry, October 15, 1981, Dallas, Texas.

What are the long-term consequences of divorce for the psychological development of the child? With the tremendous increase in the divorce rate in this country in recent years, this question has become an increasingly important mental health issue. As Wallerstein and Kelly (1980a) have pointed out, "The conventional wisdom used to be that unhappy married people should remain married 'for the good of the children'. Today's conventional wisdom holds, with equal vigor, that an unhappy couple might well *divorce* for the good of the children, that an unhappy marriage for the adults is unhappy also for the children; and that divorce that promotes the happiness of the adults will benefit the children as well" (p. 67). But which "conventional wisdom" corresponds to the facts? Or does neither?

The New York Longitudinal Study (NYLS) has had a special opportunity to investigate this issue. The subjects have now been followed anterospectively and longitudinally from early infancy to early adult life, so that data are available on childcare and parental characteristics for the age period preceding the separation and divorce. Also, the study families in which separation did not occur serve as a control population of similar demographic features, including sociocultural characteristics and age distribution, with a similar body of collected and analyzed data. Finally, special attention has been paid in the NYLS to the identification, rating, and systematic clinical evaluation of all subjects with evidence of deviant behavior at any age.

RECENT STUDIES AND LITERATURE

The most extensive and intensive study of the impact of divorce on children comes from Wallerstein and Kelly (1980b). They followed 60 divorcing families and their 131 children, with interviews with both parents and children after the separation, 18 months later, and again after 5 years. The samples was predominantly middle class, although 28% were in the lowest socioeconomic groups. Immediately after the separation more than 50% of the children were anxious and intensely preoccupied with the separation. By 18 months the symptoms of acute psychological disruption had receded or disappeared for most, though 15% still appeared overwhelmed. At 5 years much individual variation in style of coping with the divorce was evident. Overall, the authors conclude that their comparison of the children's functioning before the divorce and at the 5-year follow-up analysis "strongly suggests that the divorced family was neither more nor less beneficial or stressful for the children than the unhappy marriage" (pp. 306–307). The study, however, does not include a control group of marriages which do not end in divorce.

Hetherington and her co-workers (1978) compared a sample of 48 children of divorced middle class parents with a similar number from intact families matched by sex, age and birth order. The parents were also matched as far as possible for age, education, and length of marriage. Various behavioral measures, as well as parent interviews, were obtained at 2 months, 1 year and 2 years following the divorce. Negative behavior, especially toward the mother, appeared immediately after the divorce and included disobedience, whining, nagging and increased dependency demands. These behaviors peaked 1 year post divorce, and then declined by the 2-year followup.

Schoettle and Cantwell (1980) examined demographic variables, symptoms, and diagnostic categories in a population of 2,351 child patients consecutively presenting to the UCLA Neuropsychiatric Institute. The children of divorce represented 44.3% of the group, paralleling the divorce percentage in Los Angeles County marriages. Generally, children of divorce presented with behavior and socialization problems, while mental retardation and medical problems were more evident in the children from intact marriages.

A prospective study is reported by Block and coworkers (1981). Fifty-seven husband-wife couples independently described their child rearing values when their child was 3½ years of age, using a 91-item Q-sort. A parental agreement score was calculated by correlating the independent responses of each parental dyad. These scores were related to marital status 10 years later, and a significant difference between the intact and divorced couples found, with greater parental agreement among the intact couples. The authors also found a significant correlation between the index of parental agreement and the quality of psychological functioning in the children over a 4-year age range, from 3 to 7 years. Parental agreement was related positively to the development of ego control in the boys, but negatively to the development of ego control in the girls.

Hetherington (1979) has recently presented a systematic review of the literature concerning the child's reaction to divorce. She emphasizes that divorce must be viewed as a sequence of events, rather than a single one. The crisis model is appropriate to the short-term effects, and these are influenced by a number of factors. There is a wide variety in the responses of children to divorce, influenced by temperament, prior maladjustment, and developmental stage. The impact of marital discord and divorce appears more pervasive and enduring for boys than for girls. The author concludes that "divorce is often a positive solution to destructive family functioning; however, most children experience divorce as a difficult transition, and life in a single-parent family can be viewed as a high-risk situation for parents and children" (p. 288).

NYLS SAMPLE AND METHODS FOR CHILDHOOD PERIOD

The NYLS sample includes 133 subjects from 87 middle and upper middle class families (previous reports incorrectly gave our sample number as 136, the result of a mechanical tabulation error). The data include information gathered longitudinally and anterospectively starting in early infancy on each subject's behavioral functioning at home, in school, and in standard psychometric test situations, on parental attitudes and childcare practices, on special environmental events and subject's responses to such events, and on intellectual functioning. In the childhood years the behavioral data were obtained from parents and teachers and from periods of observation in the school and during IQ testing. The clinical evaluations involved direct play sessions or interviews, depending on the age of the subject, and a special problem oriented interview with the parents. At age 16, direct extended open-ended interviews were conducted for the first time with almost all the subjects, as well as with the parents separately. Details of data collection and data analysis methods and the findings for the childhood period have been previously reported in a number of publications and several volumes (Thomas and Chess, 1977; Thomas et al., 1963, 1968).

Of specific interest for this presentation are the parent interviews to elicit childcare practices and attitudes conducted when the child was 3 years old. These were held with each mother and father separately but simultaneously by two research staff members who had had no previous contact with the parents or the children. Immediately following the interview, the interviewer rated the parent on 99 items of information, including typical demographic and background variables and specific items relating to parental attitudes and child-care practices.

Taking these data, Cameron (1977) selected 70 items as meeting basic statistical criteria for use in correlational analyses. Only the ratings of the mothers were used, since in the overwhelming majority of cases both parents provided identical ratings. These 70 items were then subjected by Cameron to cluster analysis by means of the Tryon system. Eight oblique parental clusters were extracted: (1) parental disapproval, intolerance, and rejection; (2) parental conflict, especially regarding child rearing; (3) parental strictness versus permissiveness; (4) maternal concern and protectiveness; (5) depressed living standards; (6) limitations on the child's material supports; (7) inconsistent parental discipline; and (8) large family orientations.

EARLY ADULT PERIOD INTERVIEW

Out of the total sample of 133 subjects, 132 were interviewed at 18 to 22 years. The one subject not interviewed has not refused, but has been out of the country. The interviews were audiotaped in approximately 60% of the cases. The parents were also cooperative and were interviewed by separate staff members.

The subject interviews were with only a few exceptions conducted by one of us (A. T.) with a co-interviewer in approximately 40% ,of the cases, and separate ratings made from the audiotapes by another experienced clinical psychiatrist with no previous contact with the study. For the 132 subject interviews, there were 3 raters in 50 subjects, 2 in 29 and 1 in 54.

The subject interviews were open-ended and covered in detail the following areas: self-evaluation; medical history; life goals; immediate goals; daily routines; biological functions; athletics; special interests and hobbies; relations with family, school, work, social and sexual functioning; expressiveness and communication; adaptive patterns; substance use; and psychological and psychosomatic symptoms.

Each rater scored the subjects for each of these areas on a 7-point scale ranging from excellent to poor. An overall global adaptation score on a 9-point scale, and ratings for each of our 9 temperament categories on a 7-point scale, were also obtained from the interview Psychiatric diagnoses where indicated were also made by each rater. Interrater reliabilities were lower, being above 0.60 in only 4 categories. A high order of agreement was present among the three raters in their independent clinical evaluations and diagnoses.

For the final rating of behavioral adaptation in early adult life, the bootstrapping technique as developed at the Oregon Research Institute (Goldberg, 1970) was used. With this technique, a set of elements (our checklist items) is first subjected to an overall clinical judgment (our global adaptation score). Then, using that judgment as a criterion in a multiple regression analysis with the element scores as independent variables, the regression equation is generated that estimates the overall rating. The data finally used are not the overall global judgments but their regression estimates. The rationale for this approach is that the regression equation distills the rating policies that are implicit when the overall global score is made but, unlike the latter, are not subject to day to day variation in rater judgment. For this final adaptation score, the average of the three raters' "bootstrapped" scores was used.

SEPARATION, DIVORCE AND PARENTAL DEATH

In our sample of 132 subjects interviewed and rated in early adult life there have been permanent separations, leading in almost all cases to legal divorce, in 25 families. These involved 35 subjects. Of the 35 subjects, 22 (63%) were male and 13 (37%) were female compared with an equal distribution in the total sample (65 male, 67 female). Separation occurred when 10 subjects were 5 years or younger, none between 6 and 8, 10 between 9 and 13 years, 11 between 14 and 19, and 4 were between ages 20 and 22. There have been 2 maternal and 9 paternal deaths. Two parental deaths occurred when the subject was under 5 years; all the others occurred when the children were 12 years or older. The maternal deaths involved 2 subjects, the paternal 14 subjects. One maternal death occurred after parental separation as did one paternal death, the latter involving 2 children.

DATA ANALYSIS AND FINDINGS

A number of multiple regression analyses correlating early childhood ratings and early adult outcome have been performed. This report is concerned with the correlation of parental attitudes and childcare practices as well as parental separation-divorce or death on early adult life adaptation.

The one striking, statistically significant correlation between the 3-year maternal attitude ratings and the young adult adaptation score was with parental conflict, namely at the 0.36 level ($p < 0.01$). The correlation was in the expected direction; that is, the greater the parental conflict at 3 years the poorer the adaptation score at early adulthood of the offspring. This parental conflict cluster is composed of the following items: (1) amount of parental conflict generally, (2) amount of parental disagreement in approach to child, (3) amount of parental conflict specifically in handling child, (4) general attitude toward spouse, (5) existence of parental differences in handling discipline, and (6) self-confidence in child rearing.

In the multiple regression analysis, neither separation-divorce (correlation of 0.03) nor parental death (correlation of 0.16) showed a statistically significant relationship with early adult adaptation. Caution is indicated in interpreting the latter finding, given the small number of

TABLE 1

Correlations between Young Adult Adjustment and Parent-Related Factors

Young adult adaptation and:	
Parental conflict, year 3	0.36 ($p < 0.01$)
Separation/Divorce	0.03 NS
Parental death	0.16 NS

parental deaths and the wide variation in the child's age at the time of parental death. These findings are summarized in Table 1.

The correlation between 3-year parental conflict and later separation-divorce was found to be 0.28, statistically significant beyond the 0.01 level.

The question of subject sex differences in the relationship between predictor variables and early adult adaptation score was explored in a multiple regression analysis. The question posed was whether the interaction set; that is, sex in relationship with an independent variable (parental conflict, separation-divorce, or parental death), added significantly to the level of correlation with adult outcome produced by these independent variables and sex differences. There was no consistent relationship between the various sex-variable (conflict, divorce, death) interactions and early adult adaptations. In other words, the sex of the offspring did not influence significantly the correlations obtained in the above analyses.

The numbers in our sample subgroups were too small to permit a quantitative analysis of possible differential effects of time of parental separation-divorce on early adult outcome. Instead, a tabulation was made of the percentage of cases of separation-divorce, subdivided according to the child's age at the time this occurred (0–5 years, 9–13 years, 14–19 years, and 20–22 years), in whom the adult adaptation scores were poorer than the average for the overall sample of 132 subjects. This tabulation is presented in Table 2.

TABLE 2

Child's Age at Time of Separation/Divorce and Young Adult Adaptation

Age (yr)	N	Young Adult Adaptation; Percent below Median
0–5	10	60
6–8	0	—
9–13	10	60
14–19	11	64
20–22	4	50

As can be seen from table 2, for 10 subjects whose parents were permanently separated or divorced by age 5 years, 60% (6 out of 10) were below the median score for adult adaptation. For 10 subjects between 9 and 13 years the proportion was also 60%. For 11 subjects between 14 and 19 years the proportion was 64% (7 out of 11), and for 4 subjects between 20 and 22 years the proportion was 50% (2 out of 4). While no firm statistical conclusions can be drawn from these figures, they do not suggest any striking relationship between the child's age at the time of parental separation-divorce and early adult adaptation.

A similar tabulation was made of the cases of separation-divorce subdivided according to the child's age and the degree of parental conflict at age 3. About half (5 out of 11) of the parents with low conflict (below the median score) were separated-divorced by the time the children were 2 years of age, and about half (6 out of 11) after age 12 years. Out of 21 cases with high parental conflict (above the median score) at age 3, none were separated-divorced before the child was 2 years of age, 8 by 11 years, 11 by 19 years, and 2 by 22 years. Again, no general relationship between degree of parental conflict at age 3 years and age of the child at time of separation-divorce is suggested by this tabulation.

DISCUSSION

The above findings are relevant to the question of the long-term effects on the child of parental separation and divorce. The findings of an absence of correlation is in accord with the Wallerstein and Kelly (1980b) finding cited above that "the divorced family was neither more nor less beneficial or stressful for the children than the unhappy marriage" (pp. 306–307). Our rating of 3-year parental conflict does represent one measure of an unhappy marriage, and this rating was a significant predictor of both later separation or divorce and the level of early adult adaptation of the offspring. A simple correlative analysis would have shown an apparent relationship between parental separation-divorce and the child's functioning as a young adult. However, when the factor of 3-year parental conflict is partialled out in a multiple regression analysis, separation-divorce does not appear to have any influence as such on outcome.

The finding of a correlation between parental conflict and later divorce is in accord with the report of Block and co-workers (1981) on the predictive value of parental agreement or disagreement on subsequent divorce.

Rutter (1981a, 1981b) has also emphasized the deleterious effect on the child of parental discord as contrasted to actual separation or divorce.

Of course, the quantitative findings necessarily reflect group trends, and a different relationship may hold in any individual case. Thus, in at least several of the NYLS subjects, parental separation has appeared to represent a significant traumatic event with disturbing psychological consequences. In these cases, other factors clearly played a part, such as the young adult's temperamental characteristics, destructive legal battles over the divorce, intensely hostile interplays between the parents after the divorce from which the children could not remain aloof, etc. For the most part, however, the subjects with divorced parents have discussed this event in their early adult life interviews with equanimity and even objectivity. Parental conflict, on the other hand, was usually more distressing. The son or daughter often felt caught in the middle in the tensions and turmoil created by parental discord, with difficulty or inability to find a successful coping mechanism.

Our findings highlight the significance of parental conflict in the child's early life as a risk factor for the child's psychological development. Where such conflict is identified, parent counselling and therapy would appear to be a significant therapeutic and preventive mental health approach.

REFERENCES

Block, J. H., Block, J. & Morrison, A. (1981). Parental agreement-disagreement on child rearing orientations and gender-related personality correlates in children. *Child Developm.*, 52:965–974.

Cameron, J. R. (1977). Parental treatment, children's temperament, and the risk of childhood behavioral problems. *Amer. J. Orthopsychiat.*, 47:568–576.

Goldberg, L. R. (1970), Man versus model of man: a rationale plus evidence for a method of improving on clinical inferences. *Psychol. Bull.*, 73:422–432.

Hetherington, E. M. (1979). Divorce, a child's perspective. *Amer. Psychol.*, 34:851–858.

—— Cox, M. & Cox, R. (1978). The aftermath of divorce. In: *Mother-Child, Father-Child Relations*, ed. J. H. Stevens & M. Mathews. Washington, D.C.: National Association for the Education of Young Children.

Rutter, M. (1981a). Stress, coping and development: some issues and some questions. *J. Child Psychol. Psychiat.*, 22:323–356.

—— (1981b). Epidemiological/longitudinal strategies and causal research in child psychiatry. *This Journal*, 20:513–544.

Schoettle, V. C. & Cantwell, D. P. (1980). Children of divorce. *This Journal*, 19:453–475.

Thomas, A. & Chess, S. (1977). *Temperament and Development.* New York: Brunner/Mazel.

—— Birch, H. G., Hertzig, M. & Korn, S. (1963). *Behavioral Individuality in Early Childhood.* New York: New York University Press.

—— —— (1968). *Temperament and Behavior Disorders in Children.* New York: New York University Press.

Wallterstein, J. S. & Kelly, J. B. (1980a). California's children of divorce. *Psychol. Today*, 13:67–76.

—— —— (1980b). *Surviving the Break-up.* New York: Basic Books.

19

Bereavement Responses of Kibbutz and Non-Kibbutz Children Following the Death of the Father

Mordecai Kaffman and Esther Elizur

Kibbutz Child and Family Clinic, Tel Aviv, Israel

INTRODUCTION

This paper reports part of a larger investigation into the early effects and long-term consequences of parental bereavement on pre-adolescent children. In previous reports we have described the post-bereavement reactions of a representative sample of 25 kibbutz children, aged 2–10, who lost a father in the war of October 1973 (Kaffman and Elizur, 1979; Elizur and Kaffman, 1982). We have found a considerable amount and variety of affective grief responses and reactive behavior problems from the first months of bereavement until the fourth post-bereavement year. Among those clinical symptoms and behavior problems in which we found clear differences in comparison to the pre-bereavement condition were recurrent outbursts of crying and moodiness, overdependent behavior, separation difficulties from mother, augmented aggressive behavior, night fears and/or other anxiety states, exaggerated fear of bodily injury, regressive enuresis or encopresis, eating problems, restlessness, concentration and learning difficulties.

Although grief manifestations diminished gradually throughout the first two years of bereavement, the behavioral symptoms that indicated marked emotional disturbance continued to appear and characterize a

Reprinted with permission from the *Journal of Child Psychology and Psychiatry*, 1983, Vol. 24, No. 3, 435–442. Copyright 1983 by the Association for Child Psychology and Psychiatry.

considerable number of children for a prolonged period. Actually, in each phase of our follow-up study, 6, 18 and 42 months after the father's death, about half of the kibbutz children reacted with severe problems and maladaptive behavior during a period lasting from 6 months to over 3 yr.

Indeed, we were surprised by the high incidence, severity and persistence of clinical manifestations in a sample of normal children with no special problems before the loss. This was an unexpected finding in view of the favorable conditions in the kibbutz which assist the child and his family to cope with stressful situations (Kaffman, 1977; Kaffman and Elizur, 1977). The child in the kibbutz is not dependent on his father as a provider of material needs. Since food, lodging, clothing, daily care, and cultural and educational requirements are provided by the community, the family need not fear economic insecurity, material deprivation or any abrupt change in the routine. The setting remains stable in the children's house, and in most cases, a day or two after receiving news of his father's death the child returns to his normal daily activities. The child's contact with the mother's acute grief and with possible anxiety-provoking scenes and mourning ceremonials is rather limited compared to non-kibbutz children. Moreover, during the mourning period kibbutz children receive plenty of comfort, help and care from people around them.

It became clear to us that all these propitous conditions were not enough to protect the kibbutz child from the disruptive effect of the traumatic event. It appears that the tremendous importance of the father as a central attachment figure in the kibbutz child's emotional life by far offsets the moderating influences of environmental conditions which help the child cope with other stress situations. It is appropriate to emphasize at this point that although the father within the kibbutz setting is not the family provider nor principal supplier of its material needs, he is nevertheless highly involved instrumentally and emotionally in the care and education of the child from its earliest days. Usually both parents in the kibbutz spend the same amount of time together with their children during the family leisure hours, the father being an equal partner in daily care, in nurturing and socializing functions, and as an identification model.

Our findings regarding the serious consequences of the loss of the father appeared to confirm the centrality of the father's instrumental and affective roles in the kibbutz family. Yet we felt it imperative to compare the bereavement reactions of the group studied with those of city children raised in a regular family framework. Clearly such an investigation could amplify our observations and conclusions about the serious and extended consequences of the father's death as applied to Israeli children in general.

METHOD

Information about the child's responses and behavioral changes following death of the father was collected from two different groups of mothers: 15 mothers of the original group of 25 kibbutz children; and 13 mothers from a matched sample of 21 non-kibbutz children.

The kibbutz sample included *all* the pre-adolescent children (age 2–10) in seven kibbutzim whose fathers died in the October War. The city sample was selected from a group of Jerusalem children who had also lost a father in the same war, during the same period and under similar circumstances. Both groups were matched in terms of age, upper-middle social class background, educational standard of the child's preschool and junior school settings, family size and median years of high school education completed by the mothers. With the exception of two of the city mothers who belonged to practicing orthodox families, all of the other mothers (26) had no particular religious affiliation. Financial security and a reasonable standard of living were assured for all the bereaved families either by the community in the kibbutz setting or by a generous widow's pension provided by the Army. One and a half years after the husband's death all the city mothers were gainfully employed outside the home, as were the kibbutz mothers, who continued to play an important role in the community labor force.

The kibbutz sample consisted of 8 girls and 17 boys. Seventeen children were under the age of 6 and eight children were aged 6–10 when their fathers died. The non-kibbutz sample included 8 boys and 13 girls: 14 children between the ages of 2–6 and 7 children 6–10 years old. Only 21 non-kibbutz children were included in the final sample (instead of 25, as two city mothers refused at the last minute to be interviewed). Both the kibbutz and urban children were considered normal without any special developmental, emotional or behavioral difficulties before their father's death.

The conclusions presented in this paper are based on data obtained from semi-structured interviews with the mother of each child which took place 18 months after notification of the father's death. Details about the method for gathering of data and conduct of research can be found in our first report on this follow-up study (Kaffman and Elizur, 1979). It is sufficient to note here that the guide questionnaire for the interview included three separate sections: (1) an open-ended question exploring the current behavior and functioning of the child; (2) a structured and comprehensive check-list of 50 observable behaviors and symptoms to be used by the mother to describe the child's current emotional state, and his problems and reactions following the death of the father. The interviewer recorded and rated any symptoms reported by the mother that had persisted for at least two months; and (3) an inquiry regarding the mother's concern for the reported problems and her judgment as to the child's need for psychological or psychiatric treatment.

For the kibbutz sample separate interviews were held with the mother and teacher of each child. In the city sample, however, we could not get the cooperation of all the teachers, and so only mothers' reports were used as a source of information. It is worth noting that in our follow-up study of kibbutz bereaved children a reliability check indicated a high degree of agreement between the reports of mother and educator concerning the child's general adjustment, changes in behavior, and the nature, severity and frequency of symptomatic problems. Certain differences between the mothers' and teachers' reports stemmed basically from the particular respondent's role and the distinct quality of the interaction. Thus reactions such as remembering the dead father, expressions of longing, seeking a "substitute father," concern and worries about the mother, or devoted care of a younger sibling were more prominent in the family context and therefore more emphasized by the mothers. On the other hand, symptoms such as concentration difficulties, social withdrawal, discipline and school problems were observed and reported more by the educators.

RESULTS

Table 1 lists the comparative incidence of behavior symptoms and grief reactions reported by the mothers of kibbutz and non-kibbutz children one and a half years after the death of the father. The table shows a reasonably similar pattern of grief responses for both groups. We learned that even 1½ yr after the father's death, mothers in both kibbutz and city reported manifestations of grief. The child still looked sadder than before the loss, had recurrent periods of moodiness, cried easily in response to slight frustrations, expressed feelings of longing related to the dead father and engaged in remembering activities (looking at albums, talking to the father's picture, recalling joint experiences, reading letters, etc.). Yet in most cases mothers reported that grief symptoms

TABLE 1. FREQUENCY OF PREVALENT BEHAVIORAL PROBLEMS, GRIEF REACTIONS AND 'PATHOLOGICAL BEREAVEMENT' 18 MONTHS AFTER DEATH OF FATHER

Type of reaction or symptom	Kibbutz children (n = 25)		Non-kibbutz children (n = 21)		Altogether (n = 46)	
	(n)	%	(n)	%	(n)	%
Grief reactions						
Crying spells	(8)	32	(8)	38	(16)	35
Sadness, longing	(10)	40	(9)	43	(19)	41
Indifference, unconcern	(1)	4	(3)	14	(4)	9
Denial of death	(2)	8	(10)	48*	(12)	26
Remembering dead father	(8)	32	(10)	48	(18)	39
Avoidance of subject of death	(4)	16	(5)	24	(9)	19.5
Search for 'substitute father'	(7)	28	(14)	67†	(21)	46
Behavior symptoms						
Regressive overdependent behavior	(13)	52	(14)	67	(27)	59
Separation problems	(9)	36	(9)	43	(18)	39
Clinging to mother	(7)	28	(11)	52	(18)	39
Excessive demands for help	(5)	20	(8)	38	(13)	28
Aggressive behavior	(5)	20	(7)	33	(12)	26
Temper tantrums	(5)	20	(3)	14	(8)	17
Negativism, discipline problems	(8)	32	(9)	43	(17)	37
Restlessness	(8)	32	(9)	43	(17)	37
Fears	(12)	48	(11)	52	(23)	50
Night fears, sleeping problems	(2)	8	(10)	48‡	(12)	26
Withdrawal, social isolation	(5)	20	(7)	33	(12)	26
Rejection of strangers	(7)	28	(1)	5§	(8)	17
'Exemplary' behavior	(4)	16	(3)	14	(7)	15
Repeated complaints about health	(2)	8	(7)	33‖	(9)	19.5
Eating problems	(4)	16	(5)	24	(9)	19.5
Enuresis	(2)	8	(2)	10	(4)	9
Soiling, encopresis	(2)	8	(1)	5	(3)	6.5
Thumbsucking	(6)	24	(4)	19	(10)	22
Altogether severe disturbance: 'pathological bereavement'	(11)	48	(12)	52	(23)	50

*$P < 0.01$, $\chi^2 = 9.18$; †$P < 0.01$, $\chi^2 = 7.12$; ‡$P < 0.05$, $\chi^2 = 5.3$; §$P < 0.05$, $\chi^2 = 5.48$; ‖$P < 0.05$, $\chi^2 = 5.02$.

appear less frequently and are less noticeable than in the first 6 months after the father's death. Mothers often compared their own and their child's mourning process to a painful open wound that gradually heals.

As for the rate of behavior problems, we found a consistent trend for a higher prevalence of maladaptive responses among the non-kibbutz children. However, for most of the reported symptoms the difference did not reach statistical significance. City and kibbutz mothers gave very similar answers regarding the overall severity of the emotional impact of the loss on their children. The percentage of "pathological bereavement" characterized by the presence of multiple and persistent clinical symptoms of sufficient severity to handicap the child in his everyday life within the family, school and peer group was very high and about identical for kibbutz and non-kibbutz children, 48 (12) and 52% (11) respectively. All these findings appear to confirm our previous conclusions regarding the tremendous and lasting influence of the death of the father on the child's emotional life. It seems that in every case where the father filled a significant role in the child's life—in a city or a kibbutz family—the reaction to parental death in childhood is severe and prolonged, so much so that one and a half years after bereavement about half the children from both settings display manifest evidence of serious pathological disturbance.

A number of differences in the quality of grief and behavior reactions were found between the preschool children (age 3½–6 yr) and the school-age children (6–11½) of the kibbutz and non-kibbutz samples (Table 2). The younger children tended to be more spontaneous and actively engaged in recalling activities and talking about the dead father—with frequent use of denial regarding the finality of death. They tended to urge their mothers to get married and find a surrogate father. On the other hand, most of the older children appeared to be afraid to allow feelings of longing to emerge. They dealt with the subject of death more symbolically through play, drawing, composition of diaries and reading of selected books. Emotional restraint in verbal expression and general social withdrawal were frequently observed among the older children. Other significant differences between the two age groups were a higher frequency of night fears, separation difficulties and manifestations of overdependence and demandingness among the preschoolers. Among

TABLE 2. PREVALENT BEREAVEMENT REACTIONS ACCORDING TO AGE

		Preschool children (age 3½–6) (n = 31)		School-age children (age 6½–11½) (n = 15)	
	(n)	(n)	%	(n)	%
Remembering dead father	(18)	(13)	42	(5)	33
Denial of death	(12)	(9)	29	(3)	20
Avoidance of subject	(9)	(2)	6	(7)	46
Withdrawal, social isolation	(12)	(3)	10	(9)	60
Night fears	(12)	(10)	32	(2)	13
Separation problems	(18)	(14)	45	(4)	26
Regressive overdependent behavior	(27)	(20)	64	(7)	46
Excessive demands for help	(13)	(10)	32	(3)	20
Aggressive behavior	(12)	(7)	22	(5)	33
Restlessness	(17)	(10)	32	(7)	46
'Exemplary' behavior	(7)	(1)	3	(6)	40

the older children a higher prevalence of restlessness, aggressiveness or unexpected "exemplary behavior" was found.

Differences in Patterns of Response

We found that the differences in child-rearing methods, family functioning style and social setting influenced the type of problems which became prominent more than the overall severity of the bereavement outcome. Thus, for example, city children showed an intensified prevalence of denial of death ($x^2 = 9.18$; $P < 0.01$). About half of the city children (10), compared to only 8% (2) of the kibbutz children, still used this form of defence in the second year of bereavement. Undoubtedly, cultural factors have decisive influence in strengthening and preserving the use of denial. Kibbutz children learn to look at death more realistically, while city children are more exposed to religious ideas about the coming of the Messiah and resurrection of the dead. Four of the city children (aged 3, 4, 8 and 10) came from religious homes where the mothers explained that "father is in heaven" or "he sees us and protects us." Three other city children (aged 4, 5 and 8) held on to the idea of the Messiah which they heard at school, and still anticipated their father's return one and a half years after his death. The mothers of these children were not religious, but found it difficult to destroy the child's illusions about his father's coming back "sometime in the future," trusting that time and maturation would bring the child back to reality. Three city mothers (children aged 3½, 5 and 7) tried to get the child's mind off the subject and ignored his realistic interrogation to clarify facts and gain understanding about death as a concrete concept. One mother did not even tell her child that the father's body was buried in a grave. These examples clearly demonstrate how religious belief, or the adult's difficulty in coping with the finality of death, strengthens the child's tendency to denial and makes it difficult for him to understand the concept of irreversibility and the full meaning of death.

More city children tended to go on looking for a "father substitute" and to capriciously cling to accessible adult male figures ($x^2 = 7.12$; $P < 0.01$). We assume that in the city there are generally less opportunities of getting stable male surrogate models in the child's surroundings compared to the kibbutz, and so it may be that the city child becomes more absorbed and preoccupied in his continuous search for a substitute father figure. The kibbutz child tended to become attached to someone near and available every day who lived in the same kibbutz (grandmother, uncle, neighbor, or father of another child in his age-group). In the city the connection with the extended family or with the surroundings is often less intensive and more diffused geographically.

While there is a common denominator as to the marked degree of overall psychological disruption among bereaved children of both settings, specific differences were found regarding the nature and severity of several problem behaviors. As has been already stated, there was a consistent trend for a higher frequency of clinical symptoms among the non-kibbutz children. Thus, night fears appeared more frequently in the city children ($\chi^2 = 9.18$; $P < 0.01$). Night terrors appeared mainly in non-kibbutz preschool children; four of them had slept regularly in their mother's bed since the death of the father. At first glance it seems surprising that kibbutz children who slept in children's houses separated from their parents had less night fears than their counterparts in the city. This cannot be explained by failure to detect night fears among kibbutz children who sleep in separate dwellings. Actually, the mothers, the *metapelet* (care-giver) and the nightwatchman are very alert to recording manifestations of sleep problems and night fears in the kibbutz children's homes. Paradoxically, it appears that the setting of communal sleeping in the children's homes, the fact that the kibbutz child is less dependent on his parents and is used to remaining separated from them during the night, reduces the appearance of fears and apprehensions at night. In the city the child is, of course, more dependent on his parents for his feelings of security at night. This lower rate of night fears among kibbutz children compared to children reared in regular families has been found not only for bereaved children but also in comparative studies of samples of the general population of city and kibbutz children (Kaffman, 1961; Kaffman and Elizur, 1977).

Among city children we also found a higher frequency of overly dependent behavior [67 (14) vs 52% (13)], clinging to mother [52(11) vs 28% (6)], aggressiveness, fears, restlessness and a higher percentage of negative attention-seeking devices such as repeated health complaints without objective basis ($\varkappa^2 = 5.02$; $P < 0.05$). Another manifestation different for the two groups is the stronger tendency of kibbutz children to reject strangers who try to make contact with them ($\varkappa^2 = 5.48$; $P < 0.05$). This reaction has not been examined among kibbutz children from intact families, but our personal experience and close contact with hundreds of kibbutz youngsters make us assume that in general it is a prevalent characteristic of kibbutz children who grow up in relatively closed peer-groups until adolescence. Intrusive outsiders are not only excluded from the cohesive group but may eventually become the target of mistrust and hostility. Undoubtedly, a traumatic event of the magnitude of a father's death strengthens this tendency. It has been shown by experimental studies in the field of social psychology that states of frustration and stress often encourage animosity toward strangers (Gluetzkow and Bowman, 1946).

DISCUSSION

Our findings show that differences in terms of upbringing, system of education and family functioning do not alter the central fact that the death of the father is a severe traumatic blow to Israeli kibbutz and non-kibbutz children, causing persistent symptomatic effects and considerable emotional disturbance. A year and a half after the loss about half the children in kibbutz and city alike exhibit signs of marked distress, emotional insecurity and psychological imbalance which call for professional help.

Nevertheless, there are certain differences in the behavioral reactive style of children of the two settings—differences surely connected with cultural conditions and specific attributes of the kibbutz child-rearing methods. Thus, for example, in the city religious ideas are influential in reinforcing the young child's tendency toward denial of death. It also appears that in the city the daily setting is less stable, with greater changes in the child's routine following the father's death. Besides, the city child has a closer and more intimate contact with the acute grief reactions of the mother. All these circumstances appear to increase the level of anxiety and the child's feeling of insecurity in the post-bereavement situation, thus fostering increased dependent behavior and clinging attachment to the mother as the remaining major (or only) satisfier of the child's basic emotional and instrumental needs. The city child has more sleeping problems, night fears and clinging behavior, and is also more engrossed in seeking a "substitute father" compared with his kibbutz counterpart.

In this paper we have primarily considered the possible role of certain cultural factors which are different in the kibbutz and non-kibbutz settings. Since both kibbutz and city children showed ample evidence of serious emotional strain and psycholgical disturbance, it appears that cultural differences do not represent an exclusive or major determinant of bereavement outcome in normative Israeli families. The cultural characteristics were found, however, to play a role in determining the particular form of the bereavement reactions. Thus the overall severity of the child's mourning responses appears to be clearly influenced by the presence or absence of a supportive familial and environmental setting that enables the child and his mother to cope with the crisis with a minimum of situational disruption. Unlike the kibbutz mothers, several of the city mothers lacked a stable support network. In our experience there is a clear relation between the lack of a reliable supportive network and the magnitude of the reaction to bereavement. The relatively greater amount of psychological disturbance among the non-kibbutz children may also be partly related to the higher frequency of stressful changes in the family state of affairs following the father's death (geographic move, change of school, mother's new job)—changes which obviously add adjustment difficulties to the city child.

The fact that 18 months after the father's death we did not find any significant improvement in the marked emotional disturbance already observed in the early months of bereavement points to the severity of the traumatic blow determined by sudden and final separation from the father. Even the favorable conditions present in the kibbutz society to assure protection of the children against many stress situations fail to provide a "protective barrier" in the case of death of father.

SUMMARY

This article examines the comparative prevalence of grief reactions, behavioral symptoms and "pathological bereavement" in 25 kibbutz and 21 non-kibbutz children aged between 3½ and 11½ yr eighteen months after the death of the father in war. The findings indicate that in both kibbutz and urban settings the loss of a father becomes a serious traumatic situation for a large proportion of the children, influencing multiple areas of functioning and causing manifold behavioral symptoms. The particular differences regarding the quality of the reactive symptoms exhibited by kibbutz and non-kibbutz children appear to be related to the different sociocultural surrounding influences.

REFERENCES

Elizur, E. and Kaffman, M. (1982). Children's reactions following death of the father: the first four years. *J. Am. Acad. Child Psychiat.* In press.

Gluetzkow, H. S. and Bowman, P. H. (1946). *Men and Hunger: a Psychological Manual for Relief Workers.* Brethren, Elgin, IL.

Kaffman, M. (1961). Evaluation of emotional disturbance in 403 Israeli kibbutz children. *Am. J. Psychiat.* **117**, 732–738.

Kaffman, M. (1977). Kibbutz civilian population under war stress. *Br. J. Psychiat.* **14**, 145–154.

Kaffman, M. and Elizur, E. (1977). Infants who become enuretics: a longitudinal study of 161 kibbutz children. *Monogr. Soc. Res. Child Dev.* **42**, No. 2, Serial No. 170.

Kaffman, M. and Elizur, E. (1979). Children's bereavement reactions following death of father: the early months of bereavement. *Int. J. Family Ther.* **1**, 203–229.

20

Chowchilla Revisited: The Effects of Psychic Trauma Four Years After a School-Bus Kidnapping

Lenore C. Terr

University of California, School of Medicine, San Francisco

A 4-year follow-up study of 25 school-bus kidnapping victims and one child who narrowly missed the experience revealed that every child exhibited posttraumatic effects. Symptom severity was related to the child's prior vulnerabilities, family pathology, and community bonding. Important new findings included pessimism about the future, belief in omens and prediction, memories of incorrect perceptions, thought suppression, shame, fear of reexperiencing traumatic anxiety, trauma-specific and mundane fears, posttraumatic play, behavioral reenactment, repetitions of psychophysiological disturbances that began with the kidnapping, repeated nightmares, and dreams of personal death. Brief treatment 5–13 months after the kidnapping did not prevent symptoms and signs 4 years later.

Beginning in the spring of 1980 I conducted a 4- to 5-year follow-up study of 25 youngsters who had been kidnapped from their Chowchilla, Calif., school bus in July 1976 and of one child who had left the bus

Reprinted with permission from the *American Journal of Psychiatry*, 1983, Vol. 140, 1543–1550. Copyright 1983 by the American Psychiatric Association.

Dedicated to the memory of Selma Fraiberg, M.S.W., child psychoanalyst. Presented at the annual meeting of the American Academy of Child Psychiatry, Washington, D.C., Oct. 21, 1982.

Supported by a Rosenberg Foundation grant and by the Rockefeller Foundation Scholars-in-Residence Program.

before its capture. Originally three young kidnappers, who never explained their motives, commandeered 26 children and their bus driver at gunpoint, drove them about for 11 hours in two blackened vans, and buried them alive for 16 hours in a truck-trailer (the "hole"). Two of the kidnapped boys dug the group out. I had originally studied the 23 children who remained in Chowchilla 5–13 months after the kidnapping (1, 2), and by 1980 I located two additional kidnap victims who had moved away from Chowchilla before the 5- to 13-month study and one boy who had been let off the bus immediately before it was seized. I could not trace the 26th kidnapping victim.

Half of the group of 26 children in the 4-year follow-up volunteered, and the additional 13 joined the study after the decision was made to offer every participating child $100. (Lindy and associates [3] have outlined and discussed the problems of outreach to psychic trauma victims following the Beverly Hills Supper Club fire). There were no detectable differences in clinical features or symptom severity between the early volunteers and the latecomers to the study. Each child but Jackie, who was willing to speak with me only 1 hour, spent at least 2 hours in psychiatric interviews, and each set of parents or guardians except Bob's, who had left the community, provided at least 1 hour of history. The 4-year follow-up took 12 months to complete. The children, their parents, and their guardians understood the research and treatment objectives of the project. Their names have been uniformly disguised in each publication regarding the Chowchilla children. Ages cited in this paper are those at the time of the follow-up study. An age-, sex-, and ethnically matched control group of 25 schoolchildren at McFarland and Porterville, Calif., was studied regarding life attitudes and dreams (4).

Because group experience in sudden, unexpected, and pure terror without any concomitant mutilation or death is so rare and because it is often impossible to obtain cooperation from parents and children following a horrifying event, this follow-up was a unique opportunity to add to the psychodynamic understanding of childhood psychic trauma. The long-term follow-up of this group offered a singular chance to observe the more long-lasting effects of psychic trauma in children.

POSTTRAUMATIC AFFECTS

Residuals of Traumatic Anxiety

The Chowchilla youngsters could remember and occasionally could still feel the difference between "traumatic anxiety" and their more ordinary anxieties 4 years later. Sandra, 12, a child new to the study, remembered, "It was scarier than a scary movie—scarier than when I cut my finger with a knife. I get a lump in my throat when I go to play the bassoon for people, but this was a matter of life or death. I was horrified in a way, and also scared." Bob, 18, the group's hero, was about to embark on a career as a rodeo performer. Despite the dangers of his current work, Bob also considered the kidnapping to be associated with uniquely frightening feelings, which still occasionally bothered him. He said, "I don't like to think how weird it was I was even on that bus. It bothers me, but I can think about it . . . but when I think, I can feel how scared . . . I can feel the feeling. A few times I wake up with that feeling in morning. Rodeos, earthquakes, anything like that don't bother me a bit!" An American Indian girl, Susan, 9, taciturnly summarized this longstanding emotional state by commenting, "I'm afraid of the feeling of being afraid."

Mortification Regarding Vulnerability

A new finding in the follow-up study was the profound embarrassment demonstrated by many of the children. It was as if they felt naked, humiliated, or totally exposed when anyone knew how vulnerable they had been during the kidnapping. They preferred for no one to find out that they had been victims. Their temporary losses of personal autonomy (5) profoundly affected them 4 to 5 years after the trauma.

One of the heroes, Carl, 15, alternated between a sense of pride about his valor and a sense of mortification regarding his victimization. "Everybody makes me talk about the kidnapping, [but] I say, 'It's not true!' " Terrie, 14, who had patiently held a flashlight for the boys who dug, also expressed painful embarrassment. "It's embarrassing when people mention it," she pointed out. "I don't want people to think [that] I wanted to use it just to get attention and stuff." Sammy, 14, had resorted to evasions when strangers at Disneyland recognized him from old television clips. "No, I don't live in Chowchilla," he had responded. These embarrassed behaviors do not correspond to the happily boastful carryings-on that child psychiatrists observe in young children who have accomplished something. Even though the Chowchilla children effected their own release without a death or an injury, they hated their earlier moments of exquisite vulnerability. They could not boast. When American hostages were taken in Iran and a Chowchilla teacher asked her seventh-grade class, "What would *you* do if a gun were pointed at you?" two of the kidnapped children, Jackie and Celeste, glanced at one another and remained silent. Later, each girl told me she had been pleased to successfully avoid another public exposure.

Fears

Every one of the 25 child victims suffered from kidnap-related and/or mundane fears. Fifteen feared another kidnapping, 13 believed in the idea that a fourth kidnapper was still at large, three feared the kidnappers' friends or relatives, and four were afraid the kidnappers would return. Twenty-five feared commonly encountered, mundane things. Nineteen were intensely fearful of strangers (Benji, 10, and Mary, 9, ran whenever they saw one), 15 were afraid of the dark, seven feared vehicles (Alison, 14, made her father move the car whenever she saw a white van), 10 were afraid of the dark outside their homes, five were afraid to be alone, and three were afraid of their own bedrooms.

Despite the fact that each child remained fearful 4 years after the kidnapping, 19 children reported the spontaneous resolution of some of their fears. The extinction of classical conditioning appeared to have been the most spontaneously effective mechanism of resolution of fear. Some of the children who repeatedly exposed themselves to feared things extinguished these fears. In this way eight of 15 who had been afraid of motor vehicles the first year overcame their fears, two overcame a fear of sleeping alone, three resolved fears of being alone, and two resolved fears of the dark. Occasional panic attacks triggered by unexpected, sudden confrontations or stimuli still occurred 4 to 5 years after the kidnapping.

COGNITIVE RESTRICTIONS

Thought Suppression

By the fourth year following the traumatic event, 18 of the 25 youngsters employed suppression (6), or conscious avoidance of thoughts about the kidnapping. The children attempted to block resurgences of traumatic anxiety, shame, and fears by "not thinking or talking about it." Their parents almost uniformly aided this suppression. Interestingly, however, those few children (Leslie, Jackie, and Johnny) whose parents encouraged family discussions about the experience were not spared the effects of the trauma, nor were their clinical conditions mild 4 or 5 years later.

Thought suppression accounted for some of the difficulty I had in persuading the youngsters and their parents to embark on the long-term follow-up study. Most families and children preferred making taciturn responses to making more fully expanded explanations. Alison, 14, whose high-school teacher had asked her to admit to the class that she had been in the kidnapping, complained to me, "After that, the kids came up and talked every day about it." Alison then enumerated her responses to them. " 'Did you cry?' 'Yeah.' 'Where did they put you?' 'In the ground.' 'Did you eat?' 'Nope.' 'Were you scared?' 'Yep.' " Alison had resorted to one-word answers to protect herself from resurgences of anxiety and shame. In the same way Rachel, 16, skipped her first appointment with me to avoid the anxiety she knew would follow. "I don't know why I didn't want to come," she related. "I don't feel bothered by the kidnapping anymore. . . . I feel clear of it. . . . I don't want to be scarred by it. . . . I won't associate my fears with it. . . . I hate the feeling of helplessness more than anything else. I want to be in control, not to lose control." By day Rachel felt in control, but by night she needed to awaken one of her sisters to accompany her to the bathroom.

Denial and Repression

Four years after the kidnapping each child could give a fully detailed account of the experience, confirming the finding from the 5–13-month study that these children did not employ significant denial of external reality during their traumatic experience. Carl, 15, one of the heroes, remarked, "I can make every second, minute, and hour. I can remember every detail and I don't know how."

Although the trauma itself was etched in the children's memories, their subsequent symptoms and behaviors were often forgotten or unacknowledged 4 years later. To reremember symptoms seemed a dreaded admission of vulnerability. Several panic attacks, omens, and nightmares described in 1977 (2) simply disappeared from the children's memories. Four girls repressed so much that forgetting had become an expected process. For instance, Tania, 11, suddenly stopped her Saturday morning home interview to exclaim, "Oh, oh. I'm supposed to fix Benji's toast. I always forget everything!" Later, when Benji did not respond to a question I asked him, Tania berated him. "What's-her-name is talking to you!" Despite this forgetfulness, each of the four girls who employed ongoing repression earned excellent grades in school.

Decline in School Performance

Only four children exhibited school problems that could be connected in any way to the kidnapping. Ellen, 10, lost 8 months of reading experience because of daydreaming the year after the event, and she remained consistently one-half to 1 year behind from then on. Elizabeth, 13, missed so much school because of daydreaming and hiding from the school bus the year following the kidnapping that she repeated 1 year in school. Sandra, 12, a child new to the study who had moved from Chowchilla, "wouldn't talk or participate in class" the year afterward, but she later progressed satisfactorily. Alison's postkidnapping argumentativeness interfered with her school performance the entire 4 years. DSM-III's description of posttraumatic conditions in adults stresses the decline in work productivity that often occurs. Since so few children experienced such a decline, one might postulate that their initial absence of denial of the external events and the subsequent lack of suddenly intrusive flashbacks may have protected them from a decline in school performance.

MEMORIES

Four years afterward, the children's memories of the event remained intact and detailed. However, many of the accompanying affects had become translated into metaphors, dream-like visualizations, and psychophysiological responses; some affects had been moved to contiguous times, ideas, or people. These shifts in expression or placement of affect gave rise to screen memories (7).

Metaphor

Metaphorical expressions of remembered affect were delivered in the present tense, emphasizing the vivid immediacy of these memories. For example, Benji, 10, recalled, "It's like you're going down in a graveyard." Carl, 15, said, "I was in the bus like always. Then a nightmare begins." Bob, 18, told me, "It's like you start to get in a wreck. Here it is again—another wreck!" By creating a metaphor, the child unconsciously attempted to gain some emotional distance from the traumatic memory.

Visualization

Some children, especially when speaking of their memories of posttraumatic dreams or of hallucinations, had faraway looks as if they were leisurely visualizing. For instance, Terrie, 14, looked removed as she said, "I can still see those dreams clearly [from 4 years previously], and they're very vivid." As I interviewed Billy, 13, a child new to the study, his eyes stopped focusing on me as he spoke about a misperception, the "blue van" he believed he saw at the time of the kidnapping. Three girls shrugged their shoulders whenever they mentioned the traumatic experience. One (Mandy, 11) explained that this gesture protected her from seeing "a picture—going down at night into the 'hole.' " The children's visual memories were different from the flashbacks described in traumatized adults; they were like daydreams, and they were unaccompanied by sweating, palpitations, or other signs of acute distress.

Physiological Concomitants

A few children reported that their trauma-related memories brought on physical sensations. When Johnny, 14, spotted a kidnapper's picture in the newspaper, he recalled, "I said, 'That's him!' and I got the old chill up my back, which I get every once in a while." Four years earlier, during the first stages of the bus takeover, John had felt a "tingle" in his back. It appeared that whatever psychophysiological response appeared initially became the response when memories of the trauma were rekindled.

Displacement of Affect

Affects originally connected with memories of the kidnapping could be shifted to a related time, an associated idea, or another person, particularly the psychiatrist. Many children—and even their parents—felt afraid that their interviews would "stir things up" later. Moderate anxiety *did* follow interviews, but, in addition, sizable amounts of anxiety could precede them. Louis, 13, yelled "Help!" the day before his psychiatric appointment and never knew why. Celeste, 12, suffered with a 24-hour stomachache before her first appointment with me. Jackie, 13, had a déjà vu experience 1 hour before.

Occasionally a child shifted anxiety originally connected with memories of the events surrounding the kidnapping to a fear that the kidnapping had precipitated. Memories of the events themselves no longer brought on anxiety. For instance, Mandy had worried during the kidnapping that she would never see her mother again. Four years later, the 11-year-old was "not afraid to think about it or talk about it. . . . I don't dwell on why it happened or why it happened to me. . . . [But] whenever I can't see Mom, I get flutters in my stomach." Mandy no longer feared the kidnapping; she feared that her mother would leave her.

In several instances, affects were displaced from the kidnappers to the psychiatrist. Johnny, 15, was asked by a *Fresno Bee* reporter whether he had any fears as a result of the kidnapping. "Yes," he smiled, "fear of psychiatrists" (8). Leslie was prayed over in "tongues" at the church of a charismatic religion just so she could be strong enough to face me for an interview. Janice, 17, and her sister Barbara, 13, believed I knew about every "gruesome" incident that had occurred near Chowchilla during the 4 years. Five and one-half years after the kidnapping, Barbara, then 15, phoned me from a distant state (about 2,000 miles away) to ask if I had been slipping notes and newspaper articles about Chowchilla into her high-school locker. Her anxiety was so intense that a few hours after I had reassured her, Barbara and her mother phoned me again to double-check.

MISPERCEPTIONS

Four years after the kidnapping eight children reported newly formed memories of visual distortions, and five of the eight children who had described misperceptions during the first round of interviews had retained these images. Memories of misperceptions (9) were not simply "contagious" phenomena, although there was some spread inside families; the two children, Sandra, 12, and Billy, 13, who had quickly moved to new communities also reported misperceptions despite their isolation from the other victims.

Perceptual overgeneralizations accounted for startle reactions, suspicions, and physical discomfort. Barbara, 13, kept her radio on all night to block out any extraneous noises. Elizabeth, 13, jumped and exclaimed "Whew!" when the dog-door banged and the cat walked in. Carl, 15, noted that "sometimes in the night I feel someone is following me." An asthmatic 14-year-old, Alison, told me, "I have claustrophobia in small rooms. I can't breathe. . . . [They] cause asthma." Sandra, 12, avoided public toilet facilities because the smells reminded her of the van ride.

Most of the children could manage scheduled, expected appointments to talk about the kidnapping, but unexpected, sudden reminders that evoked sensory memories precipitated extreme anxiety.

DISRUPTIONS IN SENSE OF TIME

Time skew and omens, which were discovered in the first Chowchilla study, represent disruptions in the sense of time precipitated by pure psychic trauma. In the 1- to 4-year interval between interviews, I began a clinical study of time sense in individually traumatized adults and children (10). I found that the appreciation of duration, sequence, and temporal perspective (11) could be considerably distorted during and after psychic trauma. The 4-year Chowchilla follow-up study demonstrated that time distortions occurred regardless of the children's ages at the time of the kidnapping.

Distortions in Duration of Time

Four youngsters expressed the feeling that the kidnapping had seemed shorter than 27 hours. This finding concurs with Fraisse's citation (12) of two European mine disasters in which miners trapped 2–3 weeks estimated their underground confinement to have lasted 4–5 days.

Two additional children confused day and night during the experience. This time disorientation and the sensation of time shortening indicate two separate but strongly related causes—sensory deprivation and psychic trauma.

Time Skew (a Sequencing Disorder)

Seven children demonstrated "time skew" 4 years after the kidnapping. A total of 14 children exhibited this type of time distortion at some time following the trauma. In time skew, an event that actually came after the traumatic event is mentally reordered into a time frame preceding the trauma, leading the child to conclude that symptoms, dreams, and unrelated events had been predictive. Time skew offers powerful evidence of the inroads psychic trauma may make into previously normal cognition. For example, Leslie, 11, expressed the belief that a crank caller had actually predicted the kidnapping. In her first follow-up interview she said, "Sometimes I think someone else with those men is after me. Like the lady who called me right before." Her mother interrupted her, "After!" Her mother explained that a disturbed woman who had read the children's names in the newspaper after the kidnapping had threatened at least three of them on the phone. Leslie insisted, "I'm *sure* it was before. It seemed like a warning." The joint interview veered away to several other subjects and then concluded. Leslie said goodbye and began to walk through the doorway but suddenly wheeled around for a parting comment, "I still think she called first!"

Omen Formation (a Sequencing Disorder)

Omens are formed in retrospect by the victim, who looks back for a way he or she could have anticipated or controlled the unexpected disaster. In the 4-year follow-up interviews, 19 of the 26 children, including one who left the bus just before its takeover, described the sense that they had been given a sign or experienced a turning point before the kidnapping. The signs included events (Mary, 9: "That day I stepped in a bad luck square. . . . I think if I hadn't have stepped in that square, it would have happened, but not to me!") and fantasies (Billy, 13: "I was 8 years old when I was kidnapped. It was almost the last day of school. It was real fun. You could go swimming. That day there was a treasure hunt and candy in a box, and everybody was trying to find it. I didn't find any. I was thinking, 'Nothing ever happens to *me*.' Then I got kidnapped"). Five children blamed their parents for failing to recognize "signs." Ten believed or wondered whether they could predict the future in nonkidnap situations.

Omens are an impressive indication of how the youngster who is rendered completely helpless in an overwhelmingly frightening event tries to "solve" the event in retrospect, even though in reality such an exercise is useless. Such distortions in sequences and causalities become part of the child's developing personality. In a sense, the child chooses personal responsibility and even guilt for the event over utter helplessness and randomness.

Foreshortened Future (a Temporal Perspective Disorder)

Four years after the kidnapping 23 of 25 victims suffered from severe philosophical pessimism, the sense that their futures would be greatly limited. They expected an unusually short lifespan or a future disaster, or they were unable to envision marriage, children, or career. Some evaded answers to questions about their futures, but when pinned down, they revealed their profoundly limited life expectations. Others revealed this pessimism inadvertently. For example, Sammy, 14, in his attempt to convince me he no longer was affected by the kidnapping, said, "I never think of it now. I talk to strangers about it, and it doesn't bother me. I have a lot to tell my grandkids—*if* I ever have any." He explained that the world will end in the year 2000. His family did not share this belief.

These youngsters sounded like the disillusioned elderly as they spoke of their futures with little confidence and scant hope. Without any related questioning, Louis, 12, a Hispanic kidnap victim, said, "I worry I'm going to die when I'm young. I don't think I want a wife. If I do, I would always have to take care of her. If there was an emergency, I wouldn't have time. Only for myself." Johnny, 14, had been required to write a high-school essay about his life's purpose. He stated, "I started out in this world to give my parents something to do. Without me, they would have sat around and played Scrabble. In the future, my purpose, as far as I can see, is unknown." (8). Leslie, a pretty, bright, blond 11-year-old, declared in a matter-of-fact way, "I think I'm going to die young. I'm sure of this. Maybe 12 years old. Someone will come along and shoot me."

It is my clinical impression that depressed children do not exhibit this same sense of a foreshortened future. Further studies may indicate whether philosophical pessimism is a finding specific to psychic trauma. The McFarland-Porterville study (4) indicated that this indeed may be the case. The sense of a foreshortened future appears to be the long-term common end point of several effects of trauma: 1) the sense of foreboding and bad luck that accompanies posttraumatic time distortions, 2) longstanding fears of the mundane, 3) a firsthand knowledge of human vulnerability, and 4) dreams of personal death.

REPETITIVE PHENOMENA

Posttraumatic Dreams

The children continued to have repetitive nightmares 4 years after the kidnapping. The frequency of nightmares had decreased, but the intensity of single nightmares remained high.

The youngsters did not describe dreams that were exact repeat playbacks of the kidnapping (such dreams had been common during the first year). Instead, they reported terror dreams with no morning remembrance of the dream content (13 children), modified playback dreams (seven children), and deeply disguised dreams (12 children). This pattern did not represent the distribution of dreams over the 3-year gap between studies, however, because the group tended to report more recent dreams or earlier nightmares that were particularly vivid.

The youngsters who dreamed predominantly unremembered terror dreams also tended to walk or talk in their sleep. These children were considerably less verbal about their emotions than were those who could remember their dreams.

Dreams in which the child allowed himself or herself to die became fairly common by the fourth year after the kidnapping. Whereas five children reported such strikingly terrifying dreams in the first year, 12 described them in the follow-up interviews, for a total of 14 children with such dreams over the entire 4 years. In six of the 12 such dreams reported at follow-up, the child continued to observe himself or others after he "died"; six children's dreams blacked out entirely with the child's death. All death dreams were horrifying to the dreamers. Some death dreams were visualized at leisure during the daytime.

Eight of the Chowchilla children believed their dreams to be predictive. Their dreams assumed long-lasting significance for them (Sally, 11: "I'm worried that dreams could tell the future. They mean a lot to me."). The sense of prediction is related to posttraumatic sequencing disturbances, omens, and time skew. This "predictive" effect after a severe psychic trauma may account for society's belief that dreams foretell the future.

In 1981 I interviewed 25 "normal" children in the McFarland and Porterfield schools (4), with particular emphasis on their predictions for the world's future, their own futures, and their dreams. Eight indicated that they had dreamed of their own deaths. Six of these dreams could be linked to past episodes of severe, unexpected fright or sudden bouts of unconsciousness. Personal death dreams were more easily remembered and visualized by this normal group than were ordinary dreams. In a second group of 25 consecutive office patients aged 9–18 years who had come to me for psychiatric evaluations not related to trauma, six reported dreams of personal death. All six nightmares had occurred to children who had suffered a severe fright or had been suddenly rendered unconscious. The death dream, to my knowledge a phenomenon not described previously in the psychiatric literature, thus appears to follow psychic trauma or unconsciousness, both situations in which the individual had been utterly helpless.

Posttraumatic Play

Eighteen of the kidnapped children had played repetitively sometime during the 4 years. Five continued to play the same posttraumatic game that they had played at the time of their first interviews, 10 described new trauma-related play, and eight exhibited particularly long lag periods before the onset of any posttraumatic play. Eight had stopped playing by the time of the follow-up interviews.

Mary, 9, and her sister Elizabeth, 13, had played a tag game ever since the kidnapping, which illustrated the longevity, unconscious linkages, monotonous repetition, dangerousness, intensity, and contagiousness of posttraumatic play (13). Mary told me, "We go out to the tree. I tie Elizabeth up with the rope. I run around. Elizabeth trips me. The rope isn't really tied. I leave it loose. We play it a bunch of times. It's an important game." Elizabeth explained separately:

"Me, Mary, and Brian, my little cousin [not one of the kidnapped children], play we kidnap each other. But that don't remind me. We play it almost every day when we go over [to Brian's]. We take turns. We tie him up. We hide him from the other one. Then they break loose or stuff. We've scared each other badly with that game. We've played it in the dark. Sometimes we pretend we're leaving the person. When I'm 'kidnapper' I leave them there waiting for me!"

Reenactment

Reenactment could be distinguished from posttraumatic play only by the sense of fun that accompanied the play. Reenactment occurred in single behaviors, series of behaviors (which became habitual and thus personality changes), and recurrent psychophysiological responses. At the 4-year follow-up eight children or their parents reported episodic reenactments; 19 exhibited personality shifts, many of which were reenactment related; and 12 experienced physical disturbances that repeated sensations they had felt during the kidnapping ("psychophysiological reenactment").

Leslie, 11, ran away from home the third spring after the kidnapping. She left after midnight and hitchhiked a ride from a stranger. "He gave me enough money to go to Aunt Mary's in San Diego." The next morning Leslie's mother reported her missing daughter as kidnapped, but Leslie thought her escapade was "not at all" like the kidnapping. "The kidnapping was *they* were taking *me*," she later explained to me. "The other [the runaway] was that *I* was going." Leslie's runaway had been an episodic reenactment, firmly but unconsciously linked to the trauma.

Many personality changes were the result of repeated reenactments. Johnny presented the most memorable example of a personality shift related to the psychological effects of the kidnapping. At the time of the kidnapping Johnny, then 10, had been frustrated that he had been deemed too chubby and too weak to dig the group out of the hole. He wished to have been a hero. His previous mildly aggressive traits became substantially exaggerated after the traumatic event as he struggled to build up his muscles and to lose weight. By 1980 he had become a heavy laborer in his father's plumbing supply business. "I still work extremely hard getting strong. . . . I do a man's work—gorilla work. We're the gorillas of the bunch!" Johnny eschewed his intellect, which was formidable, and, instead, spent his time irrigating, feeding cattle, playing high-school football, and working in his father's factory. His habitual reenactments had become an integral part of his growing personality. Whether or not it accounted for the tragedy that followed is debatable.

In 1981, 15-year-old Johnny was killed in an industrial accident at his father's plant. He had been unloading a huge load when the truck hoist broke, crushing him between a wall and the heavy equipment. Whether a full-grown man would have known better how to position himself or how to avoid such a catastrophe is a haunting question.

Psychophysiological disturbances related to the kidnapping were a new finding in these studies. It will be recalled that the children were driven about in vans for 11 hours without food, water, or bathroom stops. Four years after the kidnapping, five children continued to exhibit bladder problems, two remained overweight (they had gained the weight immediately after the kidnapping), five suffered from stomachaches whenever they were anxious, and one was of extremely short stature, a finding that had not been evident 1 year after the kidnapping. In most instances medical workups for these conditions had not been done, and medical records of those children who had visited physicians were unavailable; therefore the relationship of the psychophysiological disturbances to the kidnapping could not be unequivocally proved.

TWO UNTREATED CHILDREN AND ONE WHO WAS NOT KIDNAPPED

The two children who left Chowchilla before my 5-13–month interviews were virtually indistinguishable from the original, briefly treated group of 23. Since the Chowchilla study was primarily a descriptive one, its emphasis lay in data gathering and in understanding what had happened to the children, rather than in treatment. Without a sizable untreated control group, the effects of treatment were most difficult to assess.

The brief treatment techniques that I employed in 1977 were interpretation, clarification, education, and abreaction. No massive abreactions were observed in the interviews, but the opportunity to review and describe the entire chain of events might have afforded the victims some minimal emotional release. The children often took exception to my psychiatric interpretations, but their parents also heard them, so they could have reinforced the interpretations at home. Clarification and education relieved Bob and Jackie of anxiety related to their visual misperceptions and hallucinations, but in general it appeared that the brief treatment efforts I made 5-13 months after the kidnapping had not been particularly effective in preventing symptoms and signs at 4 years.

In the initial sessions I had recommended to the parents of five youngsters that they arrange for them to work with a psychiatrist. None of these youngsters saw a psychiatrist during the interval between the studies.

The two children, Sandra, 12, and Billy, 13, who had not taken part in the first study, underwent a clinical course similar to the briefly treated group.

Tim, 9, the child who was not kidnapped, is interesting in that he also experienced posttraumatic effects. He had been let off the school bus minutes before it was taken because his mother had requested a few days before that Tim be discharged first, not last, from the bus. When the children were discovered missing, the authorities questioned Tim into the early morning hours, during a severe thunderstorm. Afterward Tim slept with his mother for months and remained overly close to her, believing her to have magical foreknowledge. He feared storms. "In my mind," he explained, "lightning and thunder is sort of like the kidnapping." He imagined up to 4 years later that the kidnappers had escaped from prison, and he repeatedly played "cops and robbers" and "Batman," monotonously rescuing kidnap victims. He became unfriendly, and he dreamed several times that he had died.

Tim was similar to the actual victims in that he too had been overwhelmingly stressed, in his case by thunder, lightning, policemen, and school officials. He experienced some of the same types of posttraumatic symptoms that the kidnapped children had, but there were two important differences. First, Tim's condition responded noticeably to three psychiatric interviews spaced over 6 months. Over that time repeated dreams lessened in frequency and intensity, posttraumatic play stopped altogether, his clinging to his mother lessened, and his fear of storms subsided considerably, although not entirely. Second and more important, Tim never exhibited a negative or pessimistic view of his future life, compared with only two of the 25 kidnapping victims. "I will live to be an old man," he declared, "maybe 83. I'll get married. I will live in Chowchilla when I'm grown up—I like how small it is, and my parents are here. I don't know what they do, but I'd like to see what they do. I want to go to college 7 long years. You *have* to, if you want to be a lawyer!"

THE FAMILIES

Every family had attempted to dampen kidnapping-related anxiety during the interval between the studies. None of them sought trauma-related counseling or psychotherapy, and they consistently downplayed the kidnapping's significance. Several parents feared additional kidnappers or conspiracies—something originally "caught" from their youngsters. Others shifted anger and anxiety to the school superintendent, bus driver, or town officials. Barbara and Janice's mother had begun, like her daughters, to fear me.

A few nonkidnapped siblings, cousins, and neighbors took part in posttraumatic play. Sheila's nonkidnapped sister played so much that she continued long after Sheila herself had stopped. Some siblings and cousins extended the kidnapped victims' visual misperceptions through family-spread tales. In general, the kidnapped children did not keep up their relationships with one another, with the exception of Susan and Ellen, who remained intimate friends. The only two mothers of kidnapped youngsters who had developed a kidnapping-related friendship abruptly and painfully ended their relationship just before the 4-year follow-up study began.

Major family problems continued to emerge during the interval between studies. Fifteen families experienced problems of enormous import, such as deaths of children or parents (three children and two families), alcoholism (five children and three families), divorce or separations (eight children and five families), violence at home (two children and one family), or two or more long-distance moves (seven children and five families). Although at 1 year there had been no correlation between symptom severity and family problems (1), at 4-5 years there was. Children from multiproblem or isolated families or from families with recent problems tended to exhibit more severe clinical manifestations on follow-up. In addition, children with prior physical or emotional vulnerabilities manifested more severe posttraumatic symptoms.

LATE VERSUS EARLY SIGNS OF PSYCHIC TRAUMA

Although this report describes many similarities between findings in school-age youngsters 1 year and 4 years after a traumatic event, certain symptoms and signs became more evident as time progressed. They included mortification, or intense shame; thought suppression; denial and repression of posttraumatic symptoms (this occurs over many years, whereas the details of the traumatic event remain clearly remembered from the first); unlinking of some memories from affect; memories of misperceptions; the sense of a foreshortened future (a striking long-term finding); death dreams; and the dangerous nature, contagion, and endless repetition of posttraumatic play and reenactment.

Even though some of the more dramatic manifestations of psychic trauma (exact repetition of dreams and some fears) disappear over time, a significant trauma continues to exert an influence on the everyday life, personality development, and future expectations of previously normal children. Four years after the Chowchilla kidnapping there were evident relationships between the clinical severity of the children's posttraumatic conditions and their preexisting family pathology, lack of community bonding, recent family problems, and individual vulnerabilities. More important, however, *every* child was found to suffer from a posttraumatic stress response syndrome as late as 4 to 5 years after the incident. The posttraumatic manifestations were strikingly similar despite the fact that the group included children of oedipal, latency, and adolescent phases of development.

DIFFERENCES BETWEEN CHILD AND ADULT RESPONSES TO TRAUMA

Despite several similarities between the findings in the Chowchilla children and some of those previously described in adults (14-18), there were significant differences between the long-term responses of children and adults to trauma: 1) The children did not become fully or partly amnesic, 2) "psychic numbing" was not observed in the children, 3) intrusive, dysphoric flashbacks were not evident in the children, 4) decline in school performance was relatively infrequent in the children, 5) posttraumatic play and reenactment were more frequently observed in the children and were more important to their personality development, 6) time skew was a more frequent posttraumatic manifestation in the children, and 7) a limited view of the future was particularly striking in the children.

From the Chowchilla studies it can be concluded that children are not more flexible than adults following a pure psychic trauma. Despite the popular wish among the public and the lay press that children will spontaneously outgrow or even improve themselves after such sudden, intense frights, the evidence from Chowchilla is to the contrary. Brief psychiatric intervention 5-13 months after the trauma did little to relieve symptoms or stem the tide of philosophical pessimism. Despite their boasts that earthquakes, world affairs, and nuclear calamities did not frighten them any longer, these children were not toughened; they simply had narrowed their spheres of concern to their own rooms at night, to the local disasters in their home towns, and to other kidnap victims around the world.

REFERENCES

1. Terr, L. (1979). Children of Chowchilla: a study of psychic trauma. Psychoanal Study Child 34:552–623.

2. Terr, L. C. (1981). Psychic trauma in children: observations following the Chowchilla school-bus kidnapping. Am J Psychiatry 138:14–19.
3. Lindy, J., Grace, M., Green, B. (1981). Survivors: outreach to a reluctant population. Am J Orthopsychiatry 51:468–478.
4. Terr, L. (1983). Life attitudes, dreams, and psychic trauma in a group of "normal" children. J Am Acad Child Psychiatry 22:221–130.
5. Erikson, E. (1950). Childhood and Society. New York, WW Norton & Co.
6. Vaillant, G. (1971). Theoretical hierarchy of adaptive ego mechanisms. Arch Gen Psychiatry 24:107–118.
7. Kennedy, H. (1950). Cover memories in formation. Psychoanal Study Child 5:275–284.
8. Tompkins, S. (1June 28, 1981). Sadly silenced. Fresno Bee, p F1.
9. Loftus, E. (1980). Memory. Reading, Mass., Addison-Wesley.
10. Terr, L. (1983). Time sense following psychic trauma: a clinical study of ten adults and twenty children. Am J Orthopsychiatry 53:244–261.
11. Ornstein, R. (1975). On the Experience of Time (1969). New York, Pelican.
12. Fraisse, P. (1963). The Psychology of Time. New York, Harper & Row.
13. Terr, L. (1981). Forbidden games: post-traumatic child's play. J Am Acad Child Psychiatry 20:741–760.
14. Erikson, K. (1976). Everything in Its Path. New York, Simon and Schuster.
15. Titchener, J. L., Kapp, F. T. (1976). Family and character change at Buffalo Creek. Am J Psychiatry 133:295–299.
16. Gleser, G., Green, B., Winget, C. (1981). Prolonged Psychosocial Effects of Disaster. New York, Academic Press.
17. Ploeger, A. (1972). A 10-year follow up of miners trapped for 2 weeks under threatening circumstances, in Stress and Anxiety. Edited by Spielberger C, Sarason J. Washington, DC, Hemisphere Publishing Corp.
18. Archibald, H., Tuddenham, R. (1965). Persistent stress reaction after combat. Arch Gen Psychiatry 12:475–481.

Part VI

CLINICAL ISSUES

In this section, Rutter presents an authoritative review of the question of cognitive deficits in the pathogenesis of autism. His survey clearly shows that children with this baffling pervasive developmental disorder have a serious cognitive deficit involving language, sequencing and abstraction. His comprehensive and systematic review suggests directions for further research and possible clues to discovering the mechanisms which may be involved in the pathogenesis of this most destructive and yet obscure mental illness of childhood. At the same time, Rutter also points to the fact that we still have much to learn about the nature of the disordered cognitive processes in autism which still remains a riddle.

The severely handicapped child has to struggle not only with the direct crippling effects of his handicap, but also with the psychological consequences these limitations impose in childhood, adolescence and adult life. The family is also caught up in a host of stresses in its struggle to accept and support its handicapped member. In her article on the psychopathology of handicap, Bicknell defines these issues with a combination of professionalism and compassion which bespeaks her commitment to these stricken children and their families. In discussing the critical issues that arise at different age-stage periods, she offers insightful recommendations and advice, which are practical, thoughtful and sensitively attuned to the needs of the youngster and the whole family.

The clinical issues involving the hyperactive child continue to present many challenging questions of etiology, prevention, treatment and prognosis. Much has been learned in recent years, but many questions still remain at best only partially solved. The two papers on childhood hyperactivity discuss two different aspects of this clinical issue. August and Stewart report two familial subtypes. In one, at least one biological parent had a diagnosis in the antisocial spectrum, and in the other subtype neither parent had such a diagnosis. The authors find correlations between the familial subtypes and the type of symptomatology exhibited by the hyperactive child. They suggest that the study of family constellations could be one fruitful method for resolving the heterogeneity of the hyperactive-child syndrome. Hechtman and Weiss undertake a review of the adolescent and early adulthood outcome of children who had been diagnosed as hyperactive (attention deficit disorder), including their own study cases. While some were found to be functioning normally as adults, a troublesome minority were experiencing substantial psychiatric problems. They leave us with the challenges to identify early in life the group with unfavorable outcomes, and to devise effective therapeutic and preventative measures for them.

Finally, Beardslee and his associates review the studies of children of parents with major affective disorders. It is clear from the relevant literature that these children are at high risk for behavior disorder development. As the authors indicate, this finding raises a number of important issues for further research. Beyond outlining these research questions, the authors emphasize the need for careful clinical attention to this group of high-risk youngsters.

21

Cognitive Deficits in the Pathogenesis of Autism

Michael Rutter

Department of Child and Adolescent Psychiatry, Institute of Psychiatry,
University of London, London

INTRODUCTION

Like all those of my generation who trained in child psychiatry at the Maudsley Hospital, I have many warm memories of Dr. Kenneth Cameron, who provided the guiding light for so many trainees over the years. He set an example of concerned clinical care with a sensitivity to the needs and feelings of children, together with an appreciation of the many difficulties faced by parents in the upbringing of those children. Perhaps it is that model of the good clinician for which Kenneth Cameron will be most remembered. But also, he was part of the birth and early growth of academic child psychiatry. His clinical research spanned a wide range of topics, but his investigations of what was then called "infantile psychosis" constituted one of the most enduring of his interests. When he wrote on the topic in the mid-'50s (Cameron, 1955, 1958) he drew attention to several issues that have been of major importance in the research that followed. He was one of the first to observe that infantile psychoses might develop on the basis of organic brain damage. Moreover, he emphasized that although straightforward mental handicap and psychosis might present as problems in differential diagnosis,

Reprinted with permission from the *Journal of Child Psychology and Psychiatry*, 1983, Vol. 24, No. 4, 513–531. Copyright 1983 by the Association for Child Psychology and Psychiatry.

Presented as the 4th Kenneth Cameron Memorial Lecture given at the 10th International Congress of the International Association for Child and Adolescent Psychiatry and Allied Professions, Dublin, 29 July, 1982.

intellectual impairments could also constitute crucial factors in the aetiology of the psychotic process. Accordingly, it seemed appropriate to
take as the topic of this memorial lecture the role of cognitive deficits
in the pathogenesis of autism—autism constituting the most important
of the pervasive developmental disorders that used to be included in the
old category of infantile psychosis.

During the last 10–15 years it has come to be accepted that autistic
children have a basic cognitive deficit (DeMyer *et al.*, 1981). Thus, in
their 1970 book *Psychological Experiments with Autistic Children*, Hermelin
and O'Connor (1970) suggested that autism stemmed from an inability
to encode stimuli meaningfully—an inability that affected what was
heard more than what was seen or felt. Somewhat similarly, in 1979 I
concluded

> There is good evidence for the existence of a basic cognitive
> deficit in autism. This deficit involves impaired language, se-
> quencing, abstraction and coding functions generally. It is
> also associated with abnormalities in language function and
> usage which are particularly characteristic of the autistic syn-
> drome. The extent and severity of the cognitive deficit are
> powerful predictors of outcome. Treatment can do much to
> reduce the social and behavioral problems shown by autistic
> children, but it does little to alter cognitive development.
> (Rutter, 1979, p. 261)

Although different researchers express their ideas on the nature of
autism in rather varied terms, and although they differ in the emphasis
placed on particular aspects of cognition, there would be little dispute
today on the general notion that autistic children have a basic cognitive
deficit.

Cognition, Conation and Affect

But just what does this mean, and what are the implications for our
understanding of the condition of autism and for our treatment of the
children with that condition? The term "cognition" refers to the mental
faculty of "knowing"—that is, the various functions by which the brain
receives, stores and processes incoming information about the environment and about the person himself. Broadly speaking, then, cognition
serves as a generic term to cover processes such as perception, attention,
learning, memory, judgment and thinking. By grouping these brain

functions together a distinction is being made between the processes involved with "knowledge" (i.e. cognition) and those concerned with "affect" (feelings, emotions and moods) or "conation" (volition, desire or willing). The differentiation of knowledge, affect and conation goes back several centuries and represents one of the earliest attempts to delineate the different types of functions served by the brain. It has proved useful to retain these terms in our conceptualization of the different aspects of human behaviour and development. Thus most textbooks on child development will have a chapter on cognitive development which is separate from those on emotional development and on social development.

However, it has been obvious for some time that although these different domains of life concern behavioral features that are indeed meaningfully different (we would all accept that an unhappy miserable mood is different from, say, the cognitive impairments shown by a mentally retarded child), nevertheless cognition, conation and affect are functionally intertwined. Their differentiation is convenient for a host of reasons, but still the separation between systems is rather artificial.

Let me illustrate this by turning to some observations on normal child development. For example, although young babies can show positive and negative emotions (they laugh, cry, whimper and chortle), they do not show *anticipatory* emotions until about the age of 9–12 months (see Rutter, 1980a). At that age they first begin to laugh in anticipation of a peek-a-boo game and also they begin to cringe and appear apprehensive when the nurse approaches with the inoculation needle. Younger infants cry when the needle is stuck into their leg, but they do not seem to incorporate the experience into their mental framework and, after the inoculation is over, they will readily return to the nurse who gave them the injection. All of that changes towards the end of the first year of life. The cognitive component of distress which characterizes fear and anxiety becomes part of emotion at that stage.

Attachment and bonding provide another example (Rutter, 1980b). Some time around 6–9 months infants ordinarily develop selective bonds or attachments to particular people. All parents are familiar with this "I want mommy" phase of development. The transition is an important one with practical consequences. In the early months of life babies admitted to hospital do not show the acute distress and protest followed by despair that is characteristic of 1- to 4-year-olds. But also, older children tend not to exhibit this pattern of emotional disturbance. Whereas the precise mechanisms underlying attachment remain a matter for controversy, it seems clear that these age changes reflect cognitive alterations. Babies readily engage in social interchanges, and it is meaningful and appropriate to talk about "dialogues" between parent and infant—it is that social quality that makes babies fun to play with. But just as they do not hold in their memory a concept of the inoculation needle, so too do they not seem to have an enduring concept of "mother" or "father" as a person. They can recognize their parents, but somehow that recognition does not yet lead to relationships with the persistence over time characteristic of bonding. When they are cognitively able to maintain that concept, then selective attachments and distress over separation from their parents develop. But that distress is a function not only of the newly acquired cognitive concept, but also of the cognitive limitation that they are not able to realize that when mummy goes away she will soon return. The acquisition of this later cognitive skill allows children to maintain the feeling of a relationship even when the person is away. It is probably for this reason that older children are much better able to cope with hospital admission and hence are less likely to show emotional disturbance when they are left in a strange environment.

These first two examples come from emotional and social development; the third may be said to represent the beginnings of moral development. Recent work by Kagan (1981) and his associates has documented the important transitions that occur towards the end of the second year, when infants first show self-awareness. The emerging set of standards, that is, the concepts of "right" and "wrong," are shown by the child's smiling and evident pleasure when he succeeds in something, as well as by his distress and concern over mistakes in his own behavior, or with objects that are flawed or broken. Most people assume that a person's moral standards reflect the way he has been brought up. This work, however, suggests that although the *particular* standards gained may well reflect patterns of upbringing, the fact that moral standards develop at all is a function of biologically determined cognitive development.

All of this research emphasizes that much of affect and conation depend on cognitive capacities of one type or another. I have somewhat labored the point because it is crucial to appreciate that these fundamental interconnections between cognition, affect and conation are part and parcel of normal behavior and development—the general idea of interconnections and the notion that cognitive deficits may underlie social or emotional features is not special to autism. Rather, it is a central tenet of developmental psychology and psychiatry.

Should we then abandon the differentiation between cognition, conation and affect if they are so closely linked? No, that would be foolish for two rather separate reasons. Firstly, although connected, they are not the same, and the factors that influence cognitive development are rather different from those that affect social and emotional development (Rutter, 1981, 1982). Secondly, if we are to understand how development proceeds and why abnormalities in development occur, we must be able to identify the specific mechanisms and processes involved. That need demands not only that we determine the precise nature of the links between cognition, conation and affect, but also that we identify the specifics of connections in particular circumstances and the directions in which the causal arrows run.

Basic Cognitive Deficits

So much for the concept of cognition as such. But the postulate that autistic children have a basic cognitive deficit involves more than an assumption that cognition and socialization may be connected. The word "deficit" implies some type of lack or deficiency in the area of cognitive functioning. Its use means that autism is being grouped with mental handicap and with the specific developmental delays rather than with mental illness. That constitutes the reason for the classification of autism under the heading of "Pervasive Developmental Disorders" in the American Psychiatric Association (1980) scheme, DSM-III, an improvement over ICD-9 in my view. The suggestion is that autism constitutes a condition in which there has been some type of interference with or abnormality of brain development such that the child has a general, or partial and specific, impairment in some aspect of cognitive functioning. Two distinctions are implicit in this application of the concept of "deficit." Firstly, it is being argued that there is some kind of inability or incapacity, as against a disordered usage of cognitive skills. That is, the problem is one of an inherent inadequacy in the child's cognitive equipment rather than performance of function that has "gone wrong" in equipment which is fundamentally sound in itself. Secondly, there is the implication that the cognitive lack represents a biological unsoundness. That does not necessarily mean that the cause of the deficit was some form of brain disease or organic pathology, but it does imply that, however caused, brain capacities have become intrinsically impaired.

The word "basic" adds the notion that these impaired cognitive capacities are in some way fundamental to the condition and not just epiphenomena or associated subsidiary or secondary problems. In other words, it is being argued that, in some respect, the cognitive deficit constitutes the core of autism; that it is an integral part of the disorder (and not just something that may or may not be present); and that it is likely to underly many of the autistic features.

Early Views of Autism as a Non-Cognitive Disorder

Before proceeding to consider some of the empirical research findings that are relevant to the hypothesis of a "basic cognitive deficit" I need to refer to some of the earlier conceptions of autism as a "non-cognitive" disorder, in order that we may bear in mind the alternatives to be considered. It is appropriate in this connection to turn to Kanner (1943), as this brilliant and incisive clinician provided the first clearly conceptualized description of the disorder as something different from other psychiatric conditions. Not surprisingly, in trying to come to terms with this puzzling disorder he emphasized different features at different times, so that his papers during the '40s and '50s seem to represent rather contradictory concepts of the nature of autism. His first paper (Kanner, 1943) concluded that: "We must, then, assume that these children have come into the world with innate inability to form the usual, biologically provided affective contact with people, just as other children come into the world with innate physical or intellectual handicaps." This certainly postulates an inborn basic deficit, although one not expressed in cognitive terms. Indeed, earlier in the same paper he argued that autistic children: " . . . are all unquestionably endowed with good cognitive potentialities," making clear that in his view the deficit was not cognitive.

During the years that followed, however, Kanner seemed to shift from his original concept of an innate deficit. Thus in 1949 he suggested that autistic children's social withdrawal ". . . seems to be an act of turning away from such a situation to seek comfort in solitude," the hypothesized situation from which they were escaping being parental coldness and mechanical care. Similarly, in 1946 Kanner argued that the linguistic processes employed by autistic children were essentially normal, apart from their lack of social intent. He quotes with approval the statement: ". . . the abnormality of the autistic person lies only in ignoring the other fellow." Again, in 1951 the obsessive manifestations are discussed in similar terms: "The patients find security in sameness, a security that is very tenuous because changes do occur constantly and the children are therefore threatened perpetually and try tensely to ward off this threat to their security." Three years later (Kanner, 1954) he stated: ". . . it should not be forgotten that the emotional refrigeration which the children experience from such parents cannot but be a highly pathogenic element in the patient's early personality development." Kanner continued to invoke a constitutional predisposition but, although he personally changed his views later, the prevailing concept had come to be one of a condition with disordered social function as a maladaptive response to a noxious environment rather than one characterized by an innate deficit.

In more recent years this concept has been espoused by the Tinbergens (1972), 1976) and by Richer (1978). The Tinbergens (1976) argue that the autistic state ". . . is characterized by an emotional imbalance, in which fear, anxiety or apprehension dominates and suppresses many forms of social and exploratory behavior . . . autistic behavior patterns can be recognized as either withdrawal from, or defense against, unfamiliar situations." They go on to suggest that the autistic child's intellectual retardation is ". . . a secondary consequence of the inhibition of social and exploratory behavior, from which normal children learn so much." Thus it is clear that the hypothesis is that the cognitive problems are purely secondary phenomena, in no way basic to autism. Moreover, the Tinbergens emphasize the parallels between normality and autism: ". . . normal children can at times show all the behavior typical of autists." According to their view, autism constitutes an extreme exaggeration of the social rather than cognitive, and there is no deficit of any kind. Richer (1978) has gone even further in asserting that the theory that autistic children cannot make sense of sensory input: ". . . is as incoherent as it is untestable." As we shall see, that view is not only silly but wrong. It is crucial that we should test the hypothesis of a "basic cognitive deficit," as it has important implications for prognosis and treatment. So, without further preamble, let me now focus on the empirical research findings that are relevant to that hypothesis.

It is convenient to begin with the question of whether autistic children's poor intellectual performance is merely a secondary consequence of their failure to make relationships. There were three reasons why Kanner supposed that their cognitive potential was normal: (a) they usually have a normal physical appearance and an alert and intelligent-looking physiognomy; (b) many have an excellent rote memory and some have unusual special talents (mostly in mathematics or music but occasionally in other areas such as drawing); and (c) a substantial proportion of the parents are intelligent professional people.

These observations have been supported by subsequent research but, of course, they do not provide an adequate test of the hypothesis that the low IQ scores are secondary to social withdrawal. In our own work we have utilized five rather different research strategies to investigate the matter (see Rutter, 1979).

Firstly, if social impairments cause intellectual backwardness, it might be predicted that all autistic children should score in the retarded range on conventional IQ tests. However, numerous studies have shown that this is not the case in that although about three-quarters of autistic children are mentally retarded, one-fifth to one-quarter are not (see, e.g., Rutter and Lockyer, 1967; DeMyer *et al.*, 1974). Severe autistic impairment is entirely compatible with high scores on at least some kinds of IQ tests. Of course, in no way does this constitute a crucial test, in that it may be that social withdrawal only causes a low IQ in certain circumstances and not in others.

The second strategy was to determine whether the IQ scores obtained by autistic children have the same predictive properties as those obtained by other children. Ordinarily, IQ tests have three obvious features: firstly, scores are moderately stable after the pre-school years and correlate fairly well with IQ scores on reaching maturity; secondly, IQ scores are moderately good predictors of scholastic attainment; and thirdly, IQ scores show a modest but positive correlation with the occupational level and level of social competence in adult life. Several investigations have shown that all three features apply in the case of autistic children. (Rutter, 1970; DeMyer *et al.*, 1973; Lotter, 1978). However, it should be added that the same research has shown that the correlations between IQ and scholastic attainment within the normal range of intelligence are lower for autistic than for normal children. We may conclude that, as judged by its predictive properties, IQ scores in the retarded range do have much the same meaning in autistic children as in other children, but that factors other than IQ play a considerable role in scholastic progress for those with normal levels of intelligence.

The third strategy was to find out whether autistic children's IQ scores varied with changes in their psychiatric state (Rutter, 1979). After all, the finding that IQ scores predict educational outcome does not necessarily mean that the scores measure cognitive capacity—rather, it could be that they reflect social impairment which in turn inhibits scholastic attainment. We tested this in two ways: initially by using naturalistic studies to determine whether IQ scores went up in those children who improved and who became more socially involved. The findings show that they did not to any substantial extent (Rutter *et al.*, 1967). Then we investigated whether intensive educational or behavioral treatments led to significant IQ gains (Rutter and Bartak, 1973; Rutter *et al.*, 1977;

Hemsley *et al.*, 1978). The results showed that they did not, even though both programs were associated with social and behavioral improvement. It appeared that changes in IQ were not particularly linked with changes in psychiatric state.

The fourth research strategy involved the investigation of possible motivational influences. Clark examined these in two different types of investigation. In the first, he studied the phenomenon of so-called "negativism"—namely, the possibility that the children know the right answers but deliberately and systematically avoid them (Clark and Rutter, 1977). No evidence of this effect was found and it was clear that this was not a usual feature of autistic children. In the second he used the board form of Raven's Progressive Matrices in order to manipulate task difficulty to see what effect that had on task performance (Clark and Rutter, 1979). The test involves a series of items utilizing a similar format of presentation going from easy to difficult, to easy again and once more from easy to difficult, and then the same reversal once more.

The findings showed the children's task performance went up and down in close relationship to the level of task difficulty. However, there were a few children who got nearly all the items correct as well as a few who got most wrong. The former subgroup was given more difficult items of the same kind and the latter subgroup similar items of a much easier variety. It was found that autistic children who had previously got items correct could be "made" to fail by using more difficult items and that those who had previously got them wrong could be "made" to get correct answers simply by giving them an easier problem, even though the overall task and test situation remained the same. The results demonstrated that autistic children's IQ scores were largely explicable in terms of cognitive factors without the need to invoke motivation. Of course, motivational factors will influence the performance of autistic children just as they do the performance of normal or mentally handicapped children, but they do not account for the low IQ scores shown by many autistic individuals.

The fifth and final strategy utilized the observation that a substantial proportion of autistic children (who previously had shown no neurological abnormality) develop epileptic seizures during adolescence. The question was whether this was related to the children's initial IQ level. The results showed that it was: whereas a third of mentally retarded autistic children developed epileptic seizures, only about one in twenty of those of normal intelligence did so (Bartak and Rutter, 1976). There is no plausible way that this could be explained in social withdrawal or motivational terms. It may be concluded that not only does the IQ in autistic children reflect cognitive capacity in much the same way that it does in other children, but also that mental retardation is associated with brain disorder—again as it is in the general population. However, there is one interesting (and possibly important) difference with respect to seizures. Whereas most mentally retarded children have their first seizure in childhood, the great majority of autistic children do not do so until adolescence (Deykin and MacMahon, 1979).

The research evidence leads to the firm conclusion that many autistic children do indeed have a general cognitive deficit which is not in any way secondary to social withdrawal. But is the deficit "basic" in the sense that it underlies the other autistic features? Two findings suggest that it might be. Firstly, epidemiological as well as clinic studies show that the risk of autism goes up as the IQ goes down (Wing and Gould, 1979), although Kanner's syndrome in its classical form is less often seen in the very most profoundly retarded—those with IQs below 20 (Wing, 1981a). Secondly, of all the clinical features the autistic child's IQ level is the most powerful predictor of psychosocial outcome (Rutter, 1970; Lotter, 1978). Both findings point to a strong and intrinsic association between a general cognitive deficit and autism. It might be added that the evidence from home movies (Rosenthal et al., 1980) suggests that autistic children's sensori-motor intelligence is already impaired during the infancy period.

On the other hand, three other findings are decisive in showing that a general cognitive deficit cannot account for the development of the autistic syndrome. As already noted, about one-fifth of autistic children have a normal non-verbal intelligence. Obviously, in those cases a general cognitive deficit cannot have been basic as it was not present. But also, the risk of autism varies not only with IQ but also with the medical condition. There are several types of mental handicap which are rarely accompanied by autism in spite of the low IQ: Down's syndrome and mental retardation with cerebral palsy provide two striking examples (Wing and Gould, 1979). The implication is that it is not any old cognitive deficit that leads to autism but rather one that differs according to medical condition. The third finding is that the IQ scores of autistic children tend to show an unusual and distinctive pattern which points to a deficit in verbal sequencing and abstraction skills rather than visuo-spatial or rote memory skills (Lockyer and Rutter, 1970; DeMyer et al., 1972; DeMyer, 1975; Tymchuk et al., 1977). This pattern suggests the importance of defects in language and language-related functions, so let us turn to the findings on these features.

LANGUAGE

From the first descriptions of autism it has been evident that language abnormalities constitute a prominent and universal (or almost universal) feature of the condition. But, as with low IQ, we have again to consider the two twin questions: are the language problems secondary to social withdrawal and, if not, do they constitute a basic cognitive deficit that might underlie the other features of autism?

Three main sets of data clearly indicate that autistic children's failure to use speech adequately is not a motivational problem (Rutter, 1979). Firstly, it is well established that the problem is not just one of little speech, but rather one of *abnormal language* (Rutter, 1979; DeMeyer *et al.*, 1981). What has to be explained in autism is not merely limited speech usage but also a serious delay in speech acquisition, and language that is markedly deviant in form. This is a quite different situation from that with elective mutism (where there is a failure to speak because of emotional disturbance) or with speech delay due to psychosocial deprivation. In neither of these conditions are there the abnormalities in spoken language seen in autism.

Secondly, autistic children's pattern of IQ scores indicates that there are cognitive problems above and beyond the failure to use speech. The point is that when autistic children are given cognitive tests that do not require them to use any kind of speech in responding, they do well at some but very badly at others. Usually the tests that show poor performance are those requiring verbal or sequencing skills (Rutter, 1979).

The third set of data comes from the experimental studies of Hermelin, O'Connor and their associates (Hermelin and O'Connor, 1970). Their investigations indicated that, in marked contrast to normal or mentally retarded children, autistic youngsters made relatively little use of *meaning* in their memory and thought processes. They showed a marked tendency to remember best what they heard last, but only a slight tendency to remember sentences better than random words. The reverse was true for normal children. Other experiments showed that autistic children's recall for words depends on their sound to a greater extent than on their meaning or grammatical usage.

The evidence is clear-cut in showing that autistic children have a serious cognitive deficit that involves language, sequencing and abstraction. It is not just a reluctance to speak, it is not a secondary consequence of social withdrawal and it involves far more than an abnormality of speech alone. The second question that had to be posed was whether such a deficit might be basic in the sense discussed earlier. But before discussing the empirical research findings relevant to that issue, it is necessary to be rather more precise on just what sort of deficit we are talking about.

A Deficit Restricted to Language Functions?

Earlier papers by a variety of workers tended to consider this question in one or other of two polar extremes. Some asked "what cognitive deficits *may* be associated with autism?" to which the answer is almost any you can think of (DeMyer *et al.*, 1981). The point is that the most seriously handicapped autistic children tend to have a multiplicity of problems, some of which are specific to autism but many of which are shared with all sorts of other children. Hence the answer that autism is due to some mixture of language, perceptual, motor and autonomic impairments (Wing and Wing, 1971) is not very helpful. The more appropriate question is "what cognitive deficits *must* be present for autism to develop?" If it is to be argued that there is a basic cognitive deficit, it is essential to determine which elements in that deficit constitute necessary features for the syndrome of autism to occur. To answer that question there is much to be said for the research strategy of studying autistic children of normal non-verbal intelligence in whom autism occurs in a "pure" form, not associated with mental retardation or other handicaps. Even though they constitute a minority of autistic children, they provide the best opportunity to delineate the cognitive deficits that are specific to autism. Of course, this strategy depends on the autism in intelligent children being similar in type to that found in mentally retarded children; research findings indicate that for the most part this seems to be so (Bartak and Rutter, 1976).

The other approach in some of the earlier papers on concepts of autism was to draw parallels between autism and developmental dysphasia and to suggest that some form of language deficit might be primary (Rutter, 1968). This hypothesis was sometimes wrongly interpreted as meaning that autism could be a consequence of a speech abnormality—a view that has never been tenable. Rather, the suggestion was that autism might be a consequence of a defect in the understanding of language and in the cognitive processes that deal with language and language-related functions. This hypothesis was tenable, but it proved to be potentially misleading in that it necessarily invoked concepts of "inner language" and of the thought processes underlying language. This constituted a problem because, although obviously there are such thought processes, there is no very straightforward way of deciding which thought processes are or are not language-related. Moreover, the hypothesis seems to require the assumption that language constitutes a distinct and separate biological entity—which it probably does not. Accordingly, rather than bother with which thought processes underlie language, it is preferable to turn directly to the key question of which specific cognitive functions have to be defective for the language abnormalities and behavioral characteristics of autism to develop.

In order to tackle that question, however, there are many advantages in comparing autistic children with non-autistic individuals with a comparable degree of impairment in spoken language. Only by rigorously controlling for level of IQ and language is it possible to investigate patterns of cognitive disability that may be specific to autism. That was the logic behind the comparison of autistic and receptive "dysphasic" children undertaken by Bartak and myself.

The findings proved to be most informative in several different respects. Firstly, it was clear that the two groups were much less alike in their social and behavioural characteristics than some of the earlier clinical descriptions had suggested (Bartak et al., 1975). There were many developmental "dysphasic" children who showed a severe defect in their understanding of spoken language but yet who were not in the least autistic. We may conclude that a receptive language disorder was not sufficient to account for the autistic syndrome. On the other hand, there was a puzzling subgroup of children with characteristics that seemed intermediate between autism and developmental receptive "dysphasia." Although the simple language hypothesis could be firmly rejected, nevertheless some overlap between the two conditions remained to be explained.

Secondly, there were some important cognitive and language features on which the autistic children were not disadvantaged compared with the "dysphasic" children. Thus the groups did not differ in non-verbal reasoning skills or in syntactic language skills, and the autistic children were actually less impaired on measures of articulation (Boucher, 1976; Cantwell et al., 1978). The findings indicate that it is most unlikely that the basis of autism lies in any general deficit in visuo-spatial or perceptual cognition, articulation or the grammatical aspects of language. The findings from other studies (DeMyer et al., 1981) lead to the same conclusions.

Thirdly, there were a number of features on which the autistic children were significantly more handicapped (Bartak et al., 1975; Cantwell et al., 1978). These included: (i) measures of the understanding of language (the language disorder of the autistic children was both more severe and more persistent); (ii) cognitive measures that required "verbal-type" skills in thought processes (the "dysphasic" children, unlike the autistic group, were not particularly impaired in so-called "inner language" functions); (iii) imaginative play and the use and understanding of gesture (the language deficit in autism was much broader than that in "dysphasia"); (iv) the use of speech for social communication (unlike "dysphasic" children, few autistic children were able to hold a proper conversation with a reciprocal and responsive to-and-fro interchange; moreover, this deficit remained even after they had gained clearly adequate language skills for the purpose); and (v) autistic children differed in showing various abnormal features of language, especially inappropriate echoing of what they themselves had just said and other forms of stereotyped and atypical language usage.

In summary, the findings showed that autism was associated with both language abnormalities and a cognitive deficit that was more severe, more widespread and somewhat different in pattern from that found in developmental "dysphasia." The cognitive abnormalities were indeed of a kind linked with language (it was striking that visuo-spatial and perceptual deficits were not associated with autism), but they extended well beyond spoken language; moreover, it appeared to be language deviance as much as language delay that was characteristic of autism.

Is This Cognitive Deficit Basic to Autism?

We must now return to the question of whether this cognitive deficit is basic to autism. Several pieces of evidence suggest that it may be. To begin with, it appears that the deficit is present in virtually all cases of autism. The possible exception is provided by some cases of so-called autistic psychopathy (Wing, 1981b), in which there is no appreciable language delay or deviance. Whether these constitute mild cases of autism or some rather different condition is not yet clear.

Secondly, there is a close association between the cognitive abnormalities and the social/behavioral features of autism. Discriminant function analyses based on Bartak's comparison of autistic and "dysphasic" children showed that autism could be diagnosed almost as well on the basis of cognitive test performance as on behavioral or linguistic grounds (Bartak et al., 1977).

Thirdly, follow-up studies have shown the very considerable prognostic importance of language measures. In our own follow-up study (Rutter et al., 1967) both a marked lack of response to sounds during the pre-school years and the failure to acquire useful speech by 5 years proved to be among the most powerful predictors of social adjustment in adolescence. Other studies have confirmed that apart from IQ, language features constitute the best predictors of psychosocial outcome (Lotter, 1978).

Fourthly, Howlin and Hemsley's intensive behavioural treatment study (Hemsley *et al.*, 1978; Rutter, 1980*c*; Howlin, 1981) showed that in both the short-term and long-term, the experimental home-based treatment group had a better outcome than their matched controls dealt with on the more conventional and less intensive outpatient basis. But, strikingly, the features least influenced by treatment were IQ and language competence. This marked resistance to treatment strongly suggests that the cognitive deficit is intrinsic and perhaps central to the autistic child's basic biological handicap.

The fifth set of findings stem from Folstein's twin study of autistic individuals (Folstein and Rutter, 1977). This was designed to examine genetic factors rather than the cognitive features, but, incidentally, it provided powerful evidence on the links between autism and cognitive deficits. Two results from Folstein's study are relevant to this issue. Firstly, it was found that whereas none of the dizygotic pairs was concordant for autism, 4 of the 11 monozygotic pairs were concordant. This difference pointed to the importance of hereditary factors. However, the second question that had to follow that finding was "what is inherited?" To answer that query it was necessary to determine whether any of the non-autistic co-twins showed any abnormalities other than autism. It was found that few of them did in the DZ pairs, but in most of the MZ pairs the co-twins showed cognitive problems. Altogether, 9 out of the 11 MZ pairs were concordant for some form of cognitive disorder, compared with only 1 of the 10 DZ pairs. The findings both strengthened the suggestion of genetic determination and indicated that what is inherited is some form of cognitive abnormality, that includes but is not restricted to autism. The cognitive abnormalities linked with autism were rather varied in type, but most involved some form of language impairment.

Folstein's conclusions on the importance of a genetic determination that applied to a broader form of cognitive deficit, of which autism is but one part, have recently been supported by a study from Iowa. August and his colleagues (1981) found that compared with the siblings of Down's syndrome individuals, the siblings of autistic probands showed a significant family clustering of cognitive disabilities. Some 15% of the sibs of autistic children, compared with 3% in the Down's syndrome group, had some form of language disorder, learning disability or mental retardation.

All of these findings are consistent in pointing to the presence of a basic cognitive deficit in autism—a deficit that is closely linked with the social and behavioral features of the condition. However, there are a few other findings that emphasize that much remains unexplained. Let me note just two of these. Among the language characteristics that I have mentioned is the autistic child's relative failure to use language for social communication. Autistic individuals may learn to talk fluently and, indeed, some autistic adults develop considerable language fluency and talk almost excessively. But still they tend to bombard their conversational partners with rather stereotyped statements and questions rather than converse in the reciprocal responsive fashion that is typical of the language interchanges of even very young normal children. It is not obvious why a cognitive deficit involving language, coding, sequencing and abstraction should lead to this lack of a social component in the use of language. The other finding is that long after autistic individuals gain fluent language and cease to show the gross cognitive deficits that characterized them when younger, they remain obviously abnormal in their social interactions (Rutter, 1970). The implication is that there is a need to focus research more explicitly on the characteristics of autistic children's social impairments and on the possible cognitive deficits that might underlie them.

SOCIAL IMPAIRMENTS

Curiously, until very recently the social abnormalities of autistic children have been the least studied of all the features of the syndrome, in spite of the fact that it is they that give rise to the name of the syndrome, autism. However, that is beginning to change. In order to examine the possibility that some form of cognitive deficit may underlie autistic children's social problems it is necessary to first determine just what the specific characteristics of the abnormalities in socialization peculiar to autism are. That requires detailed observations of autistic children's social interactions. Several studies have shown that autistic children's social development has a number of rather distinctive features (see Rutter, 1978). There is a lack of attachment behavior and a relative failure of person-specific bonding in the early years. Unlike normal toddlers, autistic children tend not to follow their parents about the house and tend not to greet them when the parents return after having been out. They also tend not to go to their parents for comfort when they are hurt or upset; however, they do not usually physically withdraw from people and may enjoy a tickle or a rough and tumble. In the first year, too, they quite often do not take up an anticipatory posture or put up their arms to be picked up in the way that normal children do.

Experimental studies, too, are needed to determine the elicitors of social behavior. For example, Clark (Clark and Rutter, 1981) exposed autistic children to four different styles of approach by an adult, the styles varying in the extent to which they made interpersonal demands of the child and in the amount of task-directed structure that was imposed. The results showed that as the demands of the situation were stepped up the children responded accordingly. That is to say, the children were most likely to make some sort of social response when the social demands made on them were increased. There was no indication at all that autistic children were motivated to avoid social encounters, as postulated by the Tinbergens (1976) and Richer (1978). In fact, the very opposite seemed to be the case. It was when the children were left to their own devices that they were most likely to be non-social and preoccupied with repetitive manipulation of the available materials. Similarly, McHale and her colleagues (1980) found that autistic children's social communication increased when a teacher interacted with them as compared to when the group of autistic children were left to initiate their own behavior. However, in each of these studies, although the amount of autistic children's interaction increased in parallel with the structuring and demands of the situation, the quality of their social interactions remained highly deviant.

Perhaps the autistic child's social abnormalities may be summarized in terms of two key features. Firstly, more than anything else it is the reciprocity of social interchange that is missing in autism (Rutter, 1978). In adolescence and early adult life autistic individuals may come to want friendships and will make social overtures. But even then they seem to lack the ability to make their social actions responsive to what the other person says or does. This observation is important if only because it forces any cognitive deficit explanation back to a very early stage in development. Even during the first six months of life normal babies will engage in responsive, reciprocal social dialogues (Rutter, 1980b). Secondly, most autistic children fail to seek bodily contact as a means of gaining security, comfort or reassurance. This is particularly striking as this non-specific, generalized attachment-seeking behavior is otherwise such a universal phenomena. In humans it may be observed in children reared in institutions with a roster of multiple ever-changing caretakers

(Rutter, 1981) or in those subject to severe physical abuse. In rhesus monkeys it is even observed in infants reared in total social isolation. Apparently it is a "social" phenomenon that is almost impossible to abolish even with the most extremely abnormal forms of upbringing. It is also true that autistic children fail to move on to the next stage of selective bonding or attachments. This failure might be thought to be due to an incapacity to differentiate between the various adults with whom they come in contact. Indeed, clinical observations do suggest that some of the most handicapped children fail to differentiate between people. But that cannot possibly account for the failure to show nonspecific, generalized attachment-seeking behavior.

So we need to focus on social capacities that in normal children are already evident in infancy. But, equally, we need to recognize that to a very large extent these social impairments persist right into adult life (Rutter, 1970). Bemporad's (1979) account of one of Kanner's cases at age 31 years is illuminating. The man was of normal intelligence and was working part-time as he completed college. However, he still showed a glaring lack of empathic relatedness; he could not appreciate how other people felt and he could not predict how they would respond. Moreover, although he had an awareness and concern that he was different from other people, there was a lack of daydreams and a paucity of sexual fantasies. Far from a withdrawal into a rich inner life, as implied by the term "autism," there was a lack of inner life into which he could withdraw—an impairment of the self as well as of social responsiveness is implied.

My own clinical experiences with autistic adults are closely similar. Several have commented that they are distressed by their inability to understand what other people are thinking or feeling. One young man who has attended the clinic for a quarter of a century since he was first referred as a non-responsive non-speaking child put it most vividly when he came back a few years ago asking for help with his social difficulties. He complained that he "couldn't mind-read." He went on to explain that other people seemed to have a special sense by which they could read other people's thought and could anticipate their responses and feelings; he knew this because they managed to avoid upsetting people whereas he was always putting his foot in it, not realizing that he was doing or saying the wrong thing until after the other person became angry or upset.

As always in the field of developmental psychopathology, it may be helpful to relate these abnormalities to the empirical findings and to the theories of normal development. Curiously, the work on attachment is of little help, largely because there is an assumption of an innate pre-disposition, without a delineation of the psychological processes involved in that predisposition (Bowlby, 1969; Rajecki *et al.*, 1978), and because the research has focused on the differentiation within qualities of security of attachment (Rutter, 1980*b*) rather than on the presence or absence of attachment *per se*. Mahler's (1968; Mahler *et al.*, 1975) theoretical perspectives on separation and individuation are equally uninformative because her account focuses on the importance of the mother rather than on the factors in the child concerned with the sense of self or with social reciprocity. Instead, we need to turn to the field of social cognition in order to gain an understanding of the possible processes that could underlie the autistic child's deficit in social relationships. Early studies of mother-infant interaction show that during the first six months there are coordinated reciprocal changes during feeding, dressing and play; at about 7–9 months the infant comes to have a greater initiating or controlling role during these interchanges (Sander, 1975). In parallel, studies of infant's self-recognition (as shown by their responses to re-flections in the mirror) indicate a regular progression in the emergence of self as both subject and object (Bertenthal and Fischer, 1978; Lewis and Brooks-Gunn, 1979). At about 5–8 months the baby shows interest in the mirror image, touching it, smiling and socializing, but apparently not responding differentially to the self and to others in the mirror. Then at around 9–12 months there is a growing awareness of cause and effect relationships between the infant's own body movements and the moving visual image; the concept of the self as an active agent in space emerges and is followed by increasing self-other differentiation. The bipolar nature of the self-other construct has come to be recognized as one of the principles of social recognition (Harter, 1983). Knowledge of the self, the differentiation of self from others and knowledge of others develop in an interlinked fashion and probably serve crucial roles in the growth of both the self-concept and also attachment and bonding. It is considered that the emergence of representational thought and the de-velopment of language aid the conceptualization of characteristics such as age and gender (Lewis and Brooks-Gunn, 1979) and that new-found perspective-taking skills begin to equip the child to imagine what other people are thinking and, in particular, what they are thinking of him (Harter, 1983). It is clear that theories of the early development of social cognition provide clues about the possible mechanism underlying both the concept of self and of social reciprocity, although it has to be added that there is little empirical evidence about how either is constructed.

With these thoughts in mind, let us return to research more directly concerned with the possible cognitive deficits that might underlie the social anomalies of autism. Piaget (1926) maintained that children's social behavior was constrained by an inability to appreciate and coordinate the perspectives of others. Hobson (1983) used an experimental approach to test the hypothesis that the autistic child's social incompetence resulted from a cognitive impairment that included an inability to recognize other people's points of view in a visuo-spatial setting. The findings showed that autistic children were not more impaired in their recognition of visuo-spatial perspectives than were normal or retarded children of a comparable intellectual level. Clearly, this does not constitute the basis of autistic children's social impairments.

Hobson (1982) went on to argue that autistic children may lack the ability to experience empathy; that is, that other people's expressions of emotions lack the emotional impact that they have for the rest of us. He has recently completed a most important set of experiments to investigate autistic children's abilities to discriminate emotional and personal cues—abilities that must be present if they are to respond with empathy. In brief, the children (both autistic, and normal or mentally retarded controls) were presented with short videotapes portraying emotions, people or things. The task for the children was the matching of the videotape with drawings depicting a range of emotions (happy, sad, angry and so forth), or of persons (man, woman, boy, girl) or of things (dog, bird, train, etc.). Each stimulus was presented in terms of visual stimuli, sound, gesture or context. The results showed that all of the groups of children were adept in choosing the appropriate pictures for "things" in each of the separate modes of presentation; there were no significant group differences and the autistic children showed no handicaps in this matching task. However, in sharp contrast, the autistic children were significantly worse than the normal and the retarded children in their appreciation of "emotions" and of "people."

The findings strongly suggest some form of cognitive deficit in the processing of stimuli relevant to affect and socialization. But what kind of deficit might that be? Obviously, it is not a matter of visuo-spatial perception as such, as the autistic children's difficulties concerned only the appreciation of sounds and shapes concerned with emotions and with people. Moreover, it cannot be a deficit restricted to visuo-spatial stimuli in that there was as much difficulty with sounds as with shapes. The findings of a separate study by Langdell (1978) provide a similar paradox. He found that autistic children differed from normal in their recognition of faces. However, it was not a straightforward matter of the autistic children being better or worse; rather, they were different and, moreover, they were different in a manner that varied with age. Normal individuals find the upper regions of the face most useful in identification, whereas young autistic children placed most reliance on the lower facial features. The older autistic children showed no particular reliance on any one area but were superior to their controls at recognizing faces when they were presented upside down. Once again, the findings are inconsistent with any hypothesis of generally inferior perception, but they do imply that autistic children process information about faces in a way that is different from normals.

Putting these findings together, we are forced to the conclusion that autistic children's social abnormalities probably do stem from some kind of "cognitive" deficit, if by that one means a deficit in dealing with social and emotional cues. But equally, the data suggest that the deficit does not lie in the processing of stimuli of any particular sensory modality or, indeed, of stimuli that are defined in terms of any particular sensory qualities. Rather, it appears that the stimuli that pose difficulties for autistic children are those that carry emotional or social "meaning." As yet it is not clear just what that might reflect in terms of brain functions or neurophysiological processes, but at least one key area that needs further systematic research has been identified.

CONCLUSIONS

In concluding, I need to return to the issue with which I started—cognitive deficits in the pathogenesis of autistic behaviour. The research findings I have considered leave no doubt that autistic children do indeed suffer from crucial cognitive deficits—that much may be regarded as established. Moreover, there is every reason to believe that these cognitive deficits are basic in the dual sense that they are not secondary to other autistic features and that they underlie many of the important handicaps of autistic children. However, the recent research findings emphasize how much remains to be explained. Clearly there are fundamental connections between the abnormalities of cognition, conation and affect found in autism, but we remain ignorant of just what those connections are and, especially, we lack knowledge about the nature of the symptoms of autism that gives the name to the syndrome. In my introductory remarks I drew attention to developmental issues and I have done so again in considering the social anomalies of autistic children. These are important, of course, for theoretical reasons, but they are also crucial for therapeutic concerns. A dozen years ago, when Sussenwein and I (Rutter and Sussenwein, 1971) discussed the rationale for the treatment of young autistic children, we emphasized that one of the prime goals must be the fostering of normal development. In that paper we sought to draw lessons from a combination of what was known about the nature of autism and what was known about normal development. It is evident that this linkage continues to pose difficulties in therapeutic planning. We have learned an enormous amount about how to modify the behavior of autistic children and there is little doubt that these gains in knowledge have led to improved treatment programs with real benefits for the children in them. Nevertheless the most crucial aspect of treatment—the facilitation of normal development—continues to wait on the solution of the riddle of the nature of the disordered cognitive processes in autism.

REFERENCES

American Psychiatric Association (1980). *Diagnostic and Statistical Manual of Mental Disorders (Third Edition)—DSM-III.* American Psychiatric Association, Washington, DC.

August, G. J., Stewart, M. A. and Tsai, L. (1981). The incidence of cognitive disabilities in the siblings of autistic children. *Br. J. Psychiat.* **138**, 416–422.

Bartak, L. and Rutter, M. (1976). Differences between mentally retarded and normally intelligent autistic children. *J. Autism child. Schizophr.* **6**, 109–120.

Bartak, L., Rutter, M. and Cox, A. (1975). A comparative study of infantile autism and specific developmental receptive language disorder. I. The children. *Br. J. Psychiat.* **126**, 127–145.

Bartak, L., Rutter, M. and Cox, A. (1977). A comparative study of infantile autism and specific developmental receptive language disorders. III. Discriminant function analysis. *J. Autism. child. Schizophr.* **7**, 383–396.

Bemporad, J. R. (1979). Adult recollections of a formerly autistic child. *J. Autism devl Dis.* **9**, 179–198.

Bertenthal, B. I. and Fischer, K. W. (1978). Development of self-recognition in the infant. *Devl Psychol.* **14**, 44–50.

Boucher, J. (1976). Articulation in early childhood autism. *J. Autism childh. Schizophr.* **6**, 297–302.

Bowlby, J. (1969). Articulation in early childhood autism. *J. Autism childh. Schizophr.* **6**, 297–302.

Bowlby, J. (1969). *Attachment and Loss: I. Attachment.* Hogarth Press, London.

Cameron, K. (1955). Psychosis in infancy and early childhood. *Med. Press* **234**, 280–283.

Cameron, K. (1958). A group of twenty-five psychotic children. *Revue Psychiat. Infantile* **25**, 117–122.

Cantwell, D., Baker, L. and Rutter, M. (1978). A comparative study of infantile autism and specific developmental receptive language disorder. IV. Analysis of syntax and language function. *J. Child Psychol. Psychiat.* **19**, 351–362.

Clark, P. and Rutter, M. (1977). Compliance and resistance in autistic children. *J. Autism childh. Schizophr.* **7**, 33–48.

Clark, P. and Rutter, M. (1979). Task difficulty and task performance in autistic children. *J. Child Psychol. Psychiat.* **20**, 271–285.

Clark, P. and Rutter, M. (1981). Autistic children's responses to structure and to inter-personal demands. *J. Autism devl Dis.* **11**, 201–217.

DeMyer, M. K. (1975). The nature of the neuropsychological disability in autistic children. *J. Autism childh. Schizophr.* **5**, 109–128.

DeMyer, M. K., Barton, S., Alpern, G. D., Kimberlin, C., Allen, J., Yang, E. and Steele, R. (1974). The measured intelligence of autistic children. *J. Autism childh. Schizophr.* **4**, 42–60.

DeMyer, M. K., Barton, S., DeMyer, W. E., Norton, J. A., Allen, J. and Steele, R. (1973). Prognosis in autism: a follow-up study. *J. Autism Childh. Schizophr.* **3**, 199–246.

DeMyer, M. K., Barton, S. and Norton, J. A. (1972). A comparison of adaptive, verbal, and motor profiles of psychotic and non-psychotic subnormal children. *J. Autism childh. Schizophr.* **2**, 359–377.

DeMyer, M. K., Hingtgen, J. N. and Jackson, R. K. (1981). Infantile autism reviewed: a decade of research. *Schizophr. Bull.* **7**, 388–451.

Deykin, E. Y. and MacMahon, B. (1979). The incidence of seizures among children with autistic symptoms. *Am. J. Psychiat.* **136**, 1310–1312.

Folstein, S. and Rutter, M. (1977). Infantile autism: a genetic study of 21 twin pairs. *J. Child Psychol Psychiat.* **18**, 297–321.

Harter, S. (1983). Developmental perspectives on the self-system. In *Social and Personality Developments.* Vol. 4. *Carmichael's Manual of Child Psychology* (Edited by Hetherington, M. E.). Wiley, New York, in press.

Hemsley, R., Howlin, P., Berger, M., Hersov, L., Holbrook, D., Rutter, M. and Yule, W. (1978). Training autistic children in a family context. In *Autism: A Reappraisal of Concepts and Treatment* (Edited by Rutter, M. and Schopler, E.), pp. 379–411. Plenum, New York.

Hermelin, B. and O'Connor, N. (1970). *Psychological Experiments with Autistic Children.* Pergamon, Oxford.

Hobson, R. P. (1982). The autistic child's concept of persons. *Proceedings of the 1981 International Conference on Autism, Boston, U.S.A.* (Edited by Park, D.). National Society for Children and Adults with Autism, Washington, DC.

Hobson, R. P. (1983). Early childhood autism and the question of egocentrism. *J. Autism devl Dis.* In press.

Howlin, P. (1981). The effectiveness of operant language training with autistic children. *J. Autism devl Dis.* **11**, 89–106.

Kagan, J. (1981). *The Emergence of Self-Awareness.* Harvard University Press, Cambridge, MA.

Kanner, L. (1943). Autistic disturbances of affective contact. *Nerv. Child* **2**, 217–250.

Kanner, L. (1946). Irrelevant and metaphorical language in early infantile autism. *Am. J. Psychiat.* **103**, 242–246.

Kanner, L. (1949). Problems of nosology and psychodynamics in early infantile autism. *Am. J. Orthopsychiat.* **19**, 416–426.

Kanner, L. (1951). The conception of wholes and parts in early infantile autism. *Am. J. Psychiat.* **108**, 23–26.

Kanner, L. (1954). To what extent is early infantile autism determined by constitutional inadequacies? In *Genetics and the Inheritance of Integrated Neurological and Psychiatric Patterns* (Edited by Hooker, D. and Hare, C. C.), pp. 378–385. Williams & Wilkins, Baltimore.

Langdell, T. (1978). Recognition of faces: an approach to the study of autism. *J. Child Psychol. Psychiat.* **19**, 255–268.

Lewis, M. and Brooks-Gunn, J. (1979). *Social Cognition and the Acquisition of Self*. Plenum, New York.

Lockyer, L. and Rutter, M. (1970). A five to fifteen year follow-up study of infantile psychosis. III. Psychological aspects. *Br. J. Psychiat.* **115**, 865–882.

Lotter, V. (1978). Follow-up studies. In *Autism: A Reappraisal of Concepts and Treatment* (Edited by Rutter, M. and Schopler, E.), pp. 475–495. Plenum, New York.

Mahler, M. S. (1968). *On Human Symbiosis and the Vicissitudes of Individuation*. Vol. 1. *Infantile Psychosis*. International Universities Press, New York.

Mahler, M. S., Pine, F. and Bergman, A. (1975). *The Psychological Birth of the Infant*. Basic Books, New York.

McHale, S. M., Simeonsson, R. J., Marcus, L. M. and Olley, J. G. (1980). The social and symbolic quality of autistic children's communication. *J. Autism devl Dis.* **10**, 299–310.

Piaget, J. (1926). *The Language and Thought of the Child* (Translation by Gabian, M.). Routledge & Kegan Paul, London.

Rajecki, D. W., Lamb, M. E. and Obmascher, P. (1978). Toward a general theory of infantile attachment: a comparative review of aspects of the social bond. *Behav. Brain Sci.* **3**, 417–464.

Richer, J. (1978). The partial noncommunication of culture to autistic children—an application of human ethology. In *Autism: A Reappraisal of Concepts and Treatment* (Edited by Rutter, M. and Schopler, E.), pp. 47–61. Plenum, New York.

Rosenthal, J., Massie, H. and Wulff, K. (1980). A comparison of cognitive development in normal and psychotic children in the first two years of life from home movies. *J. Autism devl Dis.* **10**, 433–444.

Rutter, M. (1968). Concepts of autism: a review of research. *J. Child Psychol. Psychiat.* **9**, 1–25.

Rutter, M. (1970). Autistic children: infancy to adulthood. *Semin. Psychiat.* **2**, 435–450.

Rutter, M. (1978). Diagnosis and definition. In *Autism: A Reappraisal of Concepts and Treatment* (Edited by Rutter, M. and Schopler, E.), pp. 1–25. Plenum, New York.

Rutter, M. (1979). Language, cognition and autism. In *Congenital and Acquired Cognitive Disorders* (Edited by Katzman, R.), pp. 247–264. Raven, New York.

Rutter, M. (1980a). Emotional development. In *Scientific Foundations of Developmental Psychiatry* (Edited by Rutter, M.), pp. 307–321. Heinemann Medical, London.

Rutter, M. (1980b). Attachment and the development of social relationships. In *Scientific Foundations of Developmental Psychiatry* (Edited by Rutter, M.), pp. 267–279. Heinemann Medical, London.

Rutter, M. (1980c). Language training with autistic children: how does it work and what does it achieve? In *Language and Language Disorders in Childhood* (Edited by Hersov, L. A. and Berger, M.), pp. 147–172. Pergamon, Oxford.

Rutter, M. (1981). *Maternal Deprivation Reassessed, 2nd edition*. Penguin, Harmondsworth.

Rutter, M. (1982). The family, the child and the school. In *Middle Childhood: Developmental Variation and Dysfunction Between Six and Fourteen Years* (Edited by Levine, M. D. and Satz, P.). Academic Press, New York.

Rutter, M. and Bartak, L. (1973). Special educational treatment of autistic children: a comparative study. II. Follow-up findings and implications for services. *J. Child Psychol. Psychiat.* **14**, 241–270.

Rutter, M., Greenfeld, D. and Lockyer, L. (1967). A five to fifteen year follow-up study of infantile psychosis. II. Social and behavioral outcome. *Br. J. Psychiat.* **113**, 1183–1199.

Rutter, M. and Lockyer, L. (1967). A five to fifteen year follow-up study of infantile psychosis. I. Description of sample. *Br. J. Psychiat.* **113**, 1169–1182.

Rutter, M. and Sussenwein, F. (1971). A developmental and behavioral approach to the treatment of pre-school autistic children. *J. Autism childh. Schizophr.* **1**, 376–397.

Rutter, M., Yule, W., Berger, M. and Hersov, L. (1977). An evaluation of a behavioral approach to the treatment of autistic children. Final Report to the Department of Health and Social Security, London.

Sander, L. W. (1975). Infant and caretaking environment: investigation and conceptualization of adaptive behavior in a system of increasing complexity. In *Explorations in Child Psychiatry* (Edited by Anthony, E. J.), pp. 129–165. Plenum, New York.

Tinbergen, E. A. and Tinbergen, N. (1972). Early childhood autism: an ethological approach. *Beih. z. Tierpsychol.* No. 10.

Tinbergen, E. A. and Tinbergen, N. (1976). The aetiology of childhood autism: a criticism of the Tinbergens' theory:a rejoinder. *Psychol. Med.* **6**, 545–550.

Tymchuk, A. J., Simmons, J. Q. and Neafsey, S. (1977). Intellectual characteristics of adolescent childhood psychotics with high verbal ability. *J. ment. Defic. Res.* **21**, 133–138.

Wing, L. (1981a). Language, social, and cognitive impairments in autism and severe mental retardation. *J. Autism devl Dis.* **11**, 31–44.

Wing, L. (1981b). Asperger's syndrome: a clinical account. *Psychol. Med.* **11**, 115–130.

Wing, L. and Gould, J. (1979). Severe impairments of social interaction and associated abnormalities in children: epidemiology and classification. *J. Autism devl Dis.* **9**, 11–29.

Wing, L. and Wing, J. (1971). Multiple impairments in early childhood autism. *J. Autism childh. Schizophr.* **1**, 256–266.

22

The Psychopathology of Handicap

Joan Bicknell

St. George's Hospital Medical School, London

I have chosen the psychopathology of handicap as the topic for this paper, firstly because it is an area of particular interest to me as a clinician working with mentally handicapped people. As we move away from institutional care to community care with living accommodation in small units and alternative homes, we are finding as never before that we are needing to help groups of people, parents, families and surrogate parents, in the care of mentally handicapped children and adults. Secondly, I have chosen this title because I believe it defines one role of several for the psychiatrist who works with mentally handicapped people, people with other disabilities and those with brain damage. Thirdly, this is an area of work so far little explored by clinicians and research workers.

Those of us who work with handicapped people and their families know well the following phrase: "A handicapped child is a handicapped family." We say this when we see families who are socially isolated, where the siblings are maladjusted, where the home is broken and where splitting has occurred between generations. In our more cynical moments we wonder if the handicapped person only is unscathed.

When working with these families I have been very much aware that their responses follow closely the reactions that we associate with loss, death, and dying, known usually as the *bereavement response*. I want this to be the focal point of this lecture.

Reprinted with permission from the *British Journal of Medical Psychology*, 1983, Vol. 56, 167–178. Copyright 1983 by the British Psychological Society.
Presented as Professor Joan Bicknell's Inaugural Lecture, 19 November, 1980.

A mother had a spina bifida baby and she said to me:
"Do you know when I was told that my baby was handicapped, something died in me, something that I know will never live again."
She could not explain what she meant but she continued:
"A part of me has died, a part that will never live again."
The second quotation is from a mother, who has a profoundly handicapped 12-month-old son and she said:
"Whenever I hear James cry, I hear *his* cry, but I also hear the perfect cry, of the perfect baby I never had."

So, then let us examine the reactions of parents and the extended family to the presence of a handicapped person within the family, let us look at handicapped people themselves, the siblings and then finally the decision-making times and crisis points for the whole family group.

IMPARTING BAD NEWS

There are three typical times, when the sad, bad news of handicap in the child might need to be imparted to the parents.

Firstly, at birth, when a child is born with obvious congenital handicaps. What a cruel time to impart bad news! The mother, just over the delivery, is physiologically prone to be distressed. The parents, if it is a hospital delivery, are separated for possibly the first time in their marriage. The mother is surrounded by mothers who are rejoicing in the arrival of their perfect babies. Could we choose a worse time to impart bad news? Yet we know from retrospective surveys that parents emphatically do not appreciate delay. They want to know as soon as the diagnosis is made.

Secondly, there is the situation where handicap gradually evolves during childhood. The child is perhaps an "at risk" baby—a premature baby; he is followed up by the multidisciplinary team in the Child Assessment Centre and gradually over two or three years the diagnosis becomes clear that, maybe, he has a communication defect, or a mild degree of cerebral palsy or that he is not going to be intellectually normal. When do we share that with the parents? They know why they are coming up to the clinic time and again. Sometimes in an effort to be kind we hold back until we are certain of the diagnosis but again retrospectively parents tell us they would far prefer to be involved from the moment that there are doubts in the doctor's mind.

"How the parents are told is an agonizing experience. The baby on mother's knee is special. He is loved—regardless—and to her is perfect. . . . However outwardly composed she may remain, inside she (mother) is a tigress with a cub," said one mother with an autistic son (Shrimpton, 1980).

The third typical time when handicap is diagnosed is after an illness or accident in childhood. The normal child goes off on his bicycle to visit friends, he is knocked off his bicycle and for the next six weeks he is battling for life in the Intensive Care Unit. Parents, at the end of that time, take him home, brain damaged, helpless, perhaps unable to respond. The prospect of his death has been with them since the accident. They may have thought death to be preferable to survival. They take home a different child from the one who set off on his bicycle on that fateful morning, and the perfect child before the accident becomes idealized as the only perfect reflection in the family mirror.

THE BEREAVEMENT RESPONSE

The bereavement response is the psychological work that has to be done when we come to terms with the loss of a significant object or loved person. In handicap, the bereavement response is somewhat modified; it is the mourning for the loss of the perfect child who has not arrived or who has been taken away through illness or accident.

Figure 1 shows the stages of the bereavement response as it is seen in parents who are told the diagnosis of handicap in their child.

Shock is the stage of emotional refrigeration, or emotional procrastination.

Panic: "I can't cope, I can't look after a handicapped child."

Denial: "He is not mine, the midwife has picked up the wrong baby by mistake."

Grief—the sobbing, the sleeplessness, the pain of what has happened to that family. Grief that is so powerful does not stand still. It is either taken inwards as *guilt* or it is projected outwards as *anger*.

Guilt may be *valid*, and this must be borne in mind particularly now there is more genetic counseling. For example, we may be telling the parents that they are carrying the recessive or dominant gene which has caused the handicap in their child. Guilt, however, may be *invalid*, giving rise to comments like, "it is all because my great-grandmother died in a mental hospital."

Anger may be between *relatives* coming between the generations or

anger may be of one spouse for another: "it is all on his side you know."
Even complex family trees may be produced to ensure that the one held
to blame has no escape. Anger of this nature may be powerfully divisive
when morale is low in the family.

Anger against professionals: "It is all the midwife's fault"; "Why did my
doctor allow me a home delivery?"; "Why didn't they use that stronger
antibiotic earlier?"

Then grief, guilt, anger frequently give way to *bargaining*: "I will look
after him *if* the doctors, the physiotherapists, and the nurses teach him
to be clean and dry, to walk, to speak, to earn his own living," or whatever
happens to be important at that time for that family. Bargaining gives

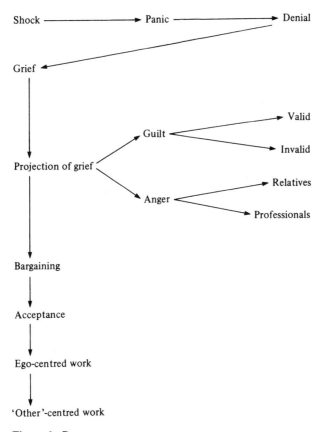

Figure 1. Bereavement response.

away to *acceptance*, when the pain subsides and love begins to take over, and reality is grasped.

Then there is *ego-centered*, or sclf-cenLered or family-centered work: "I wonder what play group he can go to, let's go and have a look at those schools they say are for mentally handicapped children. I wonder if I could meet another mother who has looked after a three-year-old incontinent child." Finally, *"other" -centered work*: the families who have had so much joy from their handicapped child may say, "We will become welfare counselors, we will visit other families, we will help run that evening club. What about that toy library? I am sure I can give two afternoons a week to help there."

Residential Care, Rejection and Abandonment

Requests for residential care are coming now far more from the stage of acceptance rather than from the stage of rejection. With the slightly better services that we are now providing families are making a positive choice of an alternative placement for their handicapped child or adult, linking their request for residential care more with the rights of the handicapped person to live elsewhere or for his special needs to be met rather than with any process of rejection. However, abandonment in residential care which has also been studied, particularly by sociologists, has surprisngly very little to do with the dynamics of rejection, but a lot to do with those who run the residential care services (Morris, 1969; Bradley, 1972). If we do not involve families, if we do not practice—although we may profess—shared care, if we do not welcome relatives who visit, then abandonment is far more likely to happen.

GENERAL POINTS ABOUT BEREAVEMENT WORK

Parents work through these stages outlined in Fig. 1 at different rates. Frequently the mother who is handling the child all day reaches the point of acceptance when the father is still very much at the point of grief or denial. Work in any stage may be incomplete and so pervades the rest of the work, for instance grief will frequently pervade acceptance. Life-events in that family that are nothing to do with the handicapped child may restart this work of grieving for the perfect child who has not arrived. Other members of the family work through the same process, grandparents frequently working through at a much slower rate. Siblings, when adolescent, are often working through for the second time, attempting to come to terms with their handicapped brother or sister with the viewpoint of the teenager. The tendency for generations to work at different rates frequently precipitates transgenerational splitting where there is a handicapped child (Lieberman, 1979).

Professional people become involved as well. None of us stands aloof from handicap when we work with these families. A family had two children, both with a fatal illness, and the children died in infancy. I could not remain aloof when the third child was born and was found to have the same disease with the same prognosis.

The bereavement process is occasionally not worked through completely and what should have been a transitional stage becomes a stage of fixation leading to metamorphosis and a different pattern of behavior, a maladaptive response which can cause endless unhappiness within the family (Evans, 1976). There is an essential difference between this bereavement response to the arrival of the handicapped child and the bereavement response as classically seen towards the loss of an object or a person. This is, of course, the continued presence of the handicapped child in that family group, a constant reminder of imperfection, its antecedents and consequences. The presence of the child also creates extra work, disturbed nights and continued disappointments as milestones fail to be achieved.

MALADAPTIVE RESPONSES IN BEREAVEMENT WORK

Figure 2 includes the same series of responses as in Fig. 1, but there are also the maladaptive responses (in italics) that parents or the family may make if they do not work through these transitional stages to the end of the psychological process.

Shopping around: Parents that are fixed in a chronic state of denial start looking around, endlessly seeking second and third opinions, perhaps selling up their home and, for example, travelling to another country attempting to find that the handicap is reversible or to find a label that for them will be acceptable; the label of autism or dyslexia seems to be far less punishing to many families than the label of mental handicap. "Shopping around" is disruptive for everybody, can be expensive and destroys any continuity of educational process. If grief is the stage at which the family becomes fixated, then over-protection and rejection may develop.

Over-protection: The child is not allowed to experience risks, to learn his daily living skills; he is made to under-function. *Overt rejection* is rare nowadays and it is related more to a failure to bond, to the expectations for that child before birth and also to the extent and sensitivity of the

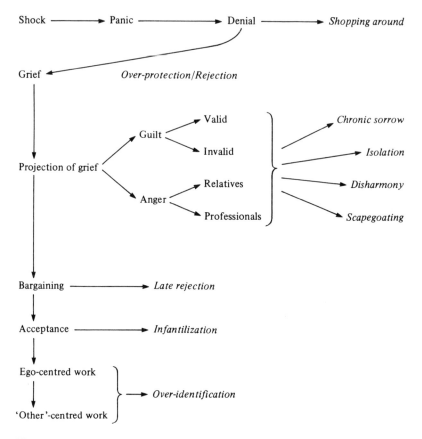

Figure 2. Bereavement response and maladaptive responses.

help that we offer to these families. Far more often than overt rejection, we see a mixture of over-protection and rejection, namely ambivalence.

Ambivalence: "I love him but he is killing me"; "Yes we will go on looking after him, but sometimes how we hate him." Ambivalence is uncomfortable for the whole family, including the handicapped child.

Guilt, anger and grief if prolonged become *chronic sorrow* (Olshansky, 1962), the sadness that pervades the family; *isolation* may occur between the generations, from one spouse to another and from professional help. *Disharmony* occurs in particular if one spouse is angry and blaming the other for the handicap. *Scapegoating* occurs when the child takes on the burden of the projected grief and the guilt, and the child is pinpointed as the cause of everything that is going wrong. *Late rejection* can occur as a result of prolonged bargaining: "We said we would look after him if he learnt to walk or to talk. He hasn't managed to do this, so you can look after him now."

Infantilization: Acceptance is usually a stage that is not blurred by maladaptive responses but occasionally the acceptance of a handicapped child is the acceptance of the child model of handicap only. The "Peter Pan and Wendy" syndrome occurs, the child is infantilized, the *child* is accepted, but the handicapped adult to come at a later date is far less easily accepted. Occasionally in family-centered and other-centered work we see an *over-identification* with handicap, frantic activity concerning handicap, covering up chronic sorrow within the family or maybe a manic defense against grief and anger.

ACCEPTANCE

Acceptance is not one stage but is at least four stages. The first stage is *fantasy*.

> Yes we love him dearly, we love him just as he is, we don't mind if he doesn't learn to walk or talk but we do cherish the hope that one day he is going to smile at us and answer to his name: Don't take that hope away from us, we know it may never happen, but it keeps us going.

This fantasy stage of acceptance is to be distinguished from the bargaining stage of potential rejection, and it is cruel to take away those fantasies. The fantasy stage leads to *duty*: "Yes he is ours, we brought him into the world and we are going to care for him." Then duty leads to *resignation*; and through resignation we come to *love*. I offer you a definition of acceptance:

> Acceptance is the death of an imaginary ideal child, and the redirection of parental love to the newly perceived child as he is in reality.

BONDING AND ATTACHMENT

Acceptance may be examined in more detail, in relation to the bonding process. The work of people such as Winnicott (1958), Bowlby (1969) and others has shown that throughout the animal kingdom the infant animal makes non-specific attachment behavior towards his caretakers. This gradually becomes specific towards the caretaker who repeatedly returns, and usually this is the mother or the surrogate mother. The mother, joyous in her mothering, responds to the attachment behavior of the baby, indeed her behavior often initiates and provokes this attachment behavior and so bonding results. Such a bond between the human mother and child withstands the testing of the toddler, creates an environment for effective discipline, withstands the testing of the adolescent and also enables the "letting go" of the young adult.

If there is a failure to bond, there is a failure to discipline from the standpoint of love, a failure in the child to develop internalized controls, leading, therefore, to a lack of self-discipline and self-esteem, and the child has failed to experience the first and most important one-to-one relationship of his life.

Many workers have indicated that non-accidental injury is likely to occur in babies who are not bonded to their mothers or surrogate mothers. Buchanan & Oliver (1977) have shown that while non-accidental injury can be a cuase of mental handicap it can also be the result of mental handicap.

All this is relevant to the development of the mentally handicapped child. Is it easy to discipline a handicapped child? Parents find it extremely difficult to get the right level of discipline partly because of the cognitive deficits in the child. Self-esteem? This has been damaged in handicapped people by many experiences of separation, failure, rejection. Bonding? If bonding were superbly good, then many of the other problems in handicap might be more easily overcome, but bonding is usually incomplete. Consider, for example, a congenitally handicapped child; his attachment behavior is likely to be very weak, he does not suck well, fixate or smile easily, he may be having apnoeic attacks, he may have fits, be intubated, or have a dreaded physical deformity that mothers look for so quickly after the birth of any baby. He might have an unusual facial appearance and he might be in an incubator. Mother for her part is mourning the loss of this perfect child who has not arrived, she may even have doubts of the viability of the child. The mother may, as a result, remain consciously unattached to her handicapped child.

> One mother who brought a severely mentally handicapped, very behavior disturbed four-year-old to me, described how when he was in an incubator, she sat there day after day practicing his death. She said that she thought she might manage that much better when his death came if she practiced

her responses over and again. She consciously held off bonding; he did not die; as a result there was no bond, mother and child were "in parallel" and the problems were enormous.

There may be, therefore, problems between parents and the handicapped child over bonding, discipline, self-esteem and separation in adolescence.

LETTING GO

Letting go of the young adult is perhaps difficult for any parent but when handicap is present the parting is complicated by skill deficits in the handicapped person and also by lack of facilities. Many a time the family has reached the point when they were ready to let go and then they have found there is nowhere for the handicapped young adult to go. Because of these difficulties, there are many mentally handicapped people who never experience the letting go process and stay with their parents, their caretakers until death inevitably separates.

But there are now more opportunities for separation as a positive growth experience. There are more vocational training units that are residential and more shared care units, and with these extra facilities we are seeing the dynamics of separation of the mentally handicapped young adult from his family for the first time. This stimulates a second bereavement work, usually far less profound than the first, but the work may be complicated if the letting go is distorted by family exhaustion, if it was no choice other than separation, if the parents disagree over the need to let go, and if the first bereavement work has not been satisfactorily completed.

THE DEATH OF A MENTALLY HANDICAPPED MEMBER OF A FAMILY

Those who remember and worked within grossly under-resourced services with, perhaps, 1000 beds in the institution and 200 people waiting for the next available bed, will perhaps be forgiven if care was directed to the family who were going to benefit by the vacant bed, rather than the family who had just lost a mentally handicapped member. Different services are now developing, locally based services, where there is more time and readily available places in residential care so that the skills may be acquired that are needed for bereavement counseling for families who have lost a handicapped member.

There are two particular pains felt by those families. Firstly, the pain of the death, and perhaps that is linked with the life that never reached the planned fulfilment. But the second pain is very often the more poignant, the pain of the relief that is felt when the handicapped person dies. That pain is often overwhelming and brings a lot of grief to the family. The term "intellectual guilt" seems to describe the situation where parents feel guilty because they think they do not feel sad enough.

THE DEVELOPMENT OF INSIGHT INTO THE PERSONAL PREDICAMENT OF HANDICAP

It was thought that insight was rarely to be found in a mentally handicapped person, but I would suggest it is present far more than we have believed. Insight is linked to the mental and chronological age of the person. There has to be some level of cognitive function for insight to develop, but that level of cognitive functioning seems to be far lower than we thought it was. The chronological age is also important. Consider the little hemiplegic child who falls over—he is picked up, cuddled, kissed, made better, and the response to his tumble is a lot of positive feedback; this boy, at 10 years, is teased by his peers and turned out of their games; that same boy when he is 19 and six feet tall is still falling because of his hemiplegia and now society is embarrassed, his caretakers are bored and tired with picking him up. Such a lad, whom I know well, fell recently and as he was picked up he said: "I wish I had be died." Insight is also linked with failure to reach self-imposed standards. The mentally handicapped child in a large sibship often self-imposes standards that are just above the younger sibling. Somebody must be less capable than him. Families can be warned that there may be problems when the younger sibling of normal intelligence overtakes the handicapped older sibling.

Insight may be linked to family environments. The academic family with the intellectually handicapped child, the cerebal palsied child in the athletic family, the deaf child in a musical family, will all learn quickly that they are not as able as others in the family and cannot share their hobbies. The peer group also matters; at one stage it was fairly fashionable, for example, to educate all spina bifida children together, but insight comes very slowly when the norm is to have spina bifida. Other parents put their handicapped child quickly into groups of normal children, hoping that they will be models for the handicapped child.

Finally, insight is linked to developmentally related needs. The deaf child has a particular need in the preschool period to be taught a system of communication, and if he does not learn then he is likely to be highly disturbed. The child with a Sturge-Weber Syndrome (the naevus or birthmark, disfiguring the face, and affecting the brain) is likely not to be too bothered in childhood, but in adolescence the birthmark becomes the excuse for failure in the job market and in peer relationships.

An awareness that a handicapped person will have insight related to these points means that there must be a much wider definition of what handicap really means. While an organic definition is a vital starting-point and that must be precise, a wider definition is required, a psycho-dynamic or an existential one.

AN EXISTENTIAL DEFINITION OF HANDICAP

What does it mean?
To this person?
To have this handicap?
At this time in his life?
With these caretakers?
In this environment?
And in this peer group?

If these questions are answered for any handicapped person there is a better understanding of his level of insight, insight that may accelerate his sense of failure, frustration, personal loss and rejection and lead itself to symptom formation.

Symptomatology of Mental Handicap

Many handicapped people develop reactions to their insight into their own handicap. The symptomatology of mental handicap has been studied. There are many cross-sectional surveys of the symptoms of mentally handicapped people. "Captive" populations in long-stay institutions, series of out-patient referrals can be studied, but the best studies are now coming from mental handicap register data, which for the first time are giving a good cross-sectional estimate of behavior problems within mental handicap (James & Snaith, 1979). These studies show that between 20 and 60 per cent of mentally handicapped people have moderate to severe behavior disorders. These are categorized according to either traditional psychiatric labels (and how much these need defining more closely in mental handicap), or by cluster analysis of symptoms. From this type of statistical approach there may be defined an over-active noisy group, a manneristic autistic group, and a multiple problem group for example (Reid *et al.*, 1978). Cluster analysis cross-sectional studies are useful for workload and staffing levels, but for the individual they give very little information of value. Far more important now is to embark upon longitudinal studies of mentally handicapped people, similar to, and taking advantage of, the important work of Paykel (1978) in "life-events." There are five life-events in mentally handicapped people that are of obvious importance.

Life-Events

First of all is the *diagnosis*. That is clearly a life-event for the family, but it is important for the person as well who has been labelled, as he may not shed that label for the rest of his life, even though it might turn out to be inappropriate. Diagnosis and labeling is the first life-event for the handicapped person.

The second are the numerous *separation experiences* imposed upon handicapped people. It is known to be important for normal children to stay with their parents, and yet mentally handicapped people are admitted and have short-term care, when their cognitive functioning does not enable them to understand the meaning of temporary loss.

Thirdly, *friendship ties may be broken* without hardly a thought. Large hospitals are now developing small residential units and returning people to their home environment, to Health Districts from whence they came, but in so doing we frequently break life-long friendships within the long-stay hospital that were tremendously important to the handicapped person.

Fourthly, a life-event is the *dawning sexuality* of the handicapped person. This for the normal young person is the time of increasing freedom, whether the parents like it or not, but for the handicapped person this is a time of decreasing freedom. A new set of dilemmas arise for the caretakers. They may have never thought about sexuality in their handicapped child who has now grown up and they deal frequently with these dilemmas by increasing the amount of restriction upon that person, sometimes linking sadly the sexuality of the handicapped teenager with their own sexuality which brought him into the world.

Fifthly, the life-event of *bereavement*. How often when there is a death in the family the handicapped person is sent to have a fortnight's holiday while the rest of the family collectively grieve the loss of say, a grandparent. The handicapped person is assumed to be unable to notice the loss but he comes back and finds that "granny" is permanently gone. He is excluded from the bereavement rituals and the family, and his need to grieve is often not acknowledged. So often for the handicapped person this is a double loss, the loss of a caretaker frequently means too the loss of a place to live. Not only do they have no chance to grieve the loss of, say, a mother or a father but at the same time they are removed from that home environment they have known so well and placed elsewhere.

Even severely and profoundly mentally handicapped people may suffer from depression related to bereavement when they are excluded from the grieving process.

REACTIONS TO INSIGHT

Adoption of the sick role
Avoidance of failure
Retreat into fantasy
Self-satisfied dependence
Breakdown of inner controls
Manipulation of inappropriate power
Extreme go-centredness
"Acting into" the label of handicap
Development of a psychiatric illness

This list shows some of the possible reactions that mentally handicapped people may develop as a result of their insight into handicap. These reactions are ways of dealing with the unhappiness that insight and life-events may bring. They are ego defence or reality avoidance mechanisms. Adoption of the sick role, avoidance of failure—we call him "stubborn"; retreat into fantasy—he is withdrawn; self-satisfied dependence—he is "lazy"; a breakdown of inner controls—he is labeled "naughty"; manipulation of inappropriate power—he "winds you round his little finger"; extreme ego-centredness—we call him "selfish"; acting into the label of handicap—"I can't do that, I am handicapped" and the development of a psychiatric illness in its more formal sense with varied symptomatology.

Whatever the reaction or symptom development, the mentally handicapped person is likely to be trapped by their symptom; "the symptom trapping effect." For example, vomiting, encopresis, self-mutilation, even stubbornness may be expressions of distress and cries for help, but so often they limit the life-style. For example, he cannot go to school any more, he is excluded from the transport, he cannot live at home and has to come into hospital, the children's home cannot cope and he is heavily sedated. An expression of distress can precipitate a downward spiral of unhappiness and life-style limitation from which the mentally handicapped person cannot free himself.

Dehumanization

So far possible reasons for unhappiness have been linked with insight, life-events that we impose upon the handicapped person and the trapping effect of symptoms.

> A man whose face is hideously deformed with the nodules of tuberose sclerosis, whose body is scarred through falls because of 40 years of unmonitored phenytoin therapy was found one day in his home with his mother dead on the kitchen floor. He came into residential care immediately and on the same day he had to part with his dog, his very dear companion. This man received help at a level of trying to enable him to find his own self-esteem again. The last time I saw him, we were chatting and he suddenly got up, took my arm formally and walked across the room and he said: "This feels like being a man and a woman."

I believe that man had been totally dehumanized by his experiences through nobody's fault and he needed help to find once more his self-esteem.

Personality Types

There is not yet a great deal of literature or skill regarding personality assessment of mentally handicapped people, but many of them have positive personality characteristics, adding greatly to the family happiness and sense of purpose; the capacity to lose, to share, to forgive, to love, to take rejection and failure and a sense of humor. But there are others who seem to have very severe personality deficits associated more with their brain damage than with life-events or insight. Examples are Kanner's syndrome and Asberger's syndrome. These people seem to have little desire to communicate, they do not develop a social conscience, nor imaginative skills and they have extreme difficulty with one-to-one relationships. They are liable to profound depressive illnesses when their sexuality develops. How much harder it is for families to accept and to love a handicapped person with such a severe personality deficit. Some parents, talking about their autistic daughter, said: "How many more years are we going to go on giving her Christmas presents when all she does is flap the paper in return?"

The Reaction of Siblings

Siblings within a family with a mentally handicapped member very broadly reflect the parental reaction, but they have problems unique to themselves (Kew, 1975). The most vulnerable sibling is the one next in birth order, either younger or older than the handicapped person. They are likely to develop symptoms of maladjustment if their own infantile needs to bond and to be cared for and to be dependent are not met, if there has been a need for them to accelerate their own process of growing up, if their need to socialize has been stifled, if their schoolwork is interfered with and particularly in adolescence if for the first time their mentally handicapped sibling is an embarrassment to them, and they will not bring their friends into the home. Siblings can also become increasingly disquieted when there are anxieties about continuing care of the handicapped person, and there is an implicit assumption in the family group that they will carry on the work of their parents. Finally they will require much help and reassurance concerning their capacity to procreate a healthy subsequent generation.

CRISIS POINTS FOR THE WHOLE FAMILY

The bad news is imparted
Bargaining fails
Educational decisions are made
Sexuality develops
Residential care is needed
Parents become elderly

There are crisis points of news receiving and decision making for the whole family: when education decisions are made and perhaps the school the parents least want is the one that is chosen, when sexuality develops, when residential care is needed (and how much professional skill is required to make this a positive experience and not a guilt-ridden one), and when parents become elderly and questions are asked about continuing care. All of us who work with handicapped people should be available, as professionals, as counselors, as friends, at the right moment to aid the decision-making process.

CONCLUSION

The diagnosis of handicap in a child stimulates bereavement work and the mourning for the perfect child who has not arrived or has been changed to imperfection. This may not be worked through to completion, and maladjusted responses by any member of the family may interfere with family happiness and cohesion.

The handicapped person develops a degree of insight into his own deficits, he may experience adverse life-events that we impose upon him and he may develop maladjusted behavioral responses including symptoms which then become a trap, further increasing personal unhappiness. Siblings develop their own reactions which if maladjusted compound the degree of family discomfort. Together the family faces times of decision making which may accentuate or relieve the stress level.

Some families with strong personal resources and with little or no help convert this potentially tragic experience of having a handicapped child into a positive growth experience for everyone involved. However, many families require our help and a full understanding of the possible stresses and traps, that is the *psychopathology of handicap* must lead to a service where sensitive intervention and a complete range of facilities meets every level of need of the handicapped person and those who care for them. Many more families will then experience the joy as well as the sadness that we more frequently associate with handicap.

REFERENCES

Bowlby, J. (1969). *Attachment and Loss*, Vol. 1. London: Hogarth Press.

Bradley, M. (1972). Problems from the parents' point of view. *Proceedings of the Royal Society of Medicine,* **65**.

Buchanan, A. & Oliver, M. E. (1977). Abuse and neglect as a cause of mental retardation. A study of 140 children admitted to subnormality hospitals in Wiltshire. *British Journal of Psychiatry,* **131**, 458–467.

Evans, E. (1976). The grief reaction of parents of the retarded and the counsellor's role. *Australian Journal of Mental Retardation,* **4** (4), 8–12.

James, F. E. & Snaith, R. P. (1979). *Psychiatric Illness and Mental Handicap.* London: Gaskell Press.

Kew, S. (1975). *Transgenerational Family Therapy.* London: Croom Helm.

Morris, P. (1969). *Put Away: A Sociological Study of Institutions for the Mentally Retarded.* London: Routledge & Kegan Paul.

Olshansky, S. (1962). Chronic sorrow, a response to having a mentally defective child. *Social Casework*, **43**, 190–193.

Paykel, E. S. (1978). Contribution of life-events to causation of psychiatric illness. *Psychological Medicine*, **8**, 245–253.

Reid, A. H., Ballinger, B. R. & Heather, B. B. (1978). Behavioural syndromes identified by cluster analysis in a sample of 100 severely and profoundly retarded adults. *Psychological Medicine*, **8**, 399–412.

Shrimpton, J. A. (1980). Personal view. *British Medical Journal*, **281**, 1487.

Winnicott, D. W. (1958). *Through Paediatrics to Psychoanalysis*. London: Tavistock.

23

Familial Subtypes of Childhood Hyperactivity

Gerald J. August

University of Texas Medical Branch, Galveston

Mark A. Stewart

University of Iowa Hospitals and Clinics, Iowa City

On the basis of family history data we defined two subtypes of childhood hyperactivity: family history-positive (FH +), in which at least one biological parent of the child had a diagnosis in the antisocial spectrum; and family history-negative (FH −), in which neither parent had such a diagnosis. While children in both subgroups were equally deviant on measures of the core components of childhood hyperactivity (e.g., inattention and reactivity), the FH + children were also deviant on dimensions of conduct disturbance and had siblings with a high prevalence of conduct disorder. FH − children showed little evidence of conduct disturbance, had more learning and academic problems, and had siblings with attentional and learning disabilities, but not conduct disorder. These findings suggest that the study of family constellations should be a fruitful method for resolving the heterogeneity of the hyperactive child syndrome.

Family studies have shown a high prevalence of sociopathy, alcoholism, and hysteria among the adult relatives of hyperactive children (9, 20),

Reprinted with permission from the *Journal of Nervous and Mental Disease*, 1983, Vol. 171, No. 6, 362–368. Copyright 1983 by The Williams & Wilkins Co.

This research was supported in part by National Institute of Mental Health Training Grant MH-14620.

while studies of adoptees (5, 6) have suggested that the familial relationship is due to genes as well as influences of the environment. Recent
research (31) has made the child's side of this relationship more specific
by showing that aggressiveness and resistance to discipline are probably
the correlates of the disorder in parents, rather than the syndrome of
hyperactivity. However, these results still have to be confirmed before
the idea of a broadly defined concept of childhood hyperactivity is abandoned altogether.

The symptoms which have been used to define childhood hyperactivity
are a loosely related set of variables. Although overactivity, inattentiveness, and impulsivity comprise the core of the syndrome, some investigators (7, 13, 28), also include aggression, non-compliance, antisocial
behavior, and learning problems. We therefore need to know whether
sociopathy and alcoholism in fathers are linked to hyperactivity in their
sons through aggressiveness, antisocial behavior, impulsivity, or some
other trait. However, even a definition of hyperactivity based on exhaustive research would not necessarily ensure that all children with the
clinical picture had the same condition. Because hyperactive children
can be divided according to associated cognitive symptoms (11), natural
history (19, 36), family history, or neurophysiological findings (27), it is
reasonable to suppose that the origins of the problem are varied. For
example, there may be several genetically distinct subgroups. Some way
to isolate homogeneous subgroups of hyperactive children is needed.
One possibility is to categorize subjects by the presence in their families
of disorders in the spectrum of antisocial personality, alcoholism, and
hysteria. We could define two familial subgroups of childhood hyperactivity: family history positive (FH +), in which at least one natural
parent has a diagnosis in the anti-social spectrum; and family history
negative (FH −), in which neither parent has such a diagnosis. In the
present study we have tested the broad hypothesis that these two
subgroups would differ on other dimensions such as the children's development, cognitive abilities, and clinical picture. Moreover, we examined the incidence and nature of behavior and/or learning problems
in their biological siblings to see whether these might further support
the familial basis of our diagnostic distinction.

SUBJECTS AND METHODS

Subjects

The study began with a review of records of the 125 patients who
served as the initial screening sample in the August and Stewart (2)

study. These subjects were taken from consecutive admissions to a child psychiatry clinic over a period of 16 months and were subsequently given a staff diagnosis of hyperkinetic syndrome of childhood (35). These staff diagnoses do not reflect current standards for the diagnosis of attentional deficit disorder, but were nevertheless utilized in order to produce a broadly defined group of hyperactive boys with or without associated conduct disturbance, as was the trend in the United States at the time the subjects were seen in the clinic. Only boys were studied because of the marked concentration of hyperactivity among boys and as a means of increasing the homogeneity of the groups studied. In addition, subjects had to meet each of the following criteria: a) an IQ greater than 70; b) the absence of any continuing medical or neurological disorder; c) the absence of psychosis; and d) were presently living with one or both parents or an immediate relative. The boys ranged in age from 5 to 13 years.

Ninety-five boys met criteria for inclusion in the study. A phone call was made to each family in which the purpose of the study was explained and permission to personally interview was requested. From the pool of 95 boys who met criteria, 72 had parents who were subsequently interviewed. Four families refused to participate and 19 could not be located due to unknown residence.[3]

Diagnoses of the Parents

A structured psychiatric interview was administered to the parents of each boy by a qualified research assistant utilizing the same interview form and procedure described in Stewart *et al.* (31). Each parent was interviewed separately following a schedule which covered the person's childhood and adolescence; their occupational, marital, and medical histories; a review of common psychiatric symptoms of adult life; and a detailed family history. One of the investigators (M.A.S.), who was blind to the child's history and specific clinical problems, reviewed the interviews and diagnosed each parent using the criteria of Feighner *et al.* (10).

On the basis of the parental diagnoses we separated out two groups. One group included those probands who had at least one parent diagnosed with a disorder in the antisocial spectrum (*i.e.*, antisocial personality, alcohol and/or drug abuse, hysteria). The second group were those probands whose biological parents were free of disorders in this antisocial spectrum. From the group of interviewees, there were 36 families in which at least one parent received a positive diagnosis (in three families there were two parents with positive diagnoses). These included nine cases of antisocial personality disorder, 15 cases of alcohol and/or drug abuse, 12 cases involving both antisocial personality disorder and alcohol and/or durg abuse, and three cases of hysteria. In the majority of cases the fathers received the positive diagnoses, although there were three mothers diagnosed with hysteria and one with alcoholism.[4] In contrast, there were 31 families in which neither parent received a positive diagnosis. There were four remaining families who were eliminated from the study due to insufficient information to make a definite diagnostic decision and one in which the only affected parent was schizophrenic.

After the probands were separated into their appropriate familial-based subgroups, data were collected from their clinical records for analysis.

Measures

Clinical assessment interview. At the child's initial visit to the psychiatry clinic the mother was given a structured interview which took about 1 hour to administer. The interview included: questions to define the age of onset (five items); and a review of common emotional and behavioral symptoms present during the past year (70 items). A detailed description of the form and reliability of this interview is provided elsewhere (32). This measure yields eight dimensions of behavioral disturbance. Each dimension consists of five behaviors, and a child's score is tabulated on the basis of the number of behaviors on which he was rated positive (Table 1).

Scores are computed from the subject's rating [1, 3, or 5] on each item in a given dimension. A perfectly normal score is 15 on each dimension; a score completely deviant in the opposite direction is 25.

Intelligence. Data on intelligence were taken from the Wechsler Intelligence Scale for Children-Revised, which was administered in the psychiatric clinic as part of the initial evaluation.

Birth history and other medical factors. Data on pregnancy, delivery, and neonatal complications were obtained from the mothers and by reviewing obstetrical charts when they were included in the medical records. Information pertaining to the presence of physical anomalies, neurological abnormalities, as well as history of medical illnesses and/or serious accidents requiring medical attention were collected as part of the child's physical examination.

TABLE 1
Dimension Items

Aggression	*Egocentricity*
Fights with peers	Excessive need for
Attacks adults	attention
Shouts at parents	Projects blame
Extremely competitive	Problems sharing
Quarrels with peers	Insensitive to others'
	feelings
Noncompliance	Lack of repentance
Ignores directions	
Resents discipline	*Reactivity*
Oppositional	Inpatient
Stays out late	Impulsive
Lacks respect for adults	Reckless
	Easily upset
Anxiety	Excitable
Worries	
Fearful	*Depression*
Nervous	Low mood
Stomach aches	Cries often
Scared of new	Sleep problem
experiences	Low self-esteem
	Few friends
Inattention	
Distractible	*Antisocial behavior*
Does not finish projects	Lies
Does not seem to listen	Steals at home
Difficulty concentrating	Steals outside home
Difficulty sticking to a	Fire setting
play activity	Vandalism

Diagnoses of the Biological Siblings

The clinical assessment interview, described above, was used to obtain information pertaining to a history of behavior and learning problems in the siblings of the probands. Only full biological siblings ranging in age from 6 to 18 years were included in the study. In addition, the mothers were specifically asked whether the child had ever been evaluated or diagnosed for a behavioral, emotional, or learning problem by a physician, school psychologist, or other health professional. When this was the case, an attempt was made to verify the presence of these problems by obtaining records from the individual sources. Upon completion of the data collection procedure all names and other identifying information were removed from the various forms. The primary investigator, who was blind to both the probands' chief clinical problems and the psychiatric diagnoses of their parents, reviewed the clinical forms and diagnosed each sibling for the following DSM-III diagnostic categories: a) attentional deficit disorders (with or without hyperactivity); b) conduct disorders (socialized or undersocialized; aggressive or nonaggressive); and c) specific developmental disorders (reading, arithmetic, or language).

The diagnoses were based on deviant dimension scores on the clinical assessment interview as well as data from clinical records provided by the individual sources. For example, a sibling was classified as having a conduct disorder when he or she scored deviant on at least two of the following four dimensions: aggression, noncompliance, egocentricity, antisocial behavior; or when parents indicated that the sib had two or more of the following problems: persistent and marked aggressiveness, resistance to discipline, destructiveness, stealing, running away, truancy, alcohol and/or drug abuse, and contacts with the police or juvenile court. The diagnostic category of conduct disorders in the present study was broadly defined to include aggressive, nonaggressive, undersocialized, and socialized subtypes. Thus, we expected not only to detect aggressive, undersocialized problems associated with younger children, but also antisocial behavior patterns such as truancy, running away, alcohol and drug abuse, and difficulties with the police, which present more frequently among adolescents (32). Attentional deficit disorders were diagnosed on the basis of deviant scores on the inattention and reactivity dimensions of the clinical assessment interview, both mandatory, and also specific confirmation from the parents or individual clinical sources that the child had problems involving attention and/or overactivity which were interfering with school or home life. Specific developmental disorders involving reading, arithmetic, and language were diagnosed on the basis of mothers' reports with supporting documentation from school sources indicating poor achievement scores relative to normal intelligence and/or placement in learning disabled or equivalent programs.

RESULTS

General Characteristics of Subjects

The 36 FH + and 31 FH − probands closely resembled each other on all background variables except the proportion living in a broken home.

TABLE 2

Background Data of Hyperactive Probands by Familial Subgroups

	FH+ Hyperactive Probands ($N = 36$)	FH− Hyperactive Probands ($N = 31$)
Age at present evaluation	9.01 ± 3.05	9.86 ± 2.67
Age at onset of initial problem	3.45 ± 2.00	2.86 ± 1.80
Age at time of first evaluation	6.61 ± 3.04	6.14 ± 2.90
Verbal WISC-R[a] IQ	97.28 ± 9.47	93.46 ± 18.07
Performance WISC-R IQ	100.12 ± 11.67	94.74 ± 20.59
Full-scale WISC-R IQ	99.76 ± 11.62	93.52 ± 20.03
Sibship size	3.11 ± 2.25	3.48 ± 1.69
Socioeconomic status[b]	3.90 ± 0.65	3.50 ± 1.32
Broken home[c] (%)	71	23

[a]Wechsler Intelligence Scale for Children-Revised.
[b]Based on the Hollingshead and Redlich Scale (15).
[c]In all cases due to divorce or separation.

This difference was statistically significant ($x^2 = 15.7, p < .001$) (Table 2).

Clinical Picture

The groups differed significantly on the dimensions of aggression, noncompliance, antisocial behavior, and egocentricity, but not attention, reactivity, anxiety, and depression. Taking a score of 19 or more as deviant (*i.e.*, two or more items out of five for a given dimension were rated positive), the FH+ group was deviant on all but anxiety, whereas the FH− group was only deviant on inattention and reactivity (Table 3).

Medical History

The groups did not differ on any of nine variables related to the index pregnancy, a child's neurological state, physical anomalies, and accidents in early childhood.

School Difficulties

Fifteen of the 31 (48 per cent) FH− probands had repeated at least one grade, compared to only eight of the 36 (22 per cent) FH+ ($x^2 =$

TABLE 3

Dimension Scores of Hyperactive Probands by Familial Subgroups
(Means ± SDs and t values)

Dimension	FH+ (N = 36)	FH− (N = 31)	t-Values
Inattention	21.83 ± 2.16	22.58 ± 2.72	(t = .70)
Reactivity	22.13 ± 2.53	22.07 ± 2.40	(t = .06)
Aggression	20.63 ± 2.85	17.30 ± 2.56	(t = 3.30)**
Noncompliance	21.25 ± 2.72	17.76 ± 2.39	(t = 3.71)***
Antisocial behavior	19.00 ± 3.57	16.53 ± 1.66	(t = 2.47)*
Egocentricity	20.75 ± 2.72	17.92 ± 2.25	(t = 3.07)**
Anxiety	16.50 ± 3.22	16.69 ± 2.15	(t = .19)
Depression	20.25 ± 3.69	18.84 ± 3.20	(t = .95)

*$p < .05$; **$p < .01$; ***$p < .001$.

4.18, $p < .05$). Similarly, 18 of the 31 (58 per cent) FH− probands were involved in special education programs, compared to 9 of 36 (25 per cent) FH+ ($x^2 = 7.57, p < .01$).

Disorders in the Siblings

In order to precisely examine the specificity of the familial linkage between parental antisocial spectrum disorders and childhood hyperactivity, the sibling data were analyzed in several different ways. In the first analysis a sibling was counted as affected if he or she satisfied the diagnostic criteria for *any one* of the three categories of childhood disorders. Sixteen of 51 (31.4 per cent) sibs of the FH+ group had at least one condition, whereas this was true for 12 of the 54 (22 per cent) FH− siblings. This difference, however, did not reach a level of statistical significance. In the second analysis, a comparison was made of the number of sibs in the two groups who met criteria for only attentional deficit disorder. Nine of the 54 (16.7 per cent) siblings from the FH− group were diagnosed with an attentional deficit disorder as compared to four of the 51 (7.8 per cent) FH+ sibs, a difference which was not significant. The third analysis featured a comparison between groups for the prevalence of conduct disorder. Twelve of the 51 (23.5 per cent) FH+ sibs satisfied criteria for conduct disorder, whereas none of the 54 sibs from the FH− group did ($x^2 = 14.35, p < .001$). No significant differences in the rates of the various diagnostic categories were obtained in the male *vs.* female siblings (Table 4).

TABLE 4
Disorders of Siblings

	Add		Conduct Disorder		Specific Developmental Disorders		Total Disorders	
	N^a	$\%^b$	N	$\%$	N	$\%$	N	$\%$
FH+								
Brothers (N = 25)	2	(8.0)	6	(24.0)	0	(0)	8	(32.0)
Sisters (N = 26)	2	(7.7)	6	(23.0)	0	(0)	8	(30.7)
Total (N = 51)	4	(7.8)	12	(23.5)	0	(0)	16	(31.4)
FH−								
Brothers (N = 24)	4	(16.7)	0	(0)	1	(4.2)	5	(20.8)
Sisters (N = 30)	5	(16.7)	0	(0)	2	(6.7)	7	(23.4)
Total (N = 54)	9	(16.7)	0	(0)	3	(5.6)	12	(22.2)

[a]Number of siblings affected.
[b]Prevalence rate of siblings affected.

DISCUSSION

Our results show that dividing hyperactive children according to their parents' psychiatric disorders leads to two relatively distinct groups. The children in one group were deviant on several dimensions of behavior, presented a clear picture of conduct disorder, and tended to have brothers and sisters with the same disorder. Not surprisingly, this was the group defined by having parents with a serious personality disorder or alcoholism. On the other hand, children whose parents did not have such disorders showed little sign of behavioral deviance beyond their difficulties with attention and impulsivity, but tended to have intellectual and academic deficits. Moreover, the brothers and sisters of the "pure hyperactive" children had similar problems themselves, or developmental learning problems, rather than conduct disturbance. Thus, a division by family history led to two clinical subtypes of childhood hyperactivity.

The present results form a mirror image of the recent finding that boys with conduct disorder tend to have parents with personality disorder and alcoholism while hyperactive boys do not (31). Earlier work (9, 20) suggested that hyperactivity was the correlate of problems in the parents, but these studies defined hyperactivity very broadly and lacked clinical controls. It now appears that children's problems correspond with those of their parents and siblings. Boys with conduct disorder tend to have siblings with the same problem and parents with related disorders, while "pure hyperactive" children have siblings with difficulties in attention or developmental learning problems.

One puzzling finding is the lack of difference in rates of attentional deficit disorder and conduct disorder in the male *vs.* female siblings of our sample of hyperactive boys. Welner *et al.* (37), for example, using a broad definition of hyperactive child syndrome, found 26 per cent of the brothers and 9 per cent of the sisters of hyperactive children to meet criteria for childhood hyperactivity, whereas Cantwell (9) reported that 22 per cent of the brothers and 8 per cent of the sisters met the same criteria. Recent research employing DSM-III criteria, however, reports approximately equal sex ratios of affected siblings. Cantwell (8) found that 24 per cent of the brothers of hyperactive children and 19 per cent of the sisters met the DSM-III criteria for attentional deficit disorder (ADD). This result, along with the finding of the present study, suggests the likelihood that the category of attentional deficit disorder picks up more girls who manifest milder variants of the hyperactive child syndrome. More specifically, girls may manifest the attentional disorder without marked features of hyperactivity, whereas boys, for a number of reasons, exhibit features of overactivity, in addition to the attentional deficit. Our criteria for diagnosing ADD were not particularly sensitive to making an unequivocal differentiation between ADD with or without attendant hyperactivity. To accomplish this will require more rigorously defined criteria. Further research is needed to help clarify both the clinical expression and etiological implications of the category of attentional deficit disorder as it pertains to sex differences.

With regard to the equal rate of conduct disorder in our brothers and sisters, this appears to be largely attributable to the age range of our probands and their siblings. Four of the six sisters meeting criteria for conduct disorders were within the age range of 16 to 18, and their problems, which included alcohol and drug abuse, running away, and criminal offenses, had only recently come to the attention of their parents. Future studies exploring familial factors in childhood hyperactivity will need to address the more refined diagnostic nomenclature of DSM-III as well as the problem of age of onset in affected relatives.

That similar disorders would be present in parents and their children raises the question of how they are transmitted. Hewitt and Jenkins (14) and Lewis (16) found that children with aggressive conduct disorder tended to have parents who had rejected them when they were very young. Many other investigators (18) have reported similar findings and Patterson's (22) work suggests that helping the parents to be more positive brings an improvement in the children's behavior. The question remains whether rejection causes a child to misbehave or a child's difficult behavior causes rejection. The latter could be associated with temperamental traits which appear in the first weeks of the child's life and which are either genetically determined or due to some biological stress such as hypoxia at birth. The available evidence argues against biological stresses being a common factor in these events (38), but leaves the question of genetic influences unanswered. Two small scale studies of adoptees (5, 6), a small half sibling study (25), and a sizable twin study (21) suggest that behavior problems of children may be partly hereditary, whereas one large adoptee study (4) leads to the opposite conclusion.

The findings of the present study confirm the work of a number of investigators (12, 26, 29, 31) who have shown that conduct disorder is the primary problem of many children who are overactive and impulsive. They also support recent reports (2, 26, 30) which point to the existence of "hyperactive" children whose problems are cognitive-attentional in nature. This distinction places in doubt the alleged specificity of hyperactive behavior in psychiatric clinic attenders, and raises the question as to the relationship between attentional deficit and conduct disturbance in hyperactive children.

On the basis of the array of aggressive and antisocial behaviors noted in our FH+ probands, and the presence of similar problems in their parents and siblings, it is reasonable to conclude that their principal disturbance is consistent with descriptions of aggressive conduct disorder (1, 3, 32, 34). The concept of this disorder, as a character disorder (33), is partially supported by its poor prognosis. Robins' (23) 30-year follow-up study of adults who were referred to a child guidance clinic as children indicates considerable continuity between childhood aggression and antisocial behavior and adult sociopathy. Our study does little, however, to advance understanding about the mechanism through which a conduct disturbance gives rise to increased activity and inattention, nor does it show how hyperactivity exhibited by conduct disordered children is different in degree or pattern from that shown by children with ADD.

Meanwhile, the clinical picture of boys in our FH − group is consistent with the definition of attention deficit disorder with hyperactivity (1), which consists of overactivity, inattention, and impulsivity, and is frequently associated with learning and academic problems. Although behavior problems such as noncompliance, stubbornness, and low frustration tolerance are often reported and aggressiveness and destructiveness may occur sporadically, persistent and repetitive disturbances of conduct and social conformity are seldom observed (17). In its pure form, ADD may be essentially characterized as a cognitive disorder involving defective arousal and attentional mechanisms (24). The construct of attention deficit offers a means of explaining a problematic aspect of these children, namely, their learning and academic difficulties. Along the same lines, amphetamines might have a beneficial effect on ADD children by improving their ability to focus and sustain attention.

The presence of several cases (8 per cent) of ADD among the siblings of our FH + probands might suggest that the two disorders are related on a continuum of etiological liability (e.g., ADD constitutes a milder manifestation of the same etiological process that underlies aggressive conduct disorder), but the prevalence rate is relatively low and not significantly different from the population risk. Furthermore, the complete absence of conduct disorder among the sibs of FH − probands also argues against a familial relationship. Thus, despite the considerable overlap which exists between ADD and conduct disorder in children, the results of our study of family constellations indicate that they most likely have independent causal factors.

REFERENCES

1. American Psychiatric Association (1980). *Diagnostic and Statistical Manual of Mental Disorders*, 3rd Ed. American Psychiatric Assoc., Washington, D.C.
2. August, G. J., and Stewart, M. A. (1982). Is there a syndrome of pure hyperactivity? Br. J. Psychiatry*140*:305–311.
3. Behar, D., and Stewart, M. A. (1982). Aggressive conduct disorder of children: The clinical history and direct observations. Acta Psychiatr. Scand., *65*:210–220.
4. Bohman, M. A. (1971). A comparative study of adopted children, foster children and children in their biological environment born after undesired pregnancies. Acta Paediatr., *221*:5–28.
5. Cadoret, R. J., Cunningham, L., Loftus, R., *et al.* (1975). Studies of adoptees from psychiatrically disturbed biological parents. J. Pediatr., *87*:301–306.
6. Cadoret, R. J., and Gath, A. (1980). Biological correlates of hyperactivity: Evidence for a genetic factor. In Sells, S., Roff, M., Strauss, J., *et al.* Eds., *Human Functioning and Longitudinal Perspective*, pp. 103–114. Williams & Wilkins, Baltimore.
7. Cantwell, D. (1977). The hyperkinetic syndrome. In Rutter, M., and Hersov, L., Eds., *Child Psychiatry: Modern Approaches*, pp. 524–555. Blackwell Scientific Publications, London.
8. Cantwell, D. (1979). Minimal brain dysfunction in adults: Evidence from studies of psychiatric illness in the families of hyperactive children. In Bellack, L., Ed., *Psychiatric Aspects of Minimal Brain Dysfunction in Adults*, pp. 37–43. Grune & Stratton, London.
9. Cantwell, D. (1972). Psychiatric illness in the families of hyperactive children. Arch. Gen. Psychiatry, *27*:414–417.
10. Feighner, J. P., Robins, E., Guze, S. B., *et al.* (1972). Diagnostic criteria for use in psychiatric research. Arch. Gen. Psychiatry, *26*:57–63.
11. Fish, B. (1971). The "one child, one drug myth" of stimulants in hyperkinesis: Importance of diagnostic categories in evaluating treatment. Arch. Gen. Psychiatry, *25*:193–203.
12. Graham, P., and Rutter, M. (1968). Organic brain dysfunction in child psychiatric disorder. Br. Med. J., *3*:695–700.
13. Greenhill, L. L., Puig-Antich, J., Chambers, W., *et al.* (1981). Hormone prolactin, and growth responses in hyperkinetic males treated with D-amphetamine. J. Am. Acad. Child Psychiatry, *20*:83–103.
14. Hewitt, L., and Jenkins, R. L. (1946). *Fundamental patterns of maladjustment*. State of Illinois, Springfield.
15. Hollingshead, A., and Redlich, F. (1958). *Social Class and Mental Illness*. John Wiley & Sons, New York.
16. Lewis, H. (1954). *Deprived Children*. Oxford University Press, London.
17. Maurer, R. G., and Stewart, M. A. (1980). Attention deficit without hyperactivity in a child psychiatry clinic. J. Clin. Psychiatry, *41*:232–233.
18. McCord, W., McCord, J., and Howard, A. (1954). Familial correlates of aggression in nondelinquent male children. J. Abnorm. Soc. Psychol., *662:79–83*.
19. Mendelson, W., Johnson, J., and Stewart, M. A. (1971). Hyperactive children as teenagers: A follow-up study. J. Nerv. Ment. Dis., *153*:273–279.
20. Morrision, J. R., and Stewart, M. A. (1971). A family study of the hyperactive child syndrome. Biol. Psychiatry, *3*:189–195.
21. O'Conner, M., Foch, T., Sherry, T., *et al.* (1980). A twin study of specific behavioral problems of socialization as viewed by parents. J. Abnorm. Child Psychol., *8*:189–199.

22. Patterson, G. R. (1974). Interventions for boys with conduct problems: Multiple settings, treatments and criteria. J. Consult. Clin. Psychol., 442:471–481.
23. Robins, L. N. (1966). Deviant Children Grown Up. Williams & Wilkins, Baltimore.
24. Rosenthal, R. H., and Allen, T. W. (1978). An examination of attention, arousal, and learning dysfunctions of hyperactive children. Psychol. Bull., 85:689–715.
25. Safer, D. J. (1973). A familial factor in minimal brain dysfunction. Behav. Genet., 3:175–186.
26. Sandberg, S. T., Rutter, M., and Taylor, E. (1978). Hyperkinetic disorder in psychiatric clinic attenders. Dev. Med. Child Neurol., 20:279–299.
27. Satterfield, J., Cantwell, D., Lesser, L., and Podosin, R. (1971). Physiological studies of the hyperkinetic child. Am. J. Psychiatry, 24:409–414.
28. Satterfield, B. T., Satterfield, J. H., and Cantwell, D. (1980). Multimodality treatment: A two year evaluation of 61 hyperactive boys. Arch. Gen. Psychiatry, 37:915–919.
29. Shaffer, D., McNamara, N., and Pincus, J. H. (1974). Controlled observations on patterns of activity, attention and impulsivity in brain damaged and psychiatrically disturbed boys. Psychol. Med., 4:4–14.
30. Stewart, M. A., Cummings, C., Singer, S., and DeBlois, C. (1981). The overlap between hyperactive and unsocialized aggressive children. J. Child Psychol. Psychiatry, 22:35–45.
31. Stewart, M. A., DeBlois, C. S., and Cummings, S. (1980). Psychiatric disorder in the parents of hyperactive boys and those with conduct disorder. J. Child Psychol. Psychiatry, 21:283–292.
32. Stewart, M. A., DeBlois, C., Meardon, J., and Cummings, S. (1980). Aggressive conduct disorder of children: The clinical picture. J. Nerv. Ment. Dis., 168:604–610.
33. Stewart, M. A., and Gath, A. (1978). Psychological Disorders of Children. Williams & Wilkins, Baltimore.
34. Stewart, M. A., and Leone, L. (1978). A family study of unsocialized aggressive boys. Biol. Psychiatry, 13:107–117.
35. Stewart, M. A., Pitts, F. N., Craig, A. G., and Dierf, W. (1966). The hyperkinetic child syndrome. Am. J. Orthopsychiatry. 36: 861–867.
36. Weiss, G., Minde, K., Werry, J. S., et al. (1971). Studies of the hyperactive child. VIII. Five year follow-up. Arch. Gen. Psychiatry, 24:409–414.
37. Welner, Z., Welner, A., Stewart, M. A., et al. (1977). A controlled study of siblings of hyperactive children. J. Nerv. Ment. Dis., 165:110–116.
38. Werner, E., Bierman, J. M., French, F. E., et al. (1968). Reproductive and environmental casualities: A report on the ten year follow-up of the children of the Kauai pregnancy study. Pediatrics, 42:112–126.

24

Long-Term Outcome of Hyperactive Children

Lily Hechtman and Gabrielle Weiss

Department of Psychiatry, Montreal Children's Hospital and McGill University, Montreal

A review of outcome studies of hyperactive children suggests that they experience significant academic, social, and conduct difficulties during adolescence, and that social, emotional, and impulse problems persist into young adulthood for the majority. While some hyperactive children were found to be functioning normally as adults, a troublesome minority were experiencing severe psychiatric or antisocial problems.

The long-term outcome of childhood conditions is of more than theoretical interest. Knowledge in this area is essential for the planning of appropriate treatment programs for children and for a better understanding of adult psychiatric disorders. Information regarding the long-term outcome of hyperactive children comes from a large number of very diverse studies that differ widely in their purposes, methodologies, and populations. This diversity in the various studies makes it difficult to arrive at an integrated picture of the outcome. However, this paper will attempt such an integration with respect to the adolescent and adult

Reprinted with permission from the *American Journal of Orthopsychiatry*, 1983, Vol. 53, No. 3, 532–541. Copyright 1983 by the American Orthopsychiatric Association, Inc.

Presented at the 1982 annual meeting of the American Orthopsychiatric Association in San Francisco. The authors' follow-up studies, referred to in this paper, were supported in part by grants (to G. Weiss) from Health and Welfare Canada and the National Institute of Mental Health, Washington, D.C.

outcomes of individuals who received childhood diagnoses of hyperactivity (attention deficit disorder).

ADOLESCENT OUTCOME

Mendelson, Johnson and Stewart[23] carried out a retrospective study of 83 children diagnosed as hyperactive from initial chart reviews. Mothers, interviewed when their children were 12–16 years of age, reported that, although 50% of the children had improved, 25% still required some form of special education, 22% had engaged in significant delinquent behavior, and 71%–84% had problems with restlessness, impulsivity, poor concentration, and discipline. In an interview study[34] of these same adolescent subjects, more than half reported that they were restless, impatient, irritable, impulsive, and found it hard to study. About 40% also had poor self-esttem.

Minde et al.[26,27,38] in a comprehensive, five-year, prospective, controlled follow-up study of 91 subjects aged 10–18 (mean 13.3 years) found that, compared to a control group matched for age, sex, IQ, and social class, hyperactive adolescents had poorer self-esteem; some 25% exhibited significant delinquent behavior, and most continued to be distractible, impulsive, and immature emotionally, although less hyperactive.

Ackerman, Dykman and Peters[1] followed up various groups of learning disabled boys, including 23 hyperactive youngsters who were also learning disabled. Their study included a matched control group. At follow-up all subjects were close to 14 years of age and had IQs of at least 80. Socioeconomic status was not specified, but none were disadvantaged. The researchers found that the hyperactive learning disabled group had significantly more adjustment problems involving oppositional or delinquent behavior. They also showed lower self-esteem; were more fidgety, impulsive, immature, and inattentive; and were less able to delay gratification. They had poorer academic performance when compared to controls but not in comparison to other learning disabled groups.

Huessy and Cohen[19] assessed, via teachers' questionnaires, some 501 children in second grade, and then again in fourth, fifth, and ninth grades. The teachers' questionnaire tapped social maturity, academic performance, general attitudes and behavior, and neuromuscular development. Those who scored in the upper (worst) 20% on these questionnaires were designated as hyperactive. Children scoring in this range in second, fourth, and fifth grades continued to have significant academic and social adjustment problems in high school.

Blouin, Bornstein and Trites[2] compared hyperactive adolescents to a group of children having difficulty in school for other reasons, but who were matched with the hyperactives for age, sex and IQ. At five-year follow-up, the hyperactives were found to drink more alcohol, be more hyperactive, and have more conduct problems than the comparison group; no differences were seen in academic achievement and intellectual ability. Ritalin treatment seems to have had no beneficial effect on these children.

In a five-year retrospective study of 81 adolescent hyperactives (mean age 15.5 years and mean IQ 99), Feldman, Denhoff and Denhoff[9] found that 57% were problem-free while 32% required stimulant medication, counseling for poor self-esteem, or special educational arrangements; another 8% had serious problems with drugs and delinquency.

We thus see that, despite significant differences in these follow-up studies of adolescent hyperactives, one is left with a uniform impression. In adolescence, those who have earlier been diagnosed as hyperactive have significant academic difficulties. They continue to have problems with restlessness, impulsivity, concentration, and immaturity. These problems often result in social and conduct difficulties with peers, teachers, and parents. In many this is accompanied by poor self-confidence and poor self-esteem, and close to 25% are involved in significant antisocial behavior.

YOUNG ADULT OUTCOME

The studies and data on adult outcome of hyperactive children can be divided into four main categories: 1) retrospective studies, 2) family studies of hyperactive children, 3) adult patients with similar current symptomatology, and 4) long-term prospective follow-up studies.

Retrospective Studies

A frequently quoted, early follow-up study was carried out by Menkes, Rowe and Menkes.[24] This was a 25-year retrospective study in which they traced 14 of 18 subjects originally seen in the Johns Hopkins Child Psychiatry Center for hyperactivity and learning difficulties. At follow-up, four subjects were psychotic, two were retarded and dependent on their families, and four of the eight who were self-sufficient had spent time in institutions. This fairly negative outcome may be related to the fact that four had initial IQs of less than 80 and six came from the poorest socioeconomic strata.

Laufer[21] reported on a 12-year questionnaire follow-up of subjects

15–26 years of age. All had been referred for hyperkenesis and treated with stimulants. Questionnaires were sent to parents of subjects, and 66 out of 100 were returned. This methodology may constitute a positive bias; however, the study showed that, while 50 of the 66 respondents required special school, 14 of 37 college-aged subjects were at college. Fifty-nine percent still reported problems with hyperactivity and 33% had required psychiatric help, though only 5% needed hospitalization. Some 30% had problems with the police, though none of the subjects were in jail at the time of the follow-up.

Borland and Hechman[3] compared 20 men (mean age 30 years), whose childhood medical records conformed to diagnostic criteria for hyperactive child syndrome 20–25 years ago, with their brothers (mean age 26 years). They found that a large majority of the men who were hyperactive had completed high school and were steadily employed and self-supporting. However, hyperactive subjects worked more hours per week, changed jobs more often, were more dissatisfied with their jobs, and had significantly lower socioeconomic status when compared to their brothers or fathers.

These hyperactive subjects also reported significantly more hyperactivity, restlessness, nervousness, impulsivity, and inclination to become upset. Nearly half had problems of a psychiatric nature and more sought psychiatric help.

Feldman, Denhoff and Denhoff[9] also carried out a 10–12 year retrospective follow-up study on 48 young adults previously diagnosed as hyperactive (mean age 21, mean IQ 104), and found that 91% were either in school or working. However, compared to their sibling controls, they had lower educational achievements and lower self-esteem. Some 10% seemed to have significant problems with drug use, inactivity, and schizoid personality disorders. Although 10% drank alcohol before work or school, compared to none of the sibling controls, the authors felt that the incidence of alcoholism and drug abuse did not differ from that found in a normal control population.

Family Studies

Morrison and Stewart[29] interviewed parents of 59 hyperactive and 41 control children and found a high prevalence of sociopathy, hysteria, and alcoholism in the parents of the hyperactive children. They also felt that significantly more parents of hyperactive than control children had themselves been hyperactive as children. This was not the case for adoptive parents of hyperactive children.[30]

In a similar study, Cantwell[4] conducted psychiatric interviews with parents of 50 hyperactive children and 50 matched control children. Again, increased prevalence rates for alcoholism, sociopathy, and hysteria were found in the parents of hyperactive children. This was particularly true among parents who were thought to have been hyperactive children themselves. These studies suggest that childhood hyperactivity may be a precursor for certain adult psychiatric illnesses.

However, Hechtman[11] compared 65 parents of young adult hyperactives with 43 parents of controls matched for age, sex, IQ, and social class. These families had been seen initially at five-year follow-up when the hyperactive subjects were adolescents and again at 10–12 year follow-up when they were young adults. Families of hyperactive young adults continued to have more difficulties when compared to the normal control families. These difficulties were in the areas of mental health of family members, marital relationships, and emotional climate of the home. The problems, however, were not as severe as those described by Morrison and Stewart[29] and by Cantwell;[4] they seemed to improve with time, particularly when the hyperactive children left home.

Evidence of Similar Adult Syndrome

Shelley and Reister[33] studied 16 adults from the U.S. Air Force who were having difficulty with fine and gross motor tasks, who showed anxiety and self-depreciation, and who had problems with impulse control and concentration. The parents reported a history of overactivity and school difficulties in childhood.

Morrison and Minkoff[28] suggested that the explosive personality characterized by sudden, intensive outbursts of verbal or physical aggression and general inability to control one's over-responsiveness to environmental pressures may be a sequel to the hyperactive child syndrome.

Mann and Greenspan[22] hypothesized that adults who had minimal brain dysfunction as children constitute a distinct diagnostic entity; Adult Brain Dysfunctio, which may exist alone or with a variety of other psychiatric syndromes. The main diagnostic characteristics include: 1) a history of early learning disorder with short attention span; 2) diffuse, severe symptoms in adulthood with elements of anxiety and depression or their equivalent; 3) a rather remarkable dramatic alteration in symptom picture with imipramine; and 4) a mental status exam characterized by rapid flow of speech and many shifts of subject but without overt indications of psychotic thinking (*e.g.*, circumstantiality, ideas of reference).

Wood *et al.*[42] also attempted to make a case for the diagnosis of minimal brain dysfunction in adults. They selected 15 adults from a psychiatric clinic population whose predominant symptoms were impulsivity, irritability, inattentiveness, restlessness, and emotional lability. The patients were given self-report forms that tapped most common characteristics of childhood MBD as well as current extensions or manifestations of this condition. Parents were given an abbreviated Conners Rating Scale to score subjects as they were at six to ten years of age. Two-thirds of these parents placed the adult patient in the 95th percentile for hyperactivity during their childhood. Some of these 15 patients responded well to stimulant or antidepressant medication.

These studies all suggest that there is a group of adult patients who present with symptoms of anxiety, irritability, poor impulse control, restlessness, inattention, and emotional lability. These individuals often have a childhood history that includes overactivity and learning or school difficulties; some of them have demonstrated a positive response to stimulant or antidepressant medication.

Long-Term Prospective Studies

Few studies have followed hyperactives prospectively into adult life. Milman[25] followed 73 patients diagnosed in childhood as having minimal brain dysfunction. In addition, 38% were classified as having development lag and 62% as having organic brain syndrome. The IQs ranged from 69 to 124, with 19% of subjects having IQs of 69. At follow up, 9–15 years after the initial assessment, subjects were 15–23 years of age, with a mean of 19.4 years. It was found that 7% were free of psychiatric disorders, 80% had various types of personality disorders, and 14% were borderline psychotic. These findings may be affected by the large number of subjects with organic brain syndrome (62%) and low IQ.

SUMMARY OF A 10–12 YEAR FOLLOW-UP STUDY

Hechtman *et al.*[14] reported on a series of outcome variables from 76 hyperactive subjects aged 17 to 24 years (mean 19.5 years) and 45 control subjects aged 17 to 24 years (mean 19.0 years). The two groups were matched with respect to age, sex, socioeconomic class, and IQ (WAIS). All the hyperactive subjects included in the study were initially assessed in the Department of Psychiatry of the Montreal Children's Hospital 10–12 years previously, at which time they were between six and 12 years of age. Children were admitted into the study if they met the following criteria: 1) restlessness and poor concentration were their main complaints, and had been present since their earliest years; 2) the complaints were a major source of problems both at home and at school; 3) all children had IQs of at least 85; 4) none of the children were psychotic, borderline psychotic, epileptic, or had cerebral palsy; and 5) all children were living at home with at least one parent.

One hundred and four hyperactive children were initially included in the study and took part in a series of drug studies determining the efficacy of chlorpromazine.[40] Ninety-one of the 104 children were reevaluated in a series of follow-up studies during their adolescence, five to six years after initial assessment.[26,27,39] In the recent 10–12 year follow-up study, 76 of these 91 subjects agreed to participate once more.

The control group was first selected at the time of the five-year follow-up study of the hyperactive children. Thirty-five children were matched with the hyperactive children on age, sex, IQ (WISC), and socioeconomic class. Criteria for inclusion in the study required that the control children had no significant academic or behavioral difficulties in the home or at school. This control group was expanded to 45 subjects at the subsequent follow-up study, using the same matching variables and criteria for inclusion.

The results of our 10–12 year follow-up study will be summarized under: 1) biographical data, 2) psychiatric assessment, 3) physiological measures, and 4) psychological tests.

Biographical Data[37]

Fewer hyperactive subjects than controls were still living with their parents (76% *vs.* 95%) and hyperactives made significantly more geographic moves during the five years before follow-up assessment. They had significantly more *car accidents* (mean 1.3 vs. 0.07), although the number of subjects in each group who had car accidents was not significantly different.

Their *school history* indicated that they had completed less education and more were still in high school at follow-up evaluation. Their average marks were lower, and more hyperactives discontinued participation in high school for this reason. They failed more grades in elementary and in high school, but no one particular subject, or subjects, was responsible for the failure.

Their *work history* indicated no difference in job status on the Hollingshead Scale[16] between the subjects working full-time in the two groups. It should be mentioned that this finding is not in agreement with that of Borland and Hechman;[3] the discrepancy can probably be accounted for by the fact that our subjects were much younger than those in Borland and Heckman's retrospective study and, in this respect, time may well be on the side of the control subjects. There was also no difference between the two groups with respect to discrepancy between the fathers' work status and that of the subjects. The vocational plans (or work aspirations) were not different between the groups as judged on the Hollingshead Scale, and there was no difference between groups on the psychiatrist's judgment of whether vocational aspirations were realistic.

With respect to *court referrals*, there was a trend for the hyperactive subjects to have more court referrals during the five years preceding follow-up (47% *vs.* 32%) but there was no difference between the groups as to the number of subjects who had court referrals during the year before follow-up. A separate analysis taking into account both the number and the seriousness (on a single three-point scale) of different kinds of court referrals showed no difference between the groups regarding the seriousness of such offenses as disturbing the peace, theft, aggression, nonmedical drug use (possession or selling), or traffic offenses committed within the five years prior to follow-up.

A significantly greater percentage (74% *vs.* 54%) of hyperactive subjects had tried some form of nonmedical drugs (mostly marijuana or hashish) in the five years preceding follow-up, but there was no difference between the groups with respect to nonmedical drug use in the year preceding follow-up. Interestingly enough, significantly more controls had used hallucinogens in the prior five years. There was no significant difference between the groups with respect to severity of drug use (three-point scale: mild, moderate, or abuse) in the five years preceding follow-up.

Psychiatric Assessment[37]

The psychiatric evaluation indicated that more hyperactive subjects were diagnosed as having a personality trait disorder, the two most frequent types being impulsive and immature-dependent personality traits. Two hyperactive subjects were diagnosed as borderline psychotic (this was not significant), but no subject in either group was diagnosed as psychotic. Significantly more hyperactive subjects felt restless than did controls, and significantly more were observed to be restless by the psychiatrist during their assessment, although actual getting up from their chairs was rare. Hyperactive subjects rated their childhood as unhappy more often than did controls. When asked what helped them most, the most frequent spontaneous response was to identify a particular parent or teacher who believed in them or to note the development of a talent. "Family fights," "feeling dumb," and "being criticized" were most frequently noted as factors that made their childhood difficult. On the Brief Psychiatric Rating Scale,[31] items such as anxiety, tension, grandiosity, and hostility were significantly more frequent among the hyperactive group.

Physiological Measures

There was no difference between the groups with respect to height, weight, blood pressure, or pulse rate.[13] Serial comparison of electroencephalograms (EEGs) of both groups at ten-year follow-up revealed no significant difference. Comparison of EEGs of hyperactive subjects at initial evaluation, five-year follow-up, and ten-year follow-up indicated that normalization of the EEG tended to occur during adolescence.[12]

Psychological Test[17,36]

Subjects rated themselves on the *California Psychological Inventory,*[10] which was designed to tap cultural ideals of self-esteem and social interaction; the SCL-90,[7] designed to tap classical psychopathology; and tests of self-esteem.[6,18,43] On both the California Psychological Inventory and on tests of self-esteem, hyperactives rated themselves as significantly inferior to controls. However, on the SCL-90, the ratings of the two groups did not differ, indicating that hyperactives do not see themselves as having classical symptoms of psychopathology. However, they do see themselves as functioning less optimally than do controls.

On *social skills tests*, hyperactives performed worse only on oral tasks, and were equal to controls on written tasks. The social skills tests used were the Situational Social Skills Inventory in written and oral form[5] and the Means-Ends Problem Solving test.[32]

Rating scales sent to employers and to teachers, containing almost identical items to be rated, showed that teachers rated hyperactives as inferior to controls on all items, whereas employers' ratings were identical for the two groups. This indicated that the demands of the social setting in which hyperactives are evaluated may significantly influence the degree to which they are considered deviant.

Cognitive style tests—Matching Familiar Figures test.[20] Embedded Figures Test,[42] and the Stroop test[35]—indicated that the problems hyperactives experience during their childhood and adolescence persist into adult life.[17]

CONCLUSIONS

This outcome study suggests that while few hyperactive children become grossly disturbed or chronic offenders of the law, the majority continue as young adults to exhibit various symptoms related to the hyperactive child syndrome. None were diagnosed as psychotic or schizophrenic, but impulsivity, low educational achievement, poorer social skills and lower self-esteem than controls, and restlessness continued to be present. At the same time, unlike the delinquency of the antisocial child in our study, the majority of hyperactives who had committed delinquent acts as adolescents had gained sufficient control by the time they were young adults, so that they did not have significantly more court referrals than normal controls.

We thus see that the various studies on adult outcomes of children who were hyperactive present a varied picture. Some of this variation is the result of the particular population studied (*e.g.*, adult psychiatric patients),[22,28] or inclusion of subjects with lower IQ[24] or organic brain syndromes.[25] Some of the variability may be the result of different methodological approaches (*e.g.*, retrospective studies, family studies, or prospective studies). However, despite these variations one can evolve a synthesized view of adult outcome of this condition. The clinical outcome of hyperactive young adults falls roughly into three categories. The first includes those hyperactive young adults whose functioning is fairly normal compared to matched controls.[3,9,15,21] Then there are the hyperactive young adults who continue to have significant concentration, social, emotional, and impulse problems. These problems often give rise to difficulties with work, interpersonal relationships, poor self-esteem, impulsivity, irritability, anxiety, and emotional lability. The vast majority of hyperactive young adults fall into this group. Almost all studies cited, irrespective of the population or methodology presented, cast some of their subjects in this light. Finally, there is a third group of hyperactive young adults who have significant psychiatric or antisocial problems. These subjects may be psychotic or borderline psychotic, severely depressed and suicidal, heavily involved in drug or alcohol abuse, or guilty of significant antisocial behavior (*e.g.*, assault, armed robbery, breaking and entering, drug dealing).[4,15,24,29,30]

We are thus left with two important challenges: 1) to identify the minority of hyperactive subjects destined to have the poorest outcomes so that special attention can be given to those at risk; and 2) to determine the types of intervention that might significantly reduce the continued morbidity of this condition. In other words, how do we modify or prevent the poor self-esteem, poor socialization, lower educational level, and impulsivity that are seen in so many young adults who were diagnosed as hyperactive in childhood?

REFERENCES

1. Ackerman, P., Dykman, R. and Peters, J. (1977). Teenage status of hyperactive and nonhyperactive learning disabled boys. Amer. J. Orthopsychiat. 47:577–596.
2. Blouin, A., Bornstein, I. and Trites, R. (1978). Teenage alcohol use among hyperactive children: a five year follow-up study. J. Pediat. Psychol. 3:188–194.
3. Borland, H. and Hechman, H. (1976). Hyperactive boys and their brothers, a twenty-five year follow-up study. Arch. Gen. Psychiat. 33:669–675.
4. Cantwell, D. (1972). Psychiatric illness in the families of hyperactive children. Arch Gen. Psychiat. 27:414–423.
5. Clark, K. (1974). Evaluation of a Group Social Skills Training Program with Psychiatric Inpatients: Training Viet Nam Veterans in Assertion, Heterosocial and Job Interview Skills Unpublished doctoral dissertation. University of Wisconsin.
6. Davidson, H. and Lang, G. (1960). Children's perceptions of their teachers' feeling towards them related to self-perception, school achievement and behavior. J. Exper. Ed. 29:107–116.
7. Derogatos, L., Lipman, R. and Iovi, I. (1973). An outpatient psychiatric rating scale: preliminary report. Psychopharmacol. Bull. 9(1):13.
8. Dykman, R. and Ackerman, P. (1980). Long term follow-up studies of hyperactive children. Advanc. Behav. Pediat. 1:97–128.
9. Feldman, S., Denhoff, E. and Denhoff, J. (1979). The attention disorders and related syndromes; outcome in adolescence and young adult life. In Minimal Brain Dysfunction: A Developmental Approach. E. Denhoff and L. Stern, eds. Masson Publishing, New York.
10. Gough, H. (1957). California Psychological Inventory. Consulting Psychologists Press. Palo Alto, Calif. (revised 1975)
11. Hechtman, L. (1981). Families of hyperactives. In Research in Community and Mental Health, Vol. 2. R. Simmons, ed. JAI Press. Greenwich, Conn.
12. Hechtman, L., Weiss, G. and Metrakos, K. (1978). Hyperactive individuals as young adults; current and longitudinal electroencephalographic evaluation and its relation to outcome. Canad. Med. Assoc. J. 118:912–923.
13. Hechtman, L., Weiss, G. and Perlman, T. (1978). Growth and cardiovascular measures in hyperactive individuals as young adults and in matched normal controls. Canad. Med. Assoc. J. 118:1247–1250.
14. Hechtman, L. et al. (1979). Hyperactive children in young adulthood; a controlled prospective ten-year follow-up. Inter. J. Ment. Hlth 8:52–66.
15. Hechtman, L. et al. (1981). Hyperactives as young adults; various clinical outcomes. Adolesc. Psychiat. 9:295–306.
16. Hollingshead, A. and Redlich, J. (1958). Social Class and Mental Illness: A Community Study. John Wiley, New York.
17. Hopkins, J. et al. (1979). Cognitive style in adults originally diagnosed as hyperactives. J. Child Psychol. Psychiat. 20:209–216.
18. Hoy, L. et al. (1978). The hyperactive child at adolescence; emotional, social and cognitive functioning. J. Abnorm. Child Psychol. 6:311–324.
19. Huessy, H. and Cohen, A. (1976). Hyperkinetic behaviors and learning disorders followed over seven years. Pediatrics 57:4–10.

20. Kagan, J. et al. (1964). Information processing in the child; significance of analytic and reflective attitudes. Psychol. Monogr. 78(1. Whole 578).

21. Laufer, M. (1971). Long term management and some follow-up findings on the use of drugs with minimal cerebral syndromes. J. Learn. Disabil. 4:55–58.

22. Mann, H. and Greenspan, S. (1976). The identification and treatment of adult brain dysfunction. Amer. J. Psychiat. 133:1013–1017.

23. Mendelson, W., Johnson, M. and Stewart, M. (1971). Hyperactive children as teenagers; a follow-up study. J. Ment. Nerv. Dis. 153:272–279.

24. Menkes, M., Rowe, J. and Menkes, J. (1967). A twenty-five year follow-up study on the hyperkinetic child with minimal brain dysfunction. Pediatrics 38:393–399.

25. Milman, D. (1979). Minimal brain dysfunction in childhood; outcome in late adolescence and early adult years. J. Clin. Psychiat. 40:371–380.

26. Minde, K. et al. (1971). The hyperactive child in elementary school; a five year controlled follow-up. Except. Child. 38:215–221.

27. Mindl, K., Weiss, G. and Mendelson, M. (1972). A five year follow-up study of 91 hyperactive school children. J. Amer. Acad. Child Psychiat. 11:595–610.

28. Morrison, J. and Minkoff, K. (1975). Explosive personality as a sequel to the hyperactive child syndrome. Comprehens. Psychiat. 16:343–348.

29. Morrison, J. and Stewart, M. (1971). A family study of the hyperactive child syndrome. Biol. Psychiat. 3:189–195.

30. Morrison, J. and Stewart, M. (1973). The psychiatric status of legal families of adopted hyperactives. Arch. Gen. Psychiat. 28:888–891.

31. Overall, J. and Gorham, D. (1962). The brief psychiatric rating scale. Psychol. Rep. 10:799.

32. Platt, J., Spivak, G. and Bloom, S. (1971). Means End Problem Solving Procedure (MEPS) Manual and Tentative Norms. Department of Mental Health Sciences, Hahnemann Medical College and Hospital, Philadelphia.

33. Shelley, E. and Reisier, A. (1972). Syndrome of minimal brain damage in young adults. Dis. Nerv. Syst. 33:335–338.

34. Stewart, M., Mendelson, W. and Johnson, S. (1973). Hyperactive children as adolescents; how they describe themselves. Child Psychiat. Hum. Devlp. 4:3–11.

35. Stroop, J. (1935). Studies in interference in serial verbal reactions. J. Exper. Psychol. 18:643–672.

36. Weiss, G., Hechtman, T. and Perlman, T. (1978). Hyperactives as young adults; school, employer, and self-rating scales obtained during ten-year follow-up evaluation. Amer. J. Orthopsychiat. 48:438–445.

37. Weiss, G. et al. (1979). Hyperactives as young adults; a controlled prospective ten-year follow-up of 75 children. Arch. Gen. Psychiat. 36:675–681.

38. Weiss, G. et al. (1971). Studies on the hyperactive child—VIII: five year follow-up. Arch. Gen. Psychiat. 24:409–414.

39. Weiss, G. et al. (1971). Comparison of the effects of chlorpromazine, dextroamphetamine, and methylphenidate on the behavior and intellectual functioning of hyperactive children. Canad. Med. Assoc. J. 104–20.

40. Werry, J. et al. (1966). Studies on the hyperactive child—III: the effect of chlorpromazine upon behavior and learning ability. J. Amer. Acad. Child Psychiat. 5:292–312.

41. Witkin, H. et al. (1962). Psychological Differentiation. John Wiley, New York.

42. Wood, D. et al. (1976). Diagnosis and treatment of minimal brain dysfunction in adults. Arch. Gen. Psychiat. 33:1453–1460.

43. Ziller, R., Hagen, J. and Smith, M. (1969). Self-esteem: a self-social construction. J. Consult. Clin. Psychol. 33:84–95.

25

Children of Parents With Major Affective Disorder: A Review

William R. Beardslee, Jules Bemporad, Martin B. Keller, and Gerald L. Klerman

Massachusetts General Hospital

The authors review published studies of the children of parents with major affective disorder and report the rates of diagnosable disorder in the children, their clinical symptoms and other behavioral disturbances, and the differing impact of parental illness at different ages and stages of development. There is significant risk to children in having parents with major affective disorder, and considerable impairment is evident in these children. The authors discuss the methodological issues in the studies and offer suggestions for future investigations.

In the last decade the hypothesis has emerged that offspring of parents with affective disorder have higher rates of affective disorder than offspring of parents without such illness. Factors contributing to the formulation of this hypothesis include documentation of a high frequency of affective disorder in adults (1); burgeoning interest in the nature of depression in childhood (2) and its diagnosis (3–5), biochemistry (6–8), and treatment (9, 10); retrospective accounts of depressed adults who

Reprinted with permission from the *American Journal of Psychiatry*, 1983, Vol. 140, 825–832. Copyright 1983 by the American Psychiatric Association.

Supported by NIMH grant MH–34780 in conjunction with the Boston Center of the NIMH-Clinical Research Brnach Collaborative Study of the Psychobiology of Depression, Clinical Studies (grant MH–25478), and by the William T. Grant Foundation, the Harris Trust (through Harvard University), the Overseas Shipholding Group, and the George Harrington Trust.

recall major difficulties with their parents (11–13); studies of clinically depressed children that reveal high rates of depression in parents (14, 15); concern with identifying vulnerable children who may develop manifest psychopathology; and the desire to devise methods of primary prevention. The literature in this area has grown sufficiently that a review is indicated.

The purposes of this article are 1) to describe the risk to children of developing psychiatric disorder by virtue of having an affectively ill parent, 2) to describe the clinical psychopathology and other disturbances the children manifest, 3) to alert clinicians who treat patients with affective disorder to these risks, and 4) to identify specific areas that need clarification through further research. We have examined 24 quantitative studies of children who are at risk because they have a parent with an affective illness. We do not review neuropsychiatric studies in this article because the methodological issues are different enough to warrant separate treatment and because such a review has been published (16). We do not review retrospective accounts about childhood from adults with affective disorder because of the possibility that such accounts may be so influenced by the subject's clinical state as to be inaccurate. The term "risk" refers to antecedent factors (for example, parental affective disorder) that increase the likelihood of difficulty in offspring. Our focus is on the difficulties manifest during childhood in children of parents with a lifetime history of affective illness.

DESIGN AND SAMPLES OF THE STUDIES

Two design approaches, cross-sectional and longitudinal, were used in the studies we reviewed. The longitudinal studies included an initial assessment and a follow-up either completed or in progress, and the cross-sectional studies involved only one assessment. Table 1 presents parental characteristics of the samples, and Table 2 gives the ages of the children, the number of children studied, and the specific outcomes assessed.

The cross-sectional studies included parents with the diagnosis of unipolar depression (29, 31, 32), those with bipolar illness (22, 26), or a combination of the two (17, 20, 24, 28). The outcomes assessed and the methods of obtaining data varied considerably among studies; very few studies employed control groups (see tables 1 and 2). Likewise, the assessment instruments varied, and there was no uniformity about what constitutes impairment. Only a few of the studies (24, 27, 28, 32) used criterion diagnoses, as most only assessed levels of impairment.

TABLE 1. Characteristics of Parents With Major Affective Disorder Reported in the Literature

Study	Diagnoses	Adult Diagnostic Criteria
Cross-sectional studies		
Conners et al. (17)	Depression, manic-depressive disorder (N=59)	Feighner et al. (18)
El-Guebaly et al. (19)	Depression (N=30), schizophrenia (N=30), alcoholism (N=30)	Feighner et al. (18)
Greenhill and Shopsin (20)	Depression (N=10), manic-depressive disorder (N=28), manic-depressive disorder (N=2)	Mayer-Gross et al. (21), DSM-II
Kuyler et al. (22)	Manic-depressive disorder (N=27)	Fieve and Dunner (23)
McKnew et al. (24)	Manic-depressive disorder (N=13), depression (N=2)	RDC (25)
O'Connell et al. (26)	Manic-depressive disorder (N=12)	RDC (25)
Orvaschel et al. (27)	Alcoholism (N=1), other (N=11); 7 also received an affective diagnosis	RDC (25)
Rutter (28) (subsection of larger study)	Schizophrenia (N=11), depression (N=43), other (N=93)	Diagnosis by clinician in record
Weissman et al. (29)a	Depression (N=40), control (N=40)	Raskin et al. (30)
Weissman and Siegel (31)a	Depression (N=16), control (N=17)	Raskin et al. (30)
Welner et al. (32)	Depression (N=29), control (N=41)	Feighner et al. (18)
Longitudinal studies		
Boston group		
Grunebaum et al. (33), Kauffman et al. (34)	Schizophrenia (N=18), depression (N=12), control (N=22)	Clinician diagnosis during hospitalization
Minnesota group		
Rolf (35)a, Rolf and Garmezy (36)a	"Internalizing" disorder (largely depression) (N=26), schizophrenia (N=31)	Diagnosis from hospital records
Rolf (37)a	"Internalizing" disorder (largely depression) (N=26), schizophrenia (N=19)	Diagnosis from hospital records
Garmezy and Devine (38)a	Not available (follow-up of samples previously studied [36, 37])	Diagnosis from hospital records
Rochester group		
Fisher and Jones (39)a	Affective psychosis (N=11), schizophrenia (N=27), other (includes "neurotic depression") (N=27)	Interview and hospital record review with DSM-III and WHO psychiatric history scales (40)
Fisher et al. (41)a, Harder et al. (42)a, Kokes et al. (43)a	Affective psychosis (N=17), schizophrenia (N=28), other (includes "neurotic depression") (N=41)	Interview and hospital record review with DSM-III and WHO psychiatric history scales (40)
Sameroff et al. (44)	Schizophrenia (N=29), depression (N=58), other (N=40), control (N=47)	CAPPS (45)
Stony Brook group		
Weintraub et al. (46)	Depression (N=17), schizophrenia (N=25), control (N=114)	CAPPS (45) and hospital records
Weintraub et al. (47)	Depression, schizophrenia, control (proportions similar to those in above study)	CAPPS (45) and hospital records

aThe sample used in this study overlaps with samples used in other studies reported here.

Garmezy (52, 53) reviewed the literature on the longitudinal studies of children who are at risk by virtue of having a schizophrenic parent. A number of such studies included the children of affectively disordered parents as a comparison group for the children of schizophrenic parents. We report on those studies that enabled conclusions to be drawn separately about the children of affectively ill parents. Studies included are those from the research groups at the University of Minnesota (35–38), the State University of New York at Stony Brook (46, 47), the University of Rochester Medical School in Rochester, N.Y. (39, 41–43), and the Cambridge Hospital and Massachusetts Mental Health Center in Boston (33, 34). A variation of the risk paradigm has been used by Sameroff and associates (44) to study mothers with mental illness (including a group with depression) during pregnancy and to follow them and their infants over 4 years.

We have not emphasized the possible differential impact on children of parental unipolar versus bipolar disorder, although we recognize the importance of the distinction. Only one study (17) contained both diagnostic entities and reported the findings on each separately enough to allow direct comparison, whereas seven others (20, 24, 27, 39, 41–43) reported combined results. The multiple sample and methodological differences among all the studies (see tables 1 and 2) led us to conclude that to distinguish between children of unipolar and bipolar parents was not yet warranted. Another reason for this decision is that many of the parents diagnosed as unipolar were relatively young when the children were assessed, and therefore an unknown proportion of them were likely to develop a bipolar illness in later life. This supports our conservative approach in not analyzing by diagnosis.

FINDINGS

Overall Rate of Psychiatric Diagnosis

Three studies presented rates of psychiatric diagnoses in children of parents with affective disorder. Orvaschel and associates (27) found psychiatric diagnoses in 43% of the 28 children studied, McKnew and associates (24) studied 30 children during their parents' hospitalization at NIMH and found the rate of psychiatric disorder to be 40%, and O'Connell and associates (26) examined 22 offspring of a wide age range and found a 45% rate of psychiatric disorder. In Orvaschel and associates' study, lifetime history of diagnosable illness was assessed, but McKnew and associates and O'Connell and associates only reported the

TABLE 2. Characteristics of Children of Parents With Major Affective Disorder Reported in the Literature

Study	Age of Children (years)	N	Outcome/Function Assessed	Source of Data About Child	Child Diagnostic Criteria
Cross-sectional studies					
Conners et al. (17)	1–18	126	Behavioral disturbance	Parent questionnaire	Absent
El-Guebaly et al. (19)	1–20	231	Behavioral disturbance	Parent questionnaire	Absent
Greenhill and Shopsin (20)	3–46	85	Behavioral disturbance	Parent questionnaire	Absent
Kuyler et al. (22)	6–18	49	Psychopathology, behavioral disturbance	Parent interview	Stewart and Gath (48), Kovacs and Beck (4)
McKnew et al. (24)	5–15	30	Psychopathology	Parent questionnaire, child interview	Children's Psychiatric Rating Scale (49), Weinberg criteria for depression (50)
O'Connell et al. (26)	5–17	22	Psychopathology	Parent interview, child interview	Children's Psychiatric Rating Scale (49)
Orvaschel et al. (27)	6–17	28	Psychopathology	Parent interview, child interview	RDC and DSM-III (25)
Rutter (28)	<1–17	137	Psychopathology, behavioral disturbance	Clinic records	O'Neal and Robins (51) (modified)
Weissman et al. (29)	1–25	109	Behavioral disturbance	Parent interview	Absent
Weissman and Siegel (31)	13–18	54	Behavioral disturbance	Parent interview	Absent
Welner et al. (32)	6–16	227	Psychopathology, behavioral disturbance, school function	Parent interview, child interview (not all subjects)	Feighner (18)
Longitudinal studies					
Boston group					
Grunebaum et al. (33), Kauffman et al. (34)	6–12	52	Competence, behavioral disturbance	Parent interview, child interview	Absent
Minnesota group					
Rolf (35), Rolf and Garmezy (36)	9–11	356[a]	Teacher evaluation, peer evaluation	Teacher rating, peer rating, school records	Absent
Rolf (37)	9–11	294[a]	Peer evaluation	Peer rating	Absent
Garmezy and Devine (38)	13–17	356	Behavioral disturbance, school performance	School records, interviews with school personnel	Absent
Rochester group					
Fisher and Jones (39)	7 and 10	65	Teacher evaluation, peer evaluation, competence	Teacher rating, peer rating, family interview, psychological tests	Absent
Fisher et al. (41), Harder et al. (42), Kokes et al. (43)	7 and 10	83	Teacher evaluation, peer evaluation, competence	Teacher rating, peer rating, family interview, psychological tests	Absent
Sameroff et al. (44)	<1–14	184	Behavioral disturbance	Parent interview, child interview, psychological tests	Absent
Stony Brook group					
Weintraub et al. (46)	5–16	215	Teacher evaluation	Teacher rating	Absent
Weintraub et al. (47)	5–16	289	Peer evaluation	Peer rating	Absent

[a]Includes classroom controls whose parents were not examined.

presence of diagnosis at the time of interview, and the diagnostic criteria were different in each of the studies (table 2).

Diagnostic and Symptomatic Pattern

The children's diagnoses and symptoms occurred in many different areas of functioning. In the course of a larger study, Rutter (28) described the children of 43 parents who received the diagnosis of depression. The diagnoses in the children were neurotic illness (N = 14), neurotic behavior disturbance (N = 14), mixed behavior disturbances (N = 8), and conduct disturbance (N = 7). The distribution of these diagnoses in the children was similar to that in children of parents with other kinds of mental illness. Kuyler and associates (22) described a variety of symptoms suggestive of personality disorders, adjustment reactions, hyperkinetic syndromes, and affective disorders. O'Connell and associates (26) reported disorders in the broad category of behavior disturbance. Two studies (26, 31) reported drug problems and two (20, 31) described sociopathy and trouble with the law. The studies by El-Guebaly and associates (19) and Conners and associates (17) confirmed the presence of wide-ranging symptoms.

Rate of Affective Diagnoses

A large percentage of the diagnoses given to the children studied were for affective disorders. In McKnew and associates' study (24) 75% (nine of 12) of the children who received psychiatric diagnoses were depressed, whereas in Orvaschel and associates' study (27) 33% (four of 12) of the diagnoses were in the affective area. In Welner and associates' study (32), designed specifically to look for depression in children, 7% (five of 75) of the experimental sample received the diagnosis of depression, but none of the control group children did.

Depressive Symptoms

In particular, depressive symptoms were reported in a high proportion of the children in many of these studies. Weissman and Siegel (31), Kuyler and associates (22), O'Connell and associates (26), and Greenhill and associates (20) all mentioned affective symptoms prominently. In Welner and associates' study (32), in addition to thise diagnosed as depressed, 8% (six of 75) of the experimental sample had four major symptoms of depression, but none of the control children did.

Comparison With Control Populations

A number of studies using peer and teacher ratings employed control groups, but because they did not yield rates of occurrence of clinical symptoms and psychopathology we report their findings in the next section. Only two studies compared rates of behavioral difficulties in experimental and control groups.

In Weissman and Siegel's study (31), depressed mothers reported having significant problems with their adolescents in 17 (74%) of the 23 cases, whereas normal mothers reported the difficulties in only three

(10%) of 31 cases. As noted, Welner and associates (32) found depression in 7% of the experimental group and none of the control group.

Developmental Perspective

Psychiatric difficulties may occur in all age groups of children. Several studies have reported findings by age in a way that allows observations about the differing psychopathological manifestations of difficulties at different ages and developmental levels.

Infancy. Sameroff and associates (44) reported a higher rate of perinatal complications and higher scores on perinatal stress measures in infants born to mothers with depression. However, mothers with other major mental illnesses also had higher levels of difficulty than controls. Those investigators found that nonspecific maternal prenatal anxiety, not diagnostic category, accounted for many of the differences in outcome among infants. Although not specific to the group of depressed mothers, the finding of impairments in the children of depressed mothers was present throughout the 4 years of the study. In early infancy, cognitive and emotional delays persisted for infants of ill mothers. Grunebaum and associates (54, 55) also found cognitive impairments in the young children of mentally ill mothers, including a group of mothers with psychotic depression. Weissman and associates (29) summarized the findings from several studies and reported that tyrannical behavior, inability to separate, and difficulties with ego boundaries existed in infancy and early childhood.

School age (6–12 years). Weissman and associates (29) reported excessive rivalry with peers and siblings for attention, feelings of isolation or depression, hyperactivity, school problems, and enuresis. Several longitudinal studies dealt primarily with this age group, employing peer and teacher ratings. Rolf and Garmezy (35, 36) reported that the children of internalizing (depressed) mothers most resembled the control population on teacher-rated measures and were different from the children of schizophrenic mothers. In contrast, investigators from the Stony Brook project (46) found differences between two groups of children with ill parents (children of schizophrenic and depressed mothers) and a control group on the following dimensions of the teacher rating scales: classroom disturbance, impatience, disrespect/defiance, and inattentiveness/withdrawal. The children of ill parents were less creative, showed less initiative and less need for closeness with teachers, and were rated lower on comprehension. In contrast, investigators in Rochester (39) reported that the sons of affectively psychotic patients were rated higher than classmates on cognitive competence and the sons of nonpsychotic hospitalized patients (including many depressive patients) were rated lower on social competence and social compliance. This latter group of children were felt to not meet expected norms of school behavior.

Studies examining peer relationships have used a class play in which all children in the class cast one another in various roles. Rolf and Garmezy (36, 37) reported that among four risk groups, the peer relationships of children of internalizing (depressed) mothers most resembled those of controls. The daughters of depressed mothers showed a tendency toward the internalizing symptoms that their mothers displayed, but the boys did not. Weintraub and associates (47), of the Stony Brook group, reported that children of schizophrenic and depressive parents differed from controls on peer rating scale dimensions of aggression and unhappiness/withdrawal. In contrast, the Rochester group (41, 42) compared the sons of affectively psychotic patients and a control group and showed that the children of ill parents had above-average scores on the peer ratings, whereas the sons of nonpsychotic hospitalized patients were perceived as experiencing difficulties.

Rolf's analysis of school records (36) showed that all risk groups in his sample had significantly poorer performance overall than the control groups.

Adolescence. In the adolescents studied by Weissman and Siegel (31), defiant behavior, rebellion, and withdrawal were the most common symptoms. Our review suggests that most difficulties of adolescents center on conflicts and disagreements with parents.

Garmezy and Devine (38) reported short-term follow-up of the children studied by Rolf and another similar group studied by Marcus in Minnesota. The outcome criteria were analysis of the cumulative school records and a brief interview with school personnel. In junior high school, the children of depressed mothers showed considerably more disturbance than had been evident from earlier reports; 22% of this group had dropped out of school, compared with only 10% of the control group, and only 43% received a positive outcome rating, compared with 69% of the control group.

Grunebaum and associates (33, 34) have followed over 15 years a group of children whose mothers were psychotic when the children were infants. In the most recent follow-up the investigators focused on competence in these children and divided the sample into those most competent and those least competent. Only one child of the six in the most competent group had a depressed mother, whereas five of the six children in the least competent group had depressed mothers (34).

DISCUSSION

The studies to date show that there is a high rate of impairment among children of parents with affective disorder. These findings are consistent with the findings from studies of children whose parents have other severe psychiatric disorders (56–59). Because of the relatively small number of subjects and the fact that only two of the studies that assessed psychopathological difficulties used a control group, it is not possible to estimate relative risk with precision. The three studies that made diagnoses for a variety of disorders found diagnosable illness in approximately 40% of the children studied, although the criteria for diagnoses were different in each study. Conclusions about prevalence rates and relative risk must await more detailed study involving control groups and prospective follow-up. The nature of the difficulties that the children experience is wide-ranging. The prevalence of depression among these children is high, particularly among the older children.

High rates of impairment were found in some of the cross-sectional studies, but relatively little impairment was found in the Minnesota and Rochester groups according to some of the data based on teacher and peer ratings. Several factors may explain the different results. The children in the Minnesota sample (ages 9–11 years) and in the Rochester sample (ages 7 and 10) were younger than the children in most of the cross-sectional studies. Also, the use of parental or child interviews is likely to generate information that is different from that obtained from teachers or peer ratings. The follow-up data in the Garmezy and Devine study (38) strongly suggest that children who were not identified as being particularly different from controls when they were 9–11 looked much more impaired as they went through high school. In the Rochester group, the sons of parents with a psychotic affective disorder were doing well, whereas the sons of nonpsychotic ill parents, who included many depressed parents, were doing very poorly. This suggests a differential impact on the young child based on the specific form of the parental illness.

The way parents have been assessed differs considerably across studies. Some studies have used hospitalized parents with only a history of illness. Some used explicit research criteria and others used clinical judgment in evaluating the parents (see Table 1). Thus, the course, duration, and severity of parental illness to which the children are exposed differ, as does the type of parental affective illness.

The rates of depression found in the studies by Welner and associates (32) and McKnew and associates (24) may have limited generalizability, since both of these studies were done after a period of parental hospitalization, and some of McKnew and associates' data were gathered while the parents were hospitalized. Thus, their depression may be a reaction to the separation from parents and may be short-lived.

This raises a question about the meaning of the impairment that was found—that is, how long does the impairment last and does it predict later difficulties? O'Connell and associates (26) commented, on the basis of face-to-face interviews aith the children in their study, that the impairments were longstanding and major, not transitory. Other investigaors generally agree, but for the most part follow-up at this point is still lacking.

From family studies of affectively ill adult patients (60) there is evidence for familial aggregation or patterning in the occurrence of affective illness. However, the studies reviewed in this article have described children who have not yet passed through the age of morbid risk for the illness of their parents. Hence, no firm conclusion can be reached about the degree of risk for affective illness as compared with other illnesses the children have. Such conclusions can be reached only when the children have been followed prospectively well into their 20s and 30s.

RECOMMENDATIONS FOR FURTHER RESEARCH

On the basis of this review, we suggest several directions that would be useful in future studies for more fully determining the influence of parental affective illness on children. There is need for cross-sectional studies, with adequate control groups and large numbers of children, that assess the impact of various affective diagnoses in the parent, the severity and chronicity of parental illness, and the influence of other risk factors. This will give a more precise estimate of the prevalence of difficulties and also help to sort out what is most deleterious about having an ill parent. For example, degree of impairment, speed of recovery from illness, or family communication difficulty may be more powerful predictors of difficulties in children than the parent's diagnostic category, as findings from the Rochester group (39, 42, 43) indicate, and long-term chronic illness may have a particularly deleterious effect, as Anthony (61) has described in the case of manic-depressive illness in parents. Similarly, factors within the child such as intelligence, presence or absence of learning disabilities, and coping capacities may contribute substantially to mediating the impact of having an ill parent. Advances (62, 63) in the study of coping and adaptation in children offer promise in this area. Longitudinal follow-up would help in determining the precursors for later illness and in assessing the risks in different age groups. Since children of varying ages and different developmental levels can be expected to react differently to the impact of parental illness, an assessment of developmental level should be part of such research.

Assuming that there is a difference between children of affectively ill parents and controls, as the weight of the evidence indicates, there is the question of etiology. Whether the observed differences are due to genetic factors or to psychosocial variables, such as marital problems or impairment in parenting ability, or to a necessary interaction between the two remains an empirical question. Further investigation of the contributions of various psychosocial variables, in conjunction with detailed family pedigree information, is needed to answer this question. The ideal design to examine the influence of genetic factors would examine the children of affectively ill parents who have been adopted away at an early age.

To resolve fundamental questions of etiology and to assist clinicians in knowing how best to treat children of ill parents, the capacity to compare findings across different studies is necessary. Essential to that effort is agreement on a standardized system of nomenclature with operationalized definitions and procedures for eliciting these data reliably. Several new semistructured interviews have been developed for the study of children—for example, the KIDDIE SADS (64), a version of the Schedule for Affective Disorders and Schizophrenia (65), and the Diagnostic Interview for Children and Adolescents (66, 67). When such instruments are used in conjunction with criterion diagnostic systems such as DSM-III, it should be possible for investigators to arrive at comparable and reliable diagnoses.

CONCLUSIONS

Despite the methodological limitations of the studies we have reported, several conclusions emerge. Children of affectively ill parents are at significant risk for developing psychopathology. Clinicians should be aware of this risk and carefully assess the children of parents with an affective disorder. The nature of the impairments in the children is wide-ranging. More efforts need to be made to determine age-specific features of children's disorders. Children of all ages and different stages of development may be affected, but early infancy and adolescence seem to be the stages in which children are particularly vulnerable. Special attention should be given to diagnosing clinical depression in these children.

REFERENCES

1. Boyd, J.H. and Weissman, M.M. (1981). Epidemiology of affective disorder. Arch Gen Psychiatry 38:1039–1049.
2. Kashani, J.H., Husain, A., Shekim, W.O., et al. (1981). Current perspectives on childhood depression: an overview. Am. J. Psychiatry 138:143–153.
3. Weinberg, W.A., Rutman, J., Sullivan, L., et al. (1973). Depression in children referred to an educational diagnostic center: diagnosis and treatment. J Pediatr. 83:1065–1072.
4. Kovacs, M., Beck, A.J. (1977). An empirical-clinical approach toward a definition of childhood depression, in Depression in Childhood: Diagnosis, Treatment, and Conceptual Models. Edited by Schulterbrand JG, Raskin A. New York, Raven Press.
5. Cytryn, L., McKnew, D.H.,JR., Brunney, W.E.,Jr. (1980). Diagnosis of depression in children: a reassessment. Am J Psychiatry 137:22–25.
6. McKnew, D.H., Cytryn, L. (1979). Urinary metabolites in chronically depressed children. J Am Acad Child Psychiatry 18:608–615.
7. Puig-Antich, J., Chambers, W., Halpern, F., et al. (1979). Cortisol hypersecretion in prepubertal depressive illness: a preliminary report. Psychoneuroendocrinology 4:191–197.
8. Puig-Antich, J., Tabrizi, M.A., Davies, M., et al. (1981). Prepubertal endogenous major depressives hyposecrete growth hormone in response to insulin-induced hypoglycemia. Biol Psychiatry 16:801–818.
9. Puig-Antich, J., Perel, J.M., Lupatkin, W., et al. (1979). Plasma levels of imipramine and desmethylimipramine and clinical response in prepubertal major depressive disorder. J Am Acad Child Psychiatry 18:616–627.
10. Bemporad, J. (1978). Psychotherapy of depression in children and adolescents, in Severe and Mild Depression: The Psychotherapeutic Approach. Edited by Arieti S, Bemporad J. New York, Basic Books.
11. Parker, G. (1979). Parental characteristics in relation to depressive disorders. Br J Psychiatry 134:138–147.
12. Jacobson, S., Fasman, J., Dimascio, A. (1975). Deprivation in the childhood of depressed women. J Nerv Ment Dis 160:5–14.
13. Raskin, A., Boothe, H.H., Reatig, N.A., et al: Factor analyses of normal and depressed patients' memories of parental behavior. Psychol Rep 29:871–879.
14. Philips, I. (1979). Childhood depression: interpersonal interactions and depressive phenomena. Am J Psychiatry 136:511–515.
15. McKnew, D.H., Cytryn, L. (1973). Historical background in children with affective disorders. Am J Psychiatry 130:178–180.
16. Garmezy, N. (1978). Attentional processes in adult schizophrenia and in children at risk. J Psychiatr Res 14:3–34.
17. Conners, C.K., Himmelhoch, J., Goyette, C.H., et al. (1979). Children of parents with affective illness. J Am Acad Child Psychiatry 18:600–607.
18. Feighner, J.P., Robins, E., Guze, S.B., et al. (1972). Diagnostic criteria for use in psychiatric research. Arch Gen Psychiatry 26:57–63.
19. El-Guebaly, N., Offord, D.R., Sullivan, K.T., et al. (1978). Psychosocial adjustment of the offspring of psychiatric inpatients: the effect of alcoholic, depressive and schizophrenic parentage. Can Psychiatr Assoc J 23:281–289.
20. Greenhill, L.L., Shopsin, B. (1979). Survey of mental disorders in the children of patients with affective disorders, in Genetic Aspects of Affective Illness. Edited by Mendlewicz J, Shopsin B. New York, Spectrum Publications.
21. Mayer-Gross, W., Slater, E., Roth, M. (1954). Clinical Psychiatry, London, Cassell.

22. Kuyler, P.L., Rosenthal, L., Igel, G., et al. (1980). Psychopathology among children of manic-depressive patients. Biol Psychiatry 15:589–597.

23. Fieve, R.R., Dunner, D.L. (1975). Unipolar and bipolar affective states, in The Nature and Treatment of Depression. Edited by Glach FF, Braghi, SC. New York, John Wiley & Sons.

24. McKnew, D.H., Cytryn, L., Effron, A.M., et al. (1979). Offspring of patients with affective disorders. Br J Psychiatry 134:148–152.

25. Spitzer, R.L., Endicott, J., Robins, E. (1977). Research Diagnostic Criteria (RDC) for a Selected Group of Functional Disorders, 3rd ed. New York, New York State Psychiatric Institute, Biometrics Research.

26. O'Connell, R.A., Mays, J.A., O'Brien, J.D., et al. (1979). Children of bipolar manic-depressives, in Genetic Aspects of Affective Illness. Edited by Mendlewicz J, Shopsin B. New York, Spectrum Publications.

27. Orvaschel, H., Weissman, M.M., Padian, N., et al. (1981). Assessing psychopathology in children of psychiatrically disturbed parents: a pilot study. J Am Acad Child Psychiatry 20:112–122.

28. Rutter, M. (1966). Children of Sick Parents: An Environmental and Psychiatric Study. Institute of Psychiatry Maudsley Monograph 16. London, Oxford University Press.

29. Weissman, M.M., Paykel, E.S., Klerman, G.L. (1972). The depressed woman as a mother. Social Psychiatry 7:98–108.

30. Raskin, A., Schulterbrandt, R.M., Rice, C.E. (1967). Factors of psychopathology in interview, ward behavior, and self-report ratings of hospitalized depressives. J Consult Psychol 31:270–278.

31. Weissman, M.M., Siegel, R. (1972). The depressed woman and her rebellious adolescent. Social Casework 53:563–570.

32. Welner, Z., Welner, A., McCrary, M.D., et al. (1977). Psychopathology in children of inpatients with depression: a controlled study. J Nerv Ment Dis 164:408–413.

33. Grunebaum, H., Cohler, B.J., Kauffman, C., et al. (1978). Children of depressed and schizophrenic mothers. Child Psychiatry Hum Dev 8:219–228.

34. Kauffman, C., Grunebaum, H., Cohler, B., et al. (1979). Superkids: competent children of psychotic mothers. Am J Psychiatry 136:1398–1402.

35. Rolf, J.E. (1972). The social and academic competence of children vulnerable to schizophrenia and other behavior pathologies. J Abnorm Psychol 80:225–243.

36. Rolf, J. E., Garmezy, N. (1974). The school performance of children vulnerable to behavior pathology, in Life History Research in Psychopathology, vol 3. Edited by Roff M. Minneapolis, University of Minnesota Press.

37. Rolf, J. E. (1976). Peer status and the directionality of symptomatic behavior: prime social competence predictors of outcome for vulnerable children. Am J Orthopsychiatry 46:74–88.

38. Garmezy, N., Devine, V. (in press). Project competence: the Minnesota studies of children vulnerable to psychopathology, in Children at Risk for Schizophrenia. Edited by Watt N, Rolf J, Anthony EJ. Cambridge, Cambridge University Press.

39. Fisher, L., Jones, J. E. (1980). Child competence and psychiatric risk, II: areas of relationship between child and family functioning. J Nerv Ment Dis 168:332–337.

40. World Health Organization (1973). The International Pilot Study of Schizophrenia, vol 1. Geneva, WHO.

41. Fisher, L., Harder, D. W., Kokes, R. F. (1980). Child competence and psychiatric risk, III: comparisons based on diagnosis of hospitalized parent. J Nerv Ment Dis 168:338–342.

42. Harder, D. W., Kokes, R. F., Fisher, L., et al. (1980). Child competence and psychiatric risk, IV: relationship of parent diagnostic classifications and parent psychopathology severity to child functioning. J Nerv Ment Dis 168:343–347.
43. Kokes, R. F., Harder, D. W., Fisher, L., et al. (1980). Child competence and psychiatric risk, V: sex of patient parent and dimensions of psychopathology. J Nerv Ment Dis 168:348–352.
44. Sameroff, A. J., Barocas, R., Seifer, R. (in press). Rochester longitudinal study progress report, in Children at Risk for Schizophrenia. Edited by Watt W, Rolf J, Anthony EJ. Cambridge, Cambridge University Press.
45. Spitzer, R., Endicott, J. (1968). Current and Past Psychopathology Scales (CAPPS). New York, New York State Department of Mental Hygiene, Biometrics Research, Evaluations Unit.
46. Weintraub, S., Neale, J. M., Liebert, D. E. (1975). Teacher ratings of children vulnerable to psychopathology. Am J Orthopsychiatry 45:839–845.
47. Weintraub, S., Prinz, R. J., Neale, G. M. (1978). Peer evaluations of the competence of children vulnerable to psychopathology. J Abnorm Child Psychol 6:461–473.
48. Stewart, M. A., Gath, A. (1978). Psychological Disorders of Children. Baltimore, Williams & Wilkins Co.
49. Children's ECDEU Battery (1973). Psychopharmacol Bull, Special Issue, pp 196–239.
50. Weinberg, W. A. (1973). Depression in children referred to an educational diagnostic center: diagnosis and treatment. J Pediatr 83:1065–1072.
51. O'Neal, P., Robins, L. N. (1958). The relation of childhood behavior problems to adult psychiatric status: a 30-year follow-up study of 150 subjects. Am J Psychiatry 114:961–969.
52. Garmezy, N. (1974). Children at risk: the search for the antecedents of schizophrenia, part II: ongoing research programs, issues, and intervention. Schizophr Bull 9:55–125.
53. Garmezy, N. (1978). Current status of a sample of other high risk research programs, in The Nature of Schizophrenia: New Approaches to Research and Treatment. Edited by Wynne L, Cromwell R, Matthysse S. New York, John Wiley & Sons.
54. Cohler, B. J., Grunebaum, H. U., Weiss, J. L., et al. (1977). Disturbance of attention among schizophrenic, depressed and well mothers and their children. J Child Psychol Psychiatry 18:115–135.
55. Gamer, E., Gallant, D., Grunebaum, H. U., et al. (1977). Children of psychotic mothers: performance of 3-year-old children on tests of attention. Arch Gen Psychiatry 34:592–597.
56. Buck, C., Laughton, K. (1959). Family patterns of illness. Acta Psychiatr Neurol Scand 39:165–175.
57. Landau, R., Harth, P., Othnay, N., et al. (1972). The influence of psychotic parents on their children's development. Am J Psychiatry 129:38–43.
58. Ekdahl, M. C., Rice, E. P., Schmidt, W. M. (1962). Children of parents hospitalized for mental illness. Am J Public Health 52:428–435.
59. Cooper, S. F., Leach, C., Storer, D., et al. (1977). The children of psychiatric patients: clinical findings. Br J Psychiatry 1321:514–522.
60. Nurnberger, J. I., Gershon, E. S. (1982). Genetics, in Handbook of Affective Disorder. Edited by Paykel ES. New York, Churchill Livingstone.
61. Anthony, E. J. (1975). The influence of a manic-depressive environment on the developing child, in Depression and Human Existence. Edited by Anthony EJ, Benedek T. Boston, Little, Brown and Co.
62. Anthony, E. J. (1974). The syndrome of the psychologically invulnerable child, in The Child in His Family, vol 3: Children at Psychiatric Risk. Edited by Anthony EJ, Kou-

pernic C. New York, John Wiley & Sons.

63. Rutter, M. (1981). Stress, coping and development: some issues and some questions. J Child Psychol Psychiatry 22:323–356.

64. Puig-Antich, J., Chambers, W. (1978). KIDDIE SADS—Schedule for Affective Disorders and Schizophrenia for School-Age Children (6–16 Years). New York, New York State Psychiatric Institute.

65. Endicott, J., Spitzer, R. L. (1978). A diagnostic interview: the Schedule for Affective Disorders and Schizophrenia. Arch Gen Psychiatry 35:837–844.

66. Herjanic, B., Reich, W. (1982). Development of a structural psychiatric interview for children, part 1: agreement between child and parent on individual symptoms. J Abnorm Child Psychiatry 10:307–324.

67. Reich, N., Herjanic, B., Welner, Z., et al. (1982). Development of a structured psychiatric interview for children, part 2: agreement on diagnoses comparing child and parent interviews. J Abnorm Child Psychiatry 10:325–336.

Part VII

EATING DISORDERS

The clinical syndrome that we label *anorexia nervosa* continues to be a most baffling and bizarre condition. Here is an illness which can affect a previously healthy teenager and lead to conscious and deliberate self-starvation that may become life-threatening. Yet, search as we do, we may find no other evidence of significant physiological or psychological pathology, past or present. It is the impression of many that its incidence is increasing, and we can only speculate about the nature and cause of this condition. The very diagnostic label is a misnomer, since the afflicted youngsters are typically not "anorectic". Quite the contrary, they are preoccupied with thoughts of food and have an avid desire to eat, and yet become involved in all kinds of complicated strategies to avoid eating. Given this puzzle, it is also no surprise that treatment is all too frequently arduous, prolonged, and uncertain in its therapeutic outcome.

The riddle of anorexia nervosa has stimulated a substantial literature on the subject. The body of literature on etiology and follow-up studies is summarized in two companion comprehensive and detailed articles from the journal *Psychological Medicine*, one by Hsü and the other by Steinhausen and Glanville. A number of suggestive findings and hypotheses are highlighted, but the need for new studies with greater methodological rigor and conceptual focus is also emphasized. Unfortunately, all too many of the published studies have suffered from gross methodological deficiences. It is hoped that as these are corrected in future investigations, meaningful subclassifications of the syndrome will become possible—a necessary precondition to an understanding of the etiology and dynamics of subgroups, and the establishment of effective methods of prevention and treatment.

In the third paper in this section, Maloney and Klykylo present an overview of bulimia, obesity and anorexia nervosa in children and adolescents. The discussion of anorexia nervosa complements the two other papers in this section by its concentration on treatment procedures, rather than etiology and follow-up. The authors point up the need for a multidimensional approach, in order to manage the medical complications of starvation, the intrapsychic character problems, and the interpersonal stresses which trouble these patients. They warn that whatever therapy is utilized, "the therapist faces a long-term, and often frustrating, treatment process."

Anorexia nervosa cases sometimes show episodes of bulimia, and Maloney and Klykylo review briefly the literature pertaining to such patients, as well as those instances in which bulimia occurs as a syndrome unassociated with anorexia nervosa. They provide a timely warning about the danger of depression and suicide in bulimia cases. Finally, the authors conclude their review of the eating disorders of childhood and adolescence with a discussion of the common syndrome of obesity. Various theories of etiology and the different approaches to treatment reported in the literature are reviewed succinctly and systematically.

26

The Aetiology of Anorexia Nervosa

L.K. George Hsu

University of Pittsburgh

Anorexia nervosa is an intriguing illness: the fact that it affects mainly attractive, intelligent young women, the wilful starvation, the near delusional insistence that they look just right, the intensive fear of becoming fat, the obsession with food and cooking, the perfectionist attitude, the secretiveness, and then the periodic gorging and vomiting. It has inspired a large number of publications recently, but there has been no consensus among the research workers on its aetiology. Currently, there are six main theories, organized along different conceptual levels, that attempt to explain this curious phenomenon. They are logically not mutually exclusive. While they overlap to some degree, their main thrust and conceptualization are distinct. This editorial will review the recent findings.

THE SOCIAL-CULTURAL THEORY

Anorexia nervosa occurs much more commonly in females than in males (Beumont *et al.* 1972; Crisp & Toms, 1972; Gull, 1874; Jones *et al.* 1980; Kendell *et al.* 1973; for a review of major series, see Hsu, 1980). It affects predominantly upper social class teenage girls in developed countries (Buhrich, 1981; Crisp *et al.* 1976; Jones *et al.* 1980; Miyai *et al.* 1975). Its incidence appears to be increasing (Duddle, 1973; Halmi, 1974; Jones *et al.* 1980; Kendell *et al.* 1973; Theander, 1970). Thus, social-cultural factors appear to be involved in the development of this disorder.

Reprinted with persmission from *Psychological Medicine*, 1983, Vol. 13, 231–237. Copyright 1983 by Cambridge University Press.

The importance of physical attractiveness in Western society is undeniable. In the female this attractiveness has taken the form of slimness. Several surveys indicated that the majority of young women are unhappy about their weight and want to be slimmer (Calden et al. 1959; Huenemann et al. 1966; Nylander, 1971). In contrast, men prefer to be bigger and heavier (Calden et al. 1959; Huenemann et al. 1966; Nylander, 1971). Garner et al. (1980), reviewing data from *Playboy* centrefolds and Miss America Pageant contestants in the last 20 years, found a significant trend towards slimness. All measurements of *Playboy* centrefold girls, except for height and waist, decreased significantly. Thus, for instance, the average Playmate in 1959 weighed 91% of average, while in 1978 they weighed only 83.5% of average. America pageant winners since 1970, with a mean weight of only 82.5% of average, weighed significantly less than the average contestant. Meanwhile, the number of diet articles in six women's magazines has increased substantially over the last 20 years. However, Garner et al. (1980) found that this emphasis on thinness and dieting occurs in a population that is becoming heavier. Weight statistics from the Society of Actuaries over the last 20 years indicated an increase in the average weight in all height categories for women below the age of 30 years. The pressure on women, particularly those of the upper social class, to diet and appear slim thus seems relentless (Goldblatt et al. 1965; Halmi et al. 1978b). That such pressure may precipitate the development of anorexia nervosa seems to be confirmed by the finding that the condition is much more common in women who must rigorously control their size and shape—such as ballerinas, modelling students and athletes (Druss & Silverman, 1979; Frisch et al. 1980; Garner & Garfinkel, 1980). Competitiveness intensifies the pressure (Garner & Garfinkel, 1980). Under such circumstances it is perhaps not surprising that Branch & Eurman (1980) found that the anorectic's friends and relatives actually admired her slimness, specialness and control. Meanwhile, Boskind-Lodahl (1976) regarded the 'cultural heritage of sexual inequality' to be directly responsible for the development of eating disorders in women. However, since such inequality presumably also exists in developing countries, it is difficult to see why the disorder is so rare in these countries (Buhrich, 1981). Palazzoli (Palazzoli, 1974; Palazzoli et al. 1977) emphasized the complex and contradictory roles which women had to play in modern society. Such role diffusion presumably increases insecurity and intensifies the striving for perfection and control.

That such social-cultural pressure generates a greater likelihod for the development of anorexia nervosa in women is probably not in dispute.

It is, however, obvious that not all women exposed to such pressure develop anorexia nervosa. Other factors must also occur to precipitate the final development of the illness.

FAMILY PATHOLOGY THEORY

The early investigators have all emphasized the family pathology in anorexia nervosa (Charcot, 1889; Gull, 1874; Lasèque, 1873). Charcot (1889) advocated the separation of the patient from her family as part of treatment. Gull (1874) found that the relatives were the worst attenders of the patient. Lasèque (1873) described the striking family enmeshment and he urged clinicians not to overlook the family pathology. Other early investigators have likewise described the adverse influence of the family on the patient (Crookshank, 1931; Young, 1931).

Attempts to identify a typical anorectic mother (Cobb, 1950; Kay & Leigh, 1954; King, 1963; Nemiah, 1950) or a typical anorectic father (Groen & Feldman-Toledo, 1966; King, 1963; Nemiah, 1950; Sours, 1981) have produced no consistent findings (Crisp et al. 1980; Kalucy et al. 1977). More recently, several authors have described a typical anorectic family interaction pathology. Bruch (1973, 1977) emphasized the facade of happiness and stability that hid a deep disillusionment and secret competition of the parents. She also found that the parents were very preoccupied with outward appearance and success. Palazzoli (1974) studied 12 anorectic families and found that a rejection of communicated message, poor conflict resolution, covert alliance of family members and blame shifting were characteristic of the anorectic family. She also emphasized their rigidity in that they tried to preserve agricultural-patriarchal values and *mores* in an urban-industrial setting. Both Palazzoli and Bruch found that the parents were overprotective but also involved the sick child in their covert competition and conflict. They seemed to use the child to discharge some of their own unfulfilled longings. Minuchin and his co-workers have written extensively on the psychosomatic family (Minuchin, 1974; Minuchin et al. 1975, 1978). They advocated an open systems model for psychosomatic illness, anorexia nervosa included. This system included parts such as extrafamilial stress, family organization and functioning, the vulnerable child, physiological and biochemical mediating mechanisms and the symptomatic child. The system could be activated at any point and the parts could affect each other. Nevertheless, these authors have emphasized almost exclusively the family pathology in this system and stated that 'When significant family interaction patterns are changed, significant changes in the symptoms of the psychosomatic illness also occur' (Minuchin *et al.* 1978, p. 21). They further hypothesized that: (1) certain family characteristics were related to the development and maintenance of psychosomatic symptoms in children; (2) the child's psychosomatic symptoms played a major role in maintaining family homeostasis. The family characteristics identified were enmeshment, overprotectiveness, rigidity and lack of conflict resolution. Meanwhile, the child was used to maintain stability and to avoid open conflict, and thus was often caught (triangulated) in the parents' covert conflict. The illness enabled the parents to submerge their conflicts in protecting or blaming the sick child, who was then defined as the sole family problem.

However, few studies exist to confirm that such family interaction pathology occurs in anorexia nervosa. Crisp *et al.* (1974) used a standardized measure (the Middlesex Hospital Questionnaire) and found that the psychoneurotic status of the parents worsened significantly as the patient's weight increased with treatment. This was particularly so if the marital relationship was poor. The six-month outcome for the patient's illness was significantly related to the initial parental psychoneurotic morbidity. Case selection factors and family therapy effects were, however, uncontrolled. Foster & Kupfer (1975) telemetrically recorded the nocturnal motility of a female patient with anorexia nervosa and found that nocturnal activity was correlated with visits by specific family members during the previous day. Visits by the father and the identical twin led to a decrease in nocturnal motility, while visits by the mother and older sister led to an increase in such 'arousal'. The extent to which such findings can be generalized is, however, questionable.

Related to the issue of family environment is the role of genetic factors in the pathogenesis of anorexia nervosa. Several large-scale studies have found an increased incidence of anorexia nervosa in the family members of the patients (Crisp *et al.* 1980; Halmi *et al.* 1977; Morgan & Russell, 1975; Theander, 1970). Monozygotic twin studies have found a concordance of about 50% (for a review, see Askevold & Heiberg, 1979) but, to the best of our knowledge, no study on dizygotic twins has been reported. Adoptive studies, however, are needed to tease out environmental *versus* genetic factors. In this connection, Crisp & Toms (1972) described a remarkable case of a male chronic anorectic whose adoptive son as well as the girl who stayed with the family as a war evacuee both developed anorexia nervosa. In sum, it remains to be substantiated that *specific* abnormal family interaction patterns occur in anorexia nervosa and that they are causally related to the development of the condition. Moreover, most of the studies quoted ignored the effect of this exasperating illness on family interaction and thus failed to distinguish between family pathology occurring as stress reactions as opposed to pre-existing patterns (Yager, 1982). The need for well-controlled direct observation studies of family interaction is obvious.

Finally, Crisp and his co-workers have suggested that family weight pathology may be specifically related to the pathogenesis of the illness (Crisp, 1977; Kalucy *et al.* 1977). In a well-controlled study of the parents of anorectic patients, Halmi *et al.* (1978*b*) failed to confirm this.

INDIVIDUAL PSYCHODYNAMIC THEORY

Psychoanalytic studies of anorexia nervosa have been reviewed by Sours (1974) and Bemis (1978). Both Bruch (1970) and Palazzoli (1974) have found that the psychoanalytic approach was relatively ineffective. In 1931, Brown observed that anorexia nervosa was a pathological manifestation of the detachment of the growing individual from parental authority. Bruch (1962, 1970, 1973, 1977) has repeatedly stated that anorexia nervosa was a struggle for a self-respecting identity. That such a struggle took the form of wilful starvation suggested serious psychological development defects. Central to such defects was the failure of the parents to regard the patients as individuals in their own right; they failed to transmit a sense of competence and self-value to their children. The youngsters were instead treated as something to complement the parents' needs. Their sense of worth and value were thus deprived from being needed by each parent. In short, they felt that they were the property of their parents. The illness thus represented an effort to escape from such a role and to establish control. Because of their disturbed perception of bodily sensation related to their lack of autonomy, and a paralysing sense of ineffectiveness, such patients misinterpreted their biological functioning and social role, and came to interpret thinness and starvation as specialness and self-control in an exaggerated and concrete way. Palazzoli (1974) and Boskind-Lodahl (1976) echoed such views.

The individual psychodynamic theory is extremely plausible, except that it has never been tested empirically. A recent single case study (Rampling, 1980) provided some evidence of abnormal mothering in a case of a male anorectic subject.

THE DEVELOPMENTAL PSYCHOBIOLOGICAL THEORY

Brown (1931) stated that a fear of growing up and assuming adult responsibility was highly characteristic of anorectics. Crisp has repeatedly stated (Crisp, 1967, 1970, 1977) that anorexia nervosa was rooted in the biological and consequently experiential aspects of normal adult weight. Starvation in the anorectic represented a phobic avoidance of adolescent/adult weight. Anorexia nervosa was thus a disorder of weight pivoting around specific maturational changes of puberty, both biological and psychological. The psychobiological regression reflected the individual's need to avoid adolescent and related family turmoil. The severe dieting was reinforced by the relief that the control and the low weight brought, as biological and related psychological childhood was re-experienced and post-pubertal experience was concurrently eliminated. Meanwhile, adolescence in the child threatened the rigid and experience-denying parents. The illness thus sometimes served to avert rekindling of buried and denied but unresolved parental conflicts and psychopathology. Needless to say, the illness brought its own problems but they were deemed to be the price that the patient and her family had to pay to avoid deeper, more fundamental discord. Crisp has repeatedly emphasized that such maturational demands of adolescence and family pathology were not specific to the condition. Indirect and partial support for this view has come from several sources: (1) the immature pattern of gonadotrophin release in anorectics which reverts to normal after weight gain (Boyar et al. 1974; Katz et al. 1978); (2) Frisch (1972, 1977) has found that puberty hinges on the individual attaining a critical amount of fatness; (3) clinical experience suggests that anorectics will often agree to eat provided that weight gain does not occur, thereby indicating that weight rather than eating is involved in the issue of control; (4) finally, Crisp et al.'s (1974) finding that the parents' psychoneurotic status worsened following the patient's recovery seems to support the notion that the illness serves to reduce family tension. Nevertheless, this theory of 'weight phobia' has never been tested empirically. One study found that anorexia nervosa patients differed from other phobic patients in terms of skin conductance changes (Salkind et al. 1980).

PRIMARY HYPOTHALAMIC DYSFUNCTION THEORY

Russell (1965, 1970, 1977a) has repeatedly suggested that a primary hypothalamic dysfunction of unknown aetiology and only partially dependent on weight loss and psychopathology occurred in anorexia nervosa. An early onset of amenorrhoea often occurs before any appreciable weight loss (for a review, see Bemis, 1978). This, in addition to the incomplete recovery of hypothalamic function and the persistent amenorrhoea despite weight gain, has been cited as evidence for a primary hypothalamic disorder (Katz et al. 1978; Russell, 1977a). Furthermore, several reports of hypothalamic tumour presenting as anorexia nervosa have appeared and the hypothalamus has traditionally been regarded as the central anatomical structure regulating feeding and satiety (for a review, see Mawson, 1974).

The role of the hypothalamus in the regulation of feeding and satiety is complex, and the importance of extra hypothalamic controls of feeding is increasingly recognized (McHugh & Moran, 1977; Morrison, 1977; Stricker, 1978). Others, however, have maintained that increased biological satiety might cause anorexia nervosa (Redmond *et al.* 1977). In fact, most anorectics experience hunger and crave food and thus to postulate that they are satiated seems contrary to existing evidence. The concurrent onset of amenorrhoea and weight loss has been reported to occur in 30–60% of patients (Beck & Brøckner-Mortensen, 1954; Dally, 1969; King, 1963; Morgan & Russell, 1975), but the figures were lower in other series (Crisp *et al.* 1980; Halmi *et al.* 1977; Theander, 1970). Amenorrhoea preceding the onset of any weight loss occurred in 7% (Theander, 1970) to 25% (Kay & Leigh, 1954; King, 1963) of cases. While such discrepancies may appear puzzling, one has to recognize the inherent difficulties involved in gathering retrospective data from anorectic patients, particularly a reliable dietary history (Crisp & Stonehill, 1971). This was well illustrated by the study of Beumont *et al.* (1981). Two patients in their series had initially indicated that amenorrhoea occurred before weight loss, but careful history-taking found that months of chaotic eating had preceded the amenorrhoea.

Various explanations have been offered for the incomplete recovery of hypothalamic function in women with apparently healthy weight following anorexia nervosa. (1) Amenorrhoea occurred in non-anorectic women who had lost 10–15% of normal weight for height (Frisch & McArthur, 1974), and menstrual cycles often failed to return unless a critical threshold weight was exceeded (Frisch, 1977). Simple weight loss itself could lead to hypothalamic dysfunction (Vigersky *et al.* 1977) and immature LH secretory pattern (Kapen *et al.* 1981). Crisp & Stonehill (1971) have suggested that the restoration of matched population mean weight rather than ideal weight was often necessary for menstruation to resume, particularly in patients who have been premorbidly obese. This view was partially supported by Knuth *et al.* (1977), who studied a group of 39 women with amenorrhoea due to loss of weight, including 24 with a diagnosis of anorexia nervosa. All patients were encouraged to gain weight and 14 who gained weight significantly (mean 3.6 kg) resumed ovulatory menstrual cycles. In contrast, there was no significant weight gain in the 25 patients who remained amenorrhoeic (mean 0.7

kg). (2) Many apparently recovered anorectics continue to starve, binge, vomit and purge (Cantwell *et al.* 1977; Hsu *et al.* 1979); Morgan & Russell, 1975). Some may selectively avoid carbohydrates. Thus dietary behaviour may determine whether hypothalamic function returns to normal (Katz *et al.* 1978). It may, of course, be argued that such dietary disturbances reflect the primary hypothalamic disorder (Russell, 1977*a*). This issue cannot be resolved on current evidence. (3) There is some evidence to suggest that the recovery of hypothalamic function occurred in sequence and full recovery took time (Wakeling *et al.* 1977). However, in the study by Wakeling *et al.* (1977) only 3 out of 7 patients who maintained their weight over a 6-month period menstruated, but it was unclear whether the patients were at or above their average weight. In sum, it remains possible that a primary hypothalamic disorder exists in anorexia nervosa. Further studies are obviously necessary to clarify the situation.

IS ANOREXIA NERVOSA RELATED TO AFFECTIVE DISORDER?

Cantwell *et al.* (1977) have recently stated that anorexia nervosa may be an atypical affective disorder occurring in an adolescent female at a time in her life when body image issues were important. Two findings in their study supported this view: an increased incidence of affective disorder in the family; and, on long-term follow-up, the anorectics were more prone to develop affective disorder than to suffer a relapse of the eating disorder. Using well-defined criteria, Winokur *et al.* (1980) found that 22% of the relatives of anorectic probands had a history of primary affective disorder, an incidence similar to that reported in families of primary affective disorder patients. A family history of alcoholism, reported to be increased in some affective disorder patients (Winokur *et al.* 1978), also appeared to be increased in anorectic patients (Cantwell *et al.* 1977). However, Winokur *et al.* (1980) failed to confirm this. Certain biological markers have recently been reported for primary affective disorder, such as high plasma cortisol level (Sachar *et al.* 1970), dexamethasone non-suppression (Carroll, 1982), and low urinary 3-methoxy-4-hydroxyphenylglycol (Schildkraut *et al.* 1973). All of these changes also occurred in some anorectics, but the abnormalities were apparently reversible with weight gain (Gerner & Gwirtsman, 1981; Gross *et al.* 1979; Halmi *et al.* 1978*a*; Walsh *et al.* 1981; Walsh, 1982). Characteristic sleep EEG findings have been reported for primary affective disorder (Kupfer *et al.* 1976; Feinberg *et al.* 1982). The changes were, however, different from those reported in anorexia nervosa patients (Neil *et al.* 1980). Meanwhile, anorectics were not as overtly depressed as patients with affective disorder (Bentovim *et al.* 1979; Crisp *et al.* 1978; Eckert *et al.* 1982). Most follow-up studies suggested that anorexia nervosa 'breeds true' (Hsu *et al.* 1979; Morgan & Russell, 1975; Russell, 1970). Cantwell *et al.*'s (1977) findings that anorexia nervosa patients were more likely to suffer from an affective disorder than anorexia nervosa at follow-up may be related to methodological issues in their study (Hsu, 1980). Finally, anecdotal reports of the usefulness of antidepressants in the treatment of anorexia nervosa (Mills, 1976; Needleman & Waber, 1977) have not been widely accepted (Crisp *et al.* 1980; Russell, 1977*b*). The complex relationship between the two disorders deserves wider study.

CONCLUSION

While it is possible that anorexia nervosa has a single discrete cause, it is equally possible that complex chains of events interact to precipitate the illness. Kendell (1975) clearly favoured the latter view for psychiatric diseases in general. He even stated that: 'The very idea of "cause" has become meaningless, other than as a convenient designation for the point in the chain of event sequences at which intervention is most practicable' (p. 64). The overlap of the theories reviewed above certainly suggests that this argument is at least plausible in the case of anorexia nervosa. If this is so, the challenge then will be to identify such events and how they interact. Needless to say, such events may include some or all of the proposed aetiological factors already reviewed, or none of them. A possible strategy may be to study prospectively and follow-up a group of youngsters considered to be at risk for developing the illness—for example, professional dance and modelling students. The logistical and ethical problems involved in such a study may, however, be prohibitive.

REFERENCES

Askevold, F. & Heiberg, A. (1979). Anorexia nervosa: two cases in discordant MZ twins. *Psychotherapy and Psychosomatics*, **32**:223–228.

Beck, J. C. & Brøchner-Mortenson, K. (1954). Observations on the prognosis in anorexia nervosa. *Acta Medica Scandinavica*, 149:409–430.

Bemis, K. M. (1978). Current approaches to the etiology and treatment of anorexia nervosa. *Psychological Bulletin*, **85**:593–617.

Bentovim, D. I., Marilov, V. & Crisp, A. H. (1979). Personality and mental state (PSE) with anorexia nervosa. *Journal of Psychosomatic Research*, **23**:321–325.

Beumont, P. J. V., Beardwood, C. J. & Russell, G. F. M. (1972). The occurrence of anorexia nervosa in male subjects. *Psychological Medicine*, **2**:216–231.

Beumont, P. J. V., Abraham, S. F. & Simson, K. G. (1981). The psychosexual histories of adolescent girls and young women with anorexia nervosa. *Psychological Medicine*, **11**:477–484.

Boskind-Lodahl, M. (1976). Cinderella's stepsisters: a feminist perspective on anorexia nervosa and bulimia. *Signs: Journal of Women in Culture and Society*, **2**:342–356.

Boyar, R. N., Katz, J., Finkelstein, J. W., Kapen, S., Weiner, H., Weitzman, E. D. & Hellman, L. (1974). Anorexia nervosa: immaturity of the 24 hour luteinizing hormone secretory pattern. *New England Journal of Medicine*, **291**:861–865.

Branch, C. H. H. & Eurman, L. K. (1980). Social attitudes toward patients with anorexia nervosa. *American Journal of Psychiatry*, **137**:632–633.

Brown, W. L. (1931). Anorexia nervosa. In *Anorexia Nervosa* (ed. W. L. Brown), pp. 11–18. C. W. Daniels: London.

Bruch, H. (1962). Perceptual and conceptual disturbances in anorexia nervosa. *Psychosomatic Medicine*, **24**:187–194.

Bruch, H. (1970). Psychotherapy in primary anorexia nervosa. *Journal of Nervous and Mental Disease*, **150**:51–67.

Bruch, H. (1973). *Eating Disorders*. Basic Books: New York.

Bruch, H. (1977). Psychological antecedents of anorexia nervosa. In *Anorexia Nervosa* (ed. R. A. Vigersky), pp. 1–10. Raven Press: New York.

Buhrich, N. (1981). Frequency of presentation of anorexia in Malaysia. *Australian and New Zealand Journal of Psychiatry*, **15**:153–155.

Calden, G., Lundy, R. M. & Schlafer, R. J. (1959). Sex differences in body concepts. *Journal of Consulting Psychiatry*, **23**:378.

Cantwell, D. P., Sturzenberger, S., Borroughs, J. Salkin, B. & Green, J. K. (1977). Anorexia nervosa—an affective disorder? *Archives of General Psychiatry*, **34**:1087–1093.

Carroll, B. J. (1982). The dexamethasone suppression test for melancholia. *British Journal of Psychiatry*, **140**:292–304.

Charcot, J. M. (1889). *Disorders of the Nervous System*. New Sydenham Society: London.

Cobb, S. (1950). *Emotions and Clinical Medicine*. Norton: New York.

Crisp, A. H. (1967). Anorexia nervosa. *Hospital Medicine*, **1**:713–718.

Crisp, A. H. (1970). Anorexia nervosa: feeding disorder, nervous malnutrition or weight phobia? *World Review of Nutrition and Diet*, **12**:452–504.

Crisp, A. H. (1977). Diagnosis and outcome of anorexia nervosa. *Proceedings of the Royal Society of Medicine*, **70**:464–470.

Crisp, A. H. & Stonehill, E. (1971). Relation between aspects of nutritional disturbance and menstrual activity in primary anorexia nervosa. *British Medical Journal* iii, 149–151.

Crisp, A. H. & Toms, D. A. (1972). Primary anorexia nervosa or weight phobia in the male. *British Medical Journal* i, 334–338.

Crisp, A. H., Harding, B. & McGuinness, B. (1974). Anorexia nervosa: psychoneurotic characteristics of parents: relationship to prognosis. *Journal of Psychosomatic Research*, **18**:167–173.

Crisp, A. H., Palmer, R. L. & Kalucy, R. S. (1976). How common is anorexia nervosa? A prevalence study. *British Journal of Psychiatry*, **128**:549–554.

Crisp, A. H., Jones, M. G. & Slater, P. (1978). The Middlesex Hospital Questionnaire, a validity study. *British Journal of Medical Psychology*, **51**:269–280.

Crisp, A. H., Hsu, L. K. G., Harding, B. & Hartshorn, J. (1980). Clinical features of anorexia nervosa. *Journal of Psychosomatic Research*, **24**:179–191.

Crookshank, F. G. (1931). Anorexia nervosa. In *Anorexia Nervosa* (ed. W. L. Brown), pp. 19–40. C. W. Daniel: London.

Dally, P. (1969). *Anorexia Nervosa.* Heinemann, London.

Druss, R. G. & Silverman, J. A (1979). Body image and perfectionism of ballerinas. *General Hospital Psychiatry,* **2**:115–121.

Duddle, M. (1973). An increase of anorexia nervosa in a university population. *British Journal of Psychiatry,* **123**:711–712.

Eckert, E. D., Goldberg, S. C., Halmi, K. A., Casper, R. C. & Davis, J. M. (1982). Depression in anorexia nervosa. *Psychological Medicine,* **12**:115–122.

Feinberg, M. Gillin, J. C., Carroll, B. J., Greden, J. F. & Zis, A. P. (1982). EEG studies of sleep in the diagnosis of depression. *Biological Psychiatry,* **17**:305–316.

Foster, F. G. & Kupfer, D. J. (1975). Anorexia nervosa: telemetric assessment of family interactions and hospital events. *Journal of Psychosomatic Research,* **12**:19–35.

Frisch, R. E. (1972). Weight in menarche. *Pediatrics,* **50**:445–450.

Frisch, R. E. (1977). Food intake, fatness and reproductive ability. In *Anorexia Nervosa* (ed. R. A. Vigersky), pp. 149–162. Raven Press: New York.

Frisch, R. E. & McArthur, J. W. (1974). Menstrual cycles: fatness as a determinant of minimum weight for the height necessary for their maintenance or onset. *Science,* **185**:949–951.

Frisch, R. E., Wyshak, G. & Vincent, L. (1980). Delayed menarche and amenorrhea in ballet dancers. *New England Journal of Medicine,* **303**:17–19.

Garner, D. M. & Garfinkel, P. E. (1980). Social cultural factors in the development of anorexia nervosa. *Psychological Medicine,* **10**:647–656.

Garner, D. M., Garfinkel, P. E., Schwartz, D. & Thompson, M. (1980). Cultural expectations of thinness in women. *Psychological Reports,* **47**:483–491.

Gerner, R. H. & Gwirstman, H. E. (1981). Abnormalities of dexamethasone suppression test and urinary MHPG in anorexia nervosa. *American Journal of Psychiatry,* **138**:650–653.

Goldblatt, P. B., Moore, M. E. & Stunkard, A. J. (1965). Social factors in obesity. *Journal of the American Medical Association,* **192**:97–102.

Groen, J. J. & Feldman-Toledano, Z. (1966). Educative treatment of patients and parents in anorexia nervosa. *British Journal of Psychiatry,* **112**:671–681.

Gross, H. A., Lake, C. R., Ebert, M. H., Hegler, M. G. & Kopin, I. J. (1979). Catecholamine metabolism in primary anorexia nervosa. *Journal of Clinical Endocrinological Metabolism,* **49**:805–809.

Gull, Sir W. (1874). Anorexia nervosa (apepsia hysterica, anorexia hysterica). *Transactions of the Clinical Society, London,* **7**:22–28.

Halmi, K. A. (1974). Anorexia nervosa: demographic and clinical features in 94 cases. *Psychosomatic Medicine,* **36**:18–26.

Halmi, K. A., Goldberg, S. C., Eckert, E. Casper, R. & Davis, J. M. (1977). Pretreatment evaluation in anorexia nervosa. In *Anorexia Nervosa* (ed. R. A. Vigersky), pp. 43–54. Raven Press: New York.

Halmi, K. A., Dekirmenjian, H., Davis, J. M., Casper, R. & Goldberg, S. C. (1978a). Catecholamine metabolism in anorexia nervosa. *Archives of General Psychiatry,* **35**:458–460.

Halmi, K. A., Struss, A. & Goldberg, S. C. (1978b). An investigation of weights in parents of anorexia nervosa patients. *Journal of Nervous and Mental Disease,* **166**:358–361.

Hsu, L. K. G. (1980). Outcome of anorexia nervosa. *Archives of General Psychiatry,* **37**:1041–1046.

Hsu, L. K. G., Crisp, A. H. & Harding, B. (1979). Outcome of anorexia nervosa. *Lancet,* i, 61–65.

Huenemann, R. L., Shapiro, L. R., Hampton, M. C. & Mitchell, B. W. (1966). A longitudinal study of gross body composition and body conformation and their association with food and activity in a teenage population. *American Journal of Clinical Nutrition,* **18**:324–338.

Jones, D. J., Fox, M. M., Babigian, H. M. & Hutton, H. E. (1980). Epidemiology of anorexia nervosa in Monroe County, New York: 1960–1976. *Psychosomatic Medicine,* **42**:551–558.

Kalucy, R., Crisp, A. H. & Harding, B. (1977). A study of 56 families with anorexia nervosa. *British Journal of Medical Psychology,* **50**:381–395.

Kapen, S., Sternthal, E. & Braverman, L. (1981). A 'pubertal' 24-hour luteinizing hormone secretory pattern following weight loss in the absence of anorexia nervosa. *Psychosomatic Medicine,* **43**:177–182.

Katz, J. L., Boyar, R., Roffwarg, H., Hellman, L. & Weiner, H. (1978). Weight and circadian luteinizing hormone secretory pattern in anorexia nervosa. *Psychosomatic Medicine,* **40**:549–567.

Kay, D. W. K. & Leigh, D. (1954). The natural history, treatment and prognosis of anorexia nervosa, based on a study of 38 patients. *Journal of Mental Science,* **100**:411–431.

Kendell, R. E. (1975). *The Role of Diagnosis in Psychiatry.* Blackwell: Oxford.

Kendell, R. E., Hall, D. J., Hailey, A. & Babigian, H. M. (1973). The epidemiology of anorexia nervosa. *Psychological Medicine,* **3**:200–203.

King, A. (1963). Primary and secondary anorexia nervosa. *British Journal of Psychiatry,* **109**:470–479.

Knuth, V. A., Hull, M. G. R. & Jacobs, H. S. (1977). Amenorrhoea and loss of weight. *British Journal of Obstetrics and Gynaecology,* **84**:801–807.

Kupfer, D. J., Thompson, K. S. & Weiss, B. (1976). EEG sleep changes as predictors in depression. *American Journal of Psychiatry,* **133**:622–626.

Lasèque, C. (1873). On hysterical anorexia. *Medical Times Gazette,* **2**:265–367.

Mawson, A. R. (1974). Anorexia nervosa and the regulation of intake: a review. *Psychological Medicine,* **4**:289–308.

McHugh, P. R. & Moran, T. H. (1977). An examination of the concept of satiety in hypothalamic hyperphagia. In *Anorexia Nervosa* (ed. R. A. Vigersky), pp. 67–74. Raven Press: New York.

Mills, I. H. (1976). Amitriptyline therapy in anorexia nervosa. *Lancet,* ii, 687.

Minuchin, S. (1974). *Families and Family Therapy.* Harvard University Press: Cambridge, Mass.

Todd, T. (1975). A conceptual model of psychosomatic illness in children. *Archives of General Psychiatry,* **32**:1031–1038.

Minuchin, S., Rosman, B. L. & Baker, L. (1978). *Psychosomatic Families: Anorexia Nervosa in Context.* Harvard University Press: Cambridge, Mass.

Miyai, K., Yamamoto, T., Azukizawa, M., Ishibashi, K. & Kumahara, Y. (1975). Serum thyroid hormones and thyrotropin in anorexia nervosa. *Journal of Clinical Endocrinology and Metabolism,* **40**:334–338.

Morgan, H. G. & Russell, G. F. M. (1975). Value of family background and clinical features as predictors of long-term outcome in anorexia nervosa: four-year follow-up study of 41 patients. *Psychological Medicine,* **5**:355–371.

Morrison, S. D. (1977). Extrahypothalamic controls of feeding. In *Anorexia Nervosa* (ed. R. A. Vigersky), pp. 75–80. Raven Press: New York.

Needleman, H. L. & Waber, D. (1977). The use of amitriptyline in anorexia nervosa. In *Anorexia Nervosa* (ed. R. A. Vigersky), pp. 357–362. Raven Press: New York.

Neil, J. F., Merikangas, J. R., Foster, F. G., Merikangas, K. R., Spiker, D. G. & Kupfer, D. J. (1980). Waking and all night EEG in anorexia nervosa. *Clinical Electroencephalography,* **11**:9–15.

Nemiah, J. C. (1950). Anorexia nervosa. *Medicine,* **29**:225–268.

Nylander, I. (1971). The feeling of being fat and dieting in a school population. *Acta Sociomedica Scandinavica,* **3**:17–26.

Palazzoli, M. S. (1974). *Self-Starvation.* Jason Aronson: New York.

Palazzoli, M. S., Boscolo, L., Cecchin, G. F. & Prata, G. (1977). Family rituals: a powerful tool in family therapy. *Family Process,* **16**:445–453.

Rampling, D. (1980). Abnormal mothering in the genesis of anorexia nervosa. *Journal of Nervous and Mental Disease,* **168**:501–504.

Redmond, D. E., Snyder, D. R. & Maas, J. W. (1977). Norepinephrine and satiety in monkeys. In *Anorexia Nervosa* (ed. R. A. Vigersky), pp. 81–96. Raven Press: New York.

Russell, G. F. M. (1965). Metabolic aspects of anorexia nervosa. *Proceedings of the Royal Society of Medicine,* **58**:811–814.

Russell, G. F. M. (1970). Anorexia nervosa—its identity as an illness and its treatment. In *Modern Trends in Psychological Medicine,* Vol. 2 (ed. J. H. Price), pp. 131–164. Butterworth: London.

Russell, G. F. M. (1977*a*). The present status of anorexia nervosa. *Psychological Medicine,* **7**:353–367.

Russell, G. F. M. (1977*b*). General management of anorexia nervosa and difficulties in assessing the efficiency of treatment. In *Anorexia Nervosa* (ed. R. A. Vigersky), pp. 277–290. Raven Press: New York.

Sachar, E. J., Hellman, L., Fukushima, D. K. & Gallagher, T. F. (1970). Cortisol production in depressive illness. *Archives of General Psychiatry,* **23**:289–298.

Salkind, M. R., Fincham, J. & Silverstone, T. (1980). Is anorexia nervosa a phobic disorder? *Biological Psychiatry,* **15**:803–808.

Schildkraut, J. J., Keeler, B. A. & Papousek, M. (1973). MHPG excretion in depressive disorders. *Science,* **181**:762–764.

Sours, J. A. (1974). The anorexia nervosa syndrome. *International Journal of Psychoanalysis,* **55**:567–576.

Sours, J. A. (1981). Depression and the anorexia nervosa syndrome. *Pediatric Clinics of North America,* **4**:145–158.

Stricker, E. (1978). Hyperphagia. *New England Journal of Medicine,* **298**:1010–1012.

Theander, S. (1970). Anorexia nervosa: a psychiatric investigation of 94 female patients. *Acta Psychiatrica Scandinavica,* Supplement 214.

Vigersky, R. A., Anderson, A. E., Thompson, R. H. & Loriaux, L. (1977). Hypothalamic dysfunction in secondary amenorrhea associated with simple weight loss. *New England Journal of Medicine,* **297**:1141–1145.

Wakeling, A., DeSouza, V. A. & Beardwood, C. J. (1977). Assessment of negative and positive feedback effects of administered oestrogen on gonadrotrophin release in patients with anorexia nervosa. *Psychological Medicine,* **7**:397–405.

Walsh, B. T. (1982). Endocrine disturbances in anorexia nervosa and depression. *Psychosomatic Medicine,* **44**:85–91.

Walsh, B. T., Katz, J. L., Levin, J., Kream, J., Fukushima, D. K., Weiner, H. & Zumoff, B. (1981). The production rate of cortisol declines during recovery from anorexia nervosa. *Journal of Clinical Endocrinology and Metabolism,* **53**:203–205.

PART VII: EATING DISORDERS

27

Follow-up Studies of Anorexia Nervosa: A Review of Research Findings

H.-C. Steinhausen and K. Glanville

Free University of Berlin

There has been a recent spate of studies on the course of anorexia nervosa which call for collation, review and analysis. The practical value of such a synopsis is related to the fact that only by means of longitudinal investigations can the efficiency of treatment be judged. As long as the aetiology of the illness remains incompletely understood therapeutic measures must be symptomatic, and the outcome of the disease may reflect its natural history as well as therapeutic intervention. This survey represents the fruits of a systematic analysis of the available literature. It presents, first, the general aspects of follow-up studies, then their results, followed by factors influencing prognosis, and some implications for further research.

GENERAL DESCRIPTION

The follow-up reports analyzed here are drawn from 45 studies in the English and German languages, published between 1953 and 1981. Their general characteristics are summarized in Table 1. In the main, the work has been concerned with two themes: the effectiveness of different methods of treatment, and the identification of prognostic factors. The number of patients examined varies between 6 and 140. Studies

Reprinted with permission from *Psychological Medicine*, 1983, Vol. 13, 239–249. Copyright 1983 by Cambridge University Press.

Table 1. *Sample characteristics of follow-up studies of anorexia nervosa*

Study	Patients at follow-up (no.)	Drop-out rate (%)	Duration of follow-up (years) I	II	III	IV	Age at onset of the disease (years)	Diagnostic criteria	Therapeutic measures
1. Kay (1953)	33	13·1	5–> 10	—	—	—	16–20	AN, AM, WL	PT, MT
2. Beck & Brøchner-Mortensen (1954)	25	10·7	—	—	1–23	—	11–31	AN, AM, WL	MT
3. Williams (1958)	42	14·3	3–21	—	—	—	13–40*	n.a.	MT
4. Lesser et al. (1960)	15	0	—	1–17	—	—	10–16	n.e.d.	MT
5. Thomä (1961)	18	40·0	—	—	0·6–7	—	13–25	AN, AM, VO	PT
6. Blitzer et al. (1961)	15	n.a.	n.a.	—	—	—	7–14	WL	PT, MT
7. Meyer (1961)	20	n.a.	—	—	10–17	—	n.e.d.	n.a.	n.e.d.
8. Tolstrup (1965)	28	0	—	—	0·5–12	—	7–24	n.a.	PT, MT
9. Frahm (1965)	30	8·8	—	—	3	—	15–18	n.a.	MT
10. Frazier (1965)	39	n.a.	—	—	5–20	—	9–35	WL, HY, NMI Distorted body image	PT, MT
11. Kay & Shapira (1965)	60	7·7	—	—	3–10	—	20–22	n.a.	MT
12. Crisp (1965, 1966)	21	n.a.	—	—	0·1–3·6	—	n.a.	n.a.	PT, MT
13. Farquharson & Hyland (1966)	15	6·2	—	—	20–30	—	13–23	n.a.	PT, MT
14. Dally & Sargant (1966)	57	n.a.	—	—	—	3–5	17–19	AN, AM, WL, NMI, NPD	MT
15. Warren (1968)	18	0	2·6–11	—	—	—	10–15	n.a.	PT, MT
16. Seidensticker & Tzagournis (1968)	53	11·7	—	—	—	1–> 10	10–59	AN, WL, NMI, NPD	PT, MT
17. Browning & Miller (1968)	36	n.a.	2–32	—	—	—	n.a.	AN, WL, NMI, NPD	PT, MT
18. Ziegler & Sours (1968)	26	77·4	—	—	1–34	—	10–15	AN, WL, NMI	n.a.
19. Dally (1969)	140	0	—	—	—	< 17	11–33	AN, AM, WL	MT
20. Theander (1970)	94	2·1	—	—	—	6	11–34	Disturbed eating attitude and body image	PT, MT
21. Valanne et al. (1972)	30	0	—	—	1–15	—	11–16	AN, AM, NMI, NPD	PT, MT
22. Halmi et al. (1973)	36	14·3	1–30	—	—	—	< 15 (N = 13) > 15 (N = 23)	Feighner et al. criteria	n.a.
23. Bruch (1973)	38	13·3	1–19	—	—	—	20–26	Distorted body image	PT, MT
24. Bhanji & Thompson (1974)	7	63·6	—	—	—	0·2–6	14–34*	n.a.	BT, MT
25. Niskanen et al. (1974)	48	n.a.	—	—	1–18	—	13–32	AN, WL, NMI, NPD	PT, MT
26. Silverman (1974)	27	6·9	—	—	—	6	9–15	n.a.	PT, MT
27. Morgan & Russell (1975)	41	0	—	—	> 4	—	11–40	AN, AM, WL, HY, LA	PT
28. Brady & Rieger (1975)	15	6·2	—	—	0·4–4	—	15–34*	AM, WL	BT
29. Pierloot et al. (1975)	32	0	—	—	—	1–6	12–25†	AN, AM, WL, NMI, NPD	PT, BT, MT
30. Niederhoff et al. (1975)	6	0	—	—	—	1–4	11–15	n.a.	MT
31. Beumont et al. (1976)	31	n.a.	—	—	—	0·3–2	Mean = 17	AN, WL, NMI, NPD	n.a.
32. Halmi et al. (1976)	79	16·8	1–50	—	—	—	< 25 (N = 69)	Feighner et al. criteria	n.a.
33. Willi & Hagemann (1976)	20	0	—	Mean = 11	—	—	Mean = 19·5	AN, AM, WL (VO, HY, LA, BU)	PT, MT
34. Rosman et al. (1976)	53	0	—	—	—	0·3–4	9–21	AN, distorted body image	FT
35. Goetz et al. (1977)	30	0	—	5–20	—	—	9–16*	WL, distorted body image, NMI	PT
36. Sturzenberger et al. (1977), Cantwell et al. (1977)	26	21·2	—	—	—	Mean = 4·9	11–16	Feighner et al. criteria	In-patient treatment
37. Stonehill & Crisp (1977)	38	13·3	—	—	—	4–7	Mean = 20*	n.a.	PT, MT

Table 1. (cont.)

Study	Sample size Patients at follow-up (no.)	Drop-out rate (%)	Duration of follow-up (years) I	II	III	IV	Age at onset of the disease (years)	Diagnostic criteria	Therapeutic measures
38. Garfinkel et al. (1977)	42	n.a.	Mean = 5	—	—	—	11–20	Feighner et al. criteria	PT, (FT, BT) MT
39. Pertschuk (1977)	27	6·9	—	—	—	0·3–3·9	14–34*	Feighner et al. criteria	BT, MT
40. Cremerius (1978)	11	15·4	—	—	—	26–29	Puberty	n.a.	PT, MT
41. Ziolko (1978)	28	0	—	—	—	5–20	14–18	n.a.	PT, MT
42. Petzold (1979)	44	4·5	—	—	—	Mean = 2·7	13–29	n.e.d.	PT (FT), MT
43. Hsu et al. (1979)	100	2·8	—	—	1–18	—	13–32	n.e.d.	PT, MT
44. Schütze (1980)	49	22·3	—	—	—	0·3–8·6	Puberty	n.a.	PT, MT
45. Rollins & Piazza (1981)	35	50·0	—	—	> 2	—	Mean = 13·7	WL, weight phobia, distorted body image	n.a.

I, related to onset of the disease; II, related to onset of therapy; III, related to termination of therapy; IV, starting point not described; * at hospital admission; † at termination.

AN = anorexia; AM = amenorrhoea; WL = weight loss; VO = vomiting; HY = hyperactivity; LA = laxative abuse; BU = bulimia; NMI = no known medical illness; NPD = no other known psychiatric disorder.

BT = behaviour therapy; FT = family therapy; MT = medical treatment; PT = psychotherapy; n.a. = not assessed; n.e.d. = not exactly described.

with the smallest number of patients (Niederhoff et al. 1975; Bhanji & Thompson, 1974) deal with tests of the effectiveness of systematically applied forms of treatment—purely medical treatment and behavior therapy. Theander (1970) and Dally (1969) studied 94 and 140 patients respectively; these larger numbers reflect the longer follow-up periods of the two investigations.

In order to gather evidence on the course of anorexia nervosa Morgan & Russell (1975) make a plea for a follow-up of at least 4 years. They assume that anorexia nervosa has a rather long duration, so that improvement and recovery may take several years. An examination of the available studies revealed some findings which meet this contention and others which were obtained too near the termination of treatment to represent stable follow-up data (e.g. Tolstrup, 1965; Crisp, 1965, 1966; Bhanji & Thompson, 1974; Brady & Rieger, 1975). Longer follow-up periods were attained in the studies of Farquharson & Hyland (1966), Theander (1970), Cremerius (1978) and Ziolko (1978).

Most of the data on the age of onset relate to the type of anorexia nervosa which begins in young adults, but a number of authors (Lesser et al. 1960; Blitzer et al. 1961; Tolstrup, 1965; Warren, 1968) have also examined patients whose illnesses began before puberty. Some workers have regarded the age of onset as a diagnostic criterion (e.g. Thomä, 1961; Dally & Sargant, 1966; Ziegler & Sours, 1968; Brady & Rieger, 1975; Feighner et al. 1972), and it may be questioned whether patients whose symptoms appear first at the age of 40 (Morgan & Russell, 1975) or even 59 (Seidensticker & Tzagournis, 1968) qualify as genuine cases of anorexia nervosa.

As can be seen from Table 1, the diagnostic criteria which are employed in many studies are often incomplete or inadequately described. This hinders comparison between findings, since it is possible that different types of patient were included. Further, the variations in approach and diagnostic criteria of those studies with more comprehensive information render comparative assessment difficult. It would clearly be desirable to adopt diagnostic criteria which are relevant to anorexia as a syndrome and also find general acceptance in clinical practice. Despite much criticism (Andersen, 1977; Fries, 1977; Rollins & Piazza, 1978), these desiderata appear to be best fulfilled by the criteria of Feighner *et al.* (1972).

Treatment regimes of internal medicine and of psychotherapy are included in the follow-up studies under survey. The two types of procedure are mostly used in combination, seldom individually. With only a few exceptions (Dally & Sargant, 1966; Rosman *et al.* 1976; Garfinkel *et al.* 1977; Petzold, 1979), the studies on the effectiveness of certain forms of treatment employed smaller patient-samples than those which concentrated on prognostic factors. This difference may have something to do with a lack of sufficient subjects on whom a particular therapeutic procedure could be systematically carried out. The psychotherapeutic procedures of behavior therapy and family therapy have been applied with increasing frequency in recent years.

The extent to which treatment programs exert a long-term positive influence on the course of anorexia nervos is assessed differently by various workers. On the basis of their follow-up results, several authors support the view that there is neither a specifically effective form of treatment for anorexia nervosa, nor any qualitative differences between therapeutic regimes (Kay, 1953; Frazier, 1965; Browning — Miller, 1968; Theander, 1970; Morgan & Russell, 1975; Bhanji & Thompson, 1974; Garfinkel *et al.* 1977; Cremerius, 1978). Others, however, have attempted to prove the effectiveness of their methods of treatment by reference to their follow-up results (e.g. Frahm, 1965; Dally & Sargant, 1966; Rosman *et al.* 1976; Niederhoff *et al.* 1975; Petzold, 1979). Most of the findings presented in these studies should be viewed critically. Either they involved too few subjects; or the follow-up periods were too short; or the evaluation of response was based on too small a number of criteria.

FOLLOW-UP RESULTS

Because of the difficulty of collecting objective information from samples of anorexic subjects, most workers appear to have limited themselves to the collection of more subjective data, basing their investigations on material obtained from former patients, supplemented in part by relatives and doctors, without employing standardized questionnaires or interviews by an independent observer. Such a method of investigation must considerably distort follow-up results and lessen their value unless the patients' veracity can be established. Very few authors used standardized tests in their follow-up investigations (e.g. Seidensticker & Tzagournis, 1968; Browning & Miller, 1968; Theander, 1970; Stonehill & Crisp, 1977; Sturzenberger *et al.* 1977). The principal results are summarized in Table 2.

With regard to *weight restoral*, there was insufficient information in many of the papers, partly because relatively few of the authors appear to have included weight as a factor to be studied (e.g. Blitzer *et al.* 1961; Halmi *et al.* 1976). In some investigations the weight as a factor to be studied (e.g. Blitzer *et al.* 1961; Halmi *et al.* 1976). In some investigations the weight of former patients is recorded, but conclusions concerning subsequent weight-levels are limited by ambiguity (Tolstrup, 1965; Farquharson & Hyland, 1966), an absence of exact data (Rosman *et al.* 1976) or a restriction of measurement to the average weight gain (Ziolko, 1978; Petzold, 1979). A large majority of the studies establish a weight restoral of between 50 and 70%, and some present increases of between 70 and 80%. Such good results are often observed in patients whose illnesses began at an early age (Sturzenberger *et al.* 1977; Rosman *et al.* 1976; Warren, 1968). The lowest figure of 15% is reported in the study by Willi & Hagemann (1976), who recorded weight restoral in only 3 of their 20 subjects, while 10 of them were described as "stably but slightly underweight." The mean weight of patients examined after treatment was 21% below average.

Goetz *et al.* (1977) reported the highest figure: at the time of their follow-up 26 patients of their total of 30 (87%) had a normal body weight, though this was not precisely defined. In relation to other assessments this statistic takes on a different significance. In terms of psychosocial adjustment, for example, 60% of the patients did well. Weight restoral alone cannot therefore be taken as sufficient evidence of recovery from anorexia nervosa. Only after a number of factors have been assessed can an assessment of the course of anorexia nervosa be properly formulated.

Amenorrhoea is widely held to be an essential diagnostic criterion in

Table 2. *Results of follow-up-studies of anorexia nervosa*

Study	Normalization of			Psychiatric status (%)	Psychosocial adaptation (%)	Chronicity (%)	Mortality rate (%)	Improvement rate (%)
	Weight (%)	Menstruation (%)	Eating behaviour (%)					
1. Kay (1953)	~50	55	35	DS = 6 NS = 40 OS = 6	Family = 9 Occupation = 3	21	18	r = 12 i = 48
2. Beck & Brøchner-Mortensen (1954)	64	68	68	n.a.	Marriage = 60 Children = 52	16	4	'Excellent health' = 80
3. Williams (1958)	55	n.a.	n.a.	n.a.	Marriage = 28 Children = 14 Occupation = 55	7	19	r = 55 i = 14
4. Lesser et al. (1960)	60	n.a.	n.a.	HP = 53 OP = 27 SP = 20	Good/fair = 87	13	0	Good/fair = 87
5. Thomä (1961)	36	73	41	n.a.	Marriage = 5 Children = 9 Occupation = 45	13	3	r/i = 33
6. Blitzer et al. (1961)	n.a.	n.a.	60	DP = 87	Improvement in general personality = 60	0	7	r = 60 i = 33
7. Meyer (1961)	n.e.d.	90	35	HP = 15 OP = 75 SC = 15	n.a.	35	15	i = 35
8. Tolstrup (1965)	n.a.	n.a.	n.a.	n.a.	Marriage = 18	14	0	Good = 22 Fair = 63
9. Frahm (1965)	n.e.d.	67	97	n.a.	100	0	0	~100
10. Frazier (1965)	n.a.	n.a.	28	SC = 28	Occupational/social relationships = 28	31	8	Markedly i = 28 Slightly i = 33
11. Kay & Shapira (1965)	~50	~40	~40	DS/OS = 27 NS = 34 SC = 3	Marriage = 34	27	17	Markedly i = 34 Partly i = 34
12. Crisp (1965, 1966)	71	44	52	DS = 4	Marriage = 28 Sexuality = 9	n.e.d.	9	43
13. Farquharson & Hyland (1966)	n.e.d.	83	87	NS = 20 SC = 7	67	7	0	r = 67
14. Dally & Sargant (1966)	60–72	69–72	55–67	DS = 3 OS = 3 SC = 3 Psychopathy = 6 Phobias = 3–7	Marriage = 33–41 Occupation = 6–15 Good = 60–72	~3–6	n.a.	60–72
15. Warren (1968)	55	55	61	DS = 5 NS = 39 SC = 5	Marriage = 5 Sexuality = 28	28	11	61
16. Seidensticker & Tzagournis (1968)	63	69	n.e.d.	n.a.	'Active and productive life' = 38	31	13	Fair = 38 Partly fair = 30
17. Browning & Miller (1968)	75	~50	50	n.a.	n.a.	16	8	i = 50 Moderately i = 25
18. Ziegler & Sours (1968)	n.e.d.	n.e.d.	n.e.d.	n.a.	Marriage = 46	11	5	n.e.d.
19. Dally (1969)	69	59	n.e.d.	DS = 24 OS = 11 SC = 1 Phobias = 10 Hypochondriasis = 23	Marriage = 31 Occupation = 25	29	3	69
20. Theander (1970)	63	76	63	DS = 29 OS = 13 SC = 1 Anxiety = 13	Marriage = 50	7	10	i = 63
21. Valanne et al. (1972)	n.e.d.	n.e.d.	47	NS = 27 PS = 13	Marriage = 13 Children = 7 Occupation = 90 Independence from the family = 23	17	0	Free of symptoms = 10
22. Halmi et al. (1973)	41	55	n.e.d.	DS = 27 NS = 61	Marriage = 34 Occupation = 36 Sexuality = 32	14	16	r = 25 i = 23 Moderately i = 23

Table 2. (*cont.*)

Study	Normalization of Weight (%)	Men- struation (%)	Eating behav- iour (%)	Psychiatric status (%)	Psychosocial adaptation (%)	Chron- icity (%)	Mortality rate (%)	Improvement rate (%)
23. Bruch (1973)	61	n.a.	~ 33	SC = 10	33	13	8	r = 33
24. Bhanji & Thompson (1974)	43	28	57	n.a.	n.a.	43	0	Good = 14 Fair = 43
25. Niskanen *et al.* (1974)	n.e.d.	n.a.	n.e.d.	BS = 2 NS = 57	Marriage = 12 Children = 10 Occupation = 48	n.a.	8	42
26. Silverman (1974)	n.e.d.	n.e.d.	n.e.d.	SC = 15	n.a.	18	0	'Well functioning' = 33
27. Morgan & Russell (1975)	68	50	33	DS = 45 OS = 23	Occupation = 73 Sexuality = 60	29	5[a]	Good = 39 Fair = 27
28. Brady & Rieger (1975)	77	36	n.a.	n.a.	Family/ occupation/ social relation- ships: good = 38	23	7	Good = 38 i = 38
29. Pierloot *et al.* (1975)	50	50	50	n.e.d.	Good social functioning = 50	34	0	r = 50 i = 16
30. Niederhoff *et al.* (1975)	66	66	66	SP and OS = 50	Normalization of life = 83	16	0	Good = 66 Fair = 16
31. Beumont *et al.* (1976)	41[b] 21[c]	n.a. n.a.	41[b] 21[c]	HP[b] = 6, OP[b] = 76 HP[c] = 50, OP[c] = 57	n.a. n.a.	29[b] 79[c]	0 0	41[b] 21[c]
32. Halmi *et al.* (1976)	n.a.	n.a.	n.a.	ED = 2 SC = 1 HP = 4	n.a.	11	21	r = 51
33. Willi & Hagemann (1976)	15	63	31	ED = 5 DS = 50 SC = 5	Marriage = 60	25	5	r = 35 i = 35
34. Rosman *et al.* (1976)	n.a.	n.a.	n.a.	n.a.	Family/school/ occupation: Good = 88	6	0	r = 86 i = 8
35. Goetz *et al.* (1977)	87	92	n.e.d.	HP = 47 OP = 40 SC = 13	Good = 60	17	0	Good = 60 Fair = 23
36. Sturzenberger *et al.* (1977), Cantwell *et al.* (1977)	77[d] 83[e]	70[d] 83[e]	81[d] 83[e]	DS = 67[d], 56[e] OS = 19[d], 44[e] Phobias = 7[d], 6[e]	Occupation/ social relation- ships/sexuality: good = 46[d], 67[e]	n.e.d.	0	Good = 67
37. Stonehill & Crisp (1977)	68	68	n.a.	n.a.	Good/fair = 71	7	n.e.d.	68
38. Garfinkel *et al.* (1977)	58	49	29	n.a.	Good = 7 Fair = 41 Occupation = 49	n.a.	2	i = 50
39. Pertschuk (1977)	67	37	n.e.d.	DS = 7	Family/ occupation/ social relation- ships: Good = 44	22	0	r = 7
40. Cremerius (1978)	n.e.d.	n.e.d.	n.e.d.	NS = 9 PS = 36	Occupation = 45 Sexuality = 18	36	18	45
41. Ziolko (1978)	n.e.d.	96	~ 50	DS = 25 PS = 3	Marriage = 35 Occupation = 89	25	3	r = 60 i = 28
42. Petzold (1979)	n.e.d.	25	54	n.a.	School/ occupation/ social relation- ships = 61	16	11	r = 27 i = 45
43. Hsu *et al.* (1979)	64	54	37	OS = 22	Marriage = 29 Children = 14 Sexuality = 83 Occupation = 82	20	2	Good = 48
44. Schütze (1980)	57	57	57	n.a.	57	21·5	0	i = 57
45. Rollins & Piazza (1981)	65	64	n.e.d.	n.e.d.	79	14	0	r/i = 69

BS = borderline symptoms; DS = depressive symptoms; NS = neurotic symptoms; OS = obsessive–compulsive symptoms; ED = endogenous depression; PS = psychosis; SC = schizophrenia; DP = depressive personality; HP = hysterical personality; OP = obsessional
personality; SP = schizoid personality.   r = recovered; i = improved; n.a. = not assessed; n.e.d. = not exactly described.
[a] Including *N* = 2 patients with death due to other causes.
[b] Patients with weight loss due to diet, food refusal, and exercising.
[c] Patients with weight loss due to habitual vomiting and abuse of purgatives.
[d] Information obtained by the parents.   [e] Information obtained by the patient.

female patients from puberty onwards. A *normalization of menstrual function* is therefore seen as an index of recovery or improvement. As with weight restoral, most studies report rates of normalization between 50 and 70%; an early onset of the disease was associated with better rates of improvement. This suggests that the criteria of change are inter-related, since a return of menstruation is usually dependent on a satisfactory weight-level (Dally, 1969). Higher rates of normalization are reported by Meyer (1961), Farquharson & Hyland (1966), Goetz *et al.* (1977) and Ziolko (1978). Bhanji & Thompson (1974), Beumont *et al.* (1976) and Petzold (1979) all present lower figures. Inspection of the studies reveals further that the higher rates are associated with longer follow-up periods, and the lower percentages with shorter periods. This correlation can be interpreted as suggesting that longer periods of observation increase the probability of a normalization of menstrual functioning.

The assessment of the *normalization of eating disorders* is particularly difficult when based on information derived from former patients, to whom food is a topic charged with emotion. This may partly explain the wide fluctuation of between 30 and 70% in published studies.

The best results (97% of normalization) were achieved by Frahm (1965), who employed purely medical treatment. It is not, however, possible to judge whether this figure would have remained at this level after a follow-up period longer than 3 years. The poorest result (21%) is reported by Beumont *et al.* (1976), who studied a group of patients among whom purgative abuse and vomiting were especially prominent symptoms. Long-term improvements of 20–50% emerge from most follow-up reports, but it was not possible to deduce the extent to which a return to normal eating patterns exerted a positive effect on weight and menstruation. The findings suggest a tendency towards no more than a limited interaction. Willi & Hagemann (1976), for example, report that while 31% of their patients showed normal eating patterns and 63% achieved regular menstruation, only 15% demonstrated weight restoral.

The varying forms of *psychiatric diagnosis* associated with anorexia nervosa make it difficult to draw general conclusions. Depression and obsessive-compulsive states or personality structure assume a prominent place in many studies. The frequency of depressive symptoms or personality traits fluctuates between 3 and 87%, with an average of 31%. The highest estimate of 87% comes from Blitzer *et al.* (1961), though the patients in this study were very young. In most studies depressive symptoms were recorded with moderate frequency (e.g. Halmi *et al.* 1973; Morgan & Russell, 1975; Willi & Hagemann, 1976; Sturzenberger *et al.* 1977) or rarely (Kay, 1953; Crisp, 1965; 1966; Dally & Sargant, 1966; Warrne, 1968; and Pertschuk, 1977). Similar differences, ranging from 3% to 83%, are reported for the frequency of obsessive-compulsive symptoms and personality traits associated with anorexia nervosa. Sturzenberger *et al.* (1977), Cantwell *et al.* (1977), Beumont *et al.* (1976) and Meyer (1961) all furnish high estimates, while the lowest come again from Dally & Sargant (1966) and Kay (1953).

The development of a psychotic disorder in cases of anorexia nervosa is recorded by most authors as occurring in fewer than 10% of cases, though some studies provide a higher estimate (Meyer, 1961; Frazier, 1965; Silverman, 1974; Goetz *et al.* 1977; Cremerius, 1978). The older notion that anorexia nervosa was in some instances a form of schizophrenic disorder has been largely abandoned. On the basis of knowledge, the emergence of a psychotic state appears to be a separate condition which develops independently, and the possibility of mis-diagnosis cannot be excluded in some cases.

The effects of anorexia nervosa extend to the patient's social environment. The *relationship to the social environment* therefore becomes another factor in the assessment of recovery, though again it is difficult to obtain relevant data on the subject's behavior in school, at work, in the family, in marriage, on their attitudes to sexuality and on their social contacts. Although it is relatively easy to assess scholastic, occupational and mental performance it is more difficult to evaluate the quality of social contacts, especially when the criteria are ill defined. Some of the information must therefore be treated with reservation. Furthermore, the varied forms in which the information is presented compounds the difficulty of integrating the studies with the aim of reaching general conclusions. In studies which grade their findings "good-fair-poor," the most common estimate of recovery is 50–80%, with younger patients exhibiting the better rates of improvement (Sturzenberger *et al.* 1977; Rosman *et al.* 1976). If other studies are included, however, then the figure of 50–80% appears to be too high.

According to Dally & Sargant (1966), patients can be said to have reached a condition of *chronicity* if they continue to display symptoms after 5 years despite suitable treatment. The rates of cases becoming chronic were less than 20% in the studies reviewed, and some workers report no chronicity (Blitzer *et al.* 1961; Frahm, 1965). These latter findings, however, are probably atypical: Blitzer *et al.*, for example, included samples of very young patients; and Frahm's follow-up period of 3 years was too short. The highest figure for chronicity (79%) is provided by Beumont *et al.* whose patients achieved weight reduction by means of vomiting and purgative abuse. The rate of less than 20% chronicity cited by the majority of studies differs from the much-quoted observation that anorexia nervosa is a chronic disease in one third of cases (Meyer, 1961; Willi & Hagemann, 1976; Cremerius, 1978).

The mortality rate for anorexia nervosa has been calculated as 7–15% (Sours, 1969). Among the studies under review there was a range of 0–21%, the highest figure coming from Halmi *et al.* (1976). The two largest sub-groups were those reporting no mortality, followed closely by those with a mortality rate of less than 10%.

Estimates of the *rate of improvement* are dependent on the criteria adopted. Some workers emphasize psychological adjustment, without reference to specifically anorexic symptoms (e.g. Lesser *et al.* 1960); others prefer the presence or absence of clinical symptoms (e.g. Thomä, 1961); all too often, no information is provided on the criteria employed (Blitzer *et al.* 1961). Some workers also demand undisturbed social behavior or the full restitution of mental health (e.g. Tolstrup, 1965).

In view of such diverse criteria, it is not surprising that the published rates of improvement vary between 10 and 86%, the majority falling between 30 and 50%. The assumption of a one third improvement, however, appears to represent an underestimate, just as the assumption of a one third chronicity rate is excessive. High rates of improvement are reported by Frahm (1965), Lesser *et al.* (1960), who relied largely on medical treatment, and Rosman *et al.* (1976) for whom family therapy was the mainstay.

PROGNOSTIC FACTORS

One of the chief aims of carrying out follow-up studies in the study of anorexia nervosa lies in the identification of possible prognostic factors, favorable or unfavorable. The more important are listed below.

(a) Age of onset

Most workers associate an early onset with a favorable prognosis (Lesser *et al.* 1960; Frazier, 1965; Theander, 1970; Halmi *et al.* 1973, 1976; Morgan & Russell, 1975; Pierloot *et al.* 1975; Willi & Hagemann, 1976; Sturzenberger *et al.* 1977; Hsu *et al.* 1979). A few authors (Tolstrup, 1965; Warren, 1968; Browning & Miller, 1968; Garfinkel *et al.* 1977), on the other hand, report no prognostic distinction between illnesses of early and late onset. Seidensticker & Tzagournis (1968) regard an onset up to the age of 30 as prognostically favorable, and Dally (1969) even claims that the prognosis of anorexia nervosa commencing before the age of 14 is unfavorable.

(b) Hysterical personality structure
This is seen as progressing with a favorable course by Lesser *et al.* 1960), Blitzer *et al.* (1961), Kay & Shapira (1965), Rollins & Blackwell (1968), Dally (1969), Kalucy *et al.* (1976) and Goetz *et al.* 1977).

(c) Parent-child relationship
Good relations between the patient and his/her parents are said to indicate a good outcome by several workers (Kay & Shapira, 1965; Dally, 1969; Crisp *et al.* 1974; Morgan & Russell, 1975; Hsu *et al.* 1979), but this is questioned by Pierloot *et al.* (1975) and Theander (1970).

(d) Duration of symptoms
A short history prior to hospitalization or a brief episode of illness augurs well according to Kay & Shapira (1965), Dally & Sargant (1966), Seidensticker & Tzagournis (1968), Pierloot *et al.* (1975), Morgan & Russell (1975) and Hsu *et al.* (1979). Browning & Miller (1968), by contrast, regard this factor as insignificant.

(e) Duration of in-patient treatment and number of readmissions
These factors emerge as unconnected with the course of the condition from the work of Browning & Miller (1968), Dally (1969) and Morgan & Russell (1975), but suggest a good prognosis according to other studies (Seidensticker & Tzagournis, 1968; Theander, 1970; Halmi *et al.* 1973, 1976; Garfinkel *et al.* 1977).

(f) Socioeconomic status
Anorexics from the upper social classes fared better in the studies of Seidensticker & Tzagournis (1968), Halmi *et al.* (1973, 1976)l Kalucy *et al.* (1976), Garfinkel *et al.* 1977) and Hsu *et al.* (1979), but carried no prognostic significance in the reports of Dally (1969) and Theander (1970).

(g) Disturbances of body perception
A diminution of these disturbances after weight increase has been reported as suggesting a good outcome by Slade & Russell (1973), Garfinkel *et al.* (1977) and Kalucy *et al.* (1977). Slade & Russell (1973) and

Kalucy *et al.* (1977) report that a good outcome is related to a correction of such perceptual disturbances as a result of weight increase.

(h) Hyperactivity and dieting
    The exclusive use of these methods to reduce weight is regarded as pointing to a favorable outcome by Beumont *et al.* (1976), but as unimportant prognostically by Halmi *et al.* (1973, 1976) and Pierloot *et al.* (1975).

(i) Specifically unfavorable prognostic factors
    These include *vomiting* during the onset and course of anorexia nervosa (Theander, 1970; Halmi *et al.* 1973; Crisp *et al.* 1974; Beumont *et al.* 1976; Garfinkel *et al.* 1977; Hsu *et al.* 1979); *purgative abuse* and *bulimia* during the onset and course of the condition (Theander, 1970; Halmi *et al.* 1973; Beumont *et al.* 1976; Willi & Hagemann, 1976; Kalucy *et al.* 1976; Hsu *et al.* 1979); *extreme loss of weight* (Dally, 1969; Morgan & Russell, 1975; Hsu *et al.* 1979); *depressive* and *obsessive-compulsive symptoms* (Halmi *et al.* 1973); *chronicity*, associated particularly with obsessive-compulsive personality traits (Lesser *et al.* 1960; Kay & Shapira, 1965; Dally, 1969; Bhanji & Thompson, 1974; Kalucy *et al.* 1976; Goetz *et al.* 1977); *older maternal age* (Dally, 1969; Theander, 1970; Halmi *et al.* 1973); *premorbid developmental and clinical abnormal phenomena* (Dally, 1969; Morgan & Russell, 1975); *high rates of physical complaints* (Halmi *et al.* 1973; Stonehill & Crisp, 1977); *acute body perception disturbances* (Garfinkel *et al.* 1977; Kalucy *et al.* 1977); *neuroticism* (Dally, 1969; Pierloot *et al.* 1975); *psychological test-results suggestive of psychosis* Pierloot *et al.* 1975); the *masculine sex* (Kalucy *et al.* 1977); and *marriage* (Seidensticker & Tzagournis, 1968; Kalucy *et al.* 1976; Hsu *et al.* 1979; except for the study of Willi & Hagemann, 1976).

CONCLUSIONS

In toto, research on the course of anorexia nervosa does not constitute a unified whole. In addition to the numerous methodological problems, many of the conclusions are probably drawn from atypical samples. Furthermore, the proportion of dropouts during re-examination, which reaches a maximum figure of 77% with an average of 77%, has not been subjected to a systematic test of trends in respect of individual characteristics. The extent to which certain findings are representative has therefore remained insufficiently analyzed. It could be that the methods used for re-examination exercised a strong influence on the proportion of drop-outs. It is even possible that it is precisely the least reliable examinations—those relying on information obtained from telephone enquiries or from relatives—which actually lead to lower drop-out rates than structured examinations carried out in direct contact with the patient. The inadequate sampling of follow-up data is also indicated by the contradictory assessment of some prognostic factors. In view of the fact that most of these factors are described in relative isolation from one another, it cannot be determined which of them is the more significant.

In the light of these considerations we may formulate the needs of any future research dealing with the course of anorexia nervosa. First, the diagnostic classification of symptoms must be documented unequivocally in order to enable changes to be assessed and studies to be compared with one another. In addition, future studies should not rely on restrictive categories of patient populations.

It is necessary to record not only syndrome-specific variables but also aspects of general psychopathology and psychosocial adjustment, both at the onset as well as during the course of the illness. For these reasons, uni-dimensional follow-up studies which restrict themselves, for example, to the criterion of body weight are relatively useless. Furthermore, the criteria of psychosocial adjustment, if such are to be evaluated, must be operational so that crossvalidation and verification become feasible.

Whether they are retrospective or prospective, follow-up studies must specify not only the proportion of drop-outs but also ascertain whether these subjects differ in any essential respects from other patients and so make it possible to judge to what extent the studies are representative. Since the natural history of anorexia nervosa cannot be assessed in less than 4 years, it is necessary to observe patients for at least this period or to establish that it is possible to achieve an equally reliable forecast within a shorter time.

Follow-up results should be based on a direct re-examination and not on indirect questions to relatives and friends or on telephone calls. At the same time, the reliability of any procedures must be documented or demonstrated. For this purpose use should be made of standardized procedures, i.e. interviews and questionnaires.

A multidimensional strategy of evaluation would facilitate an assessment of the determinants of prognosis. An adequate number of samples must be obtained, and the data should be analyzed by appropriate multivariate techniques. Research into anorexia nervosa which employs these criteria will be in a better position than hitherto to report more accurately on the course of the condition.

REFERENCES

Andersen, A. E. (1977). Atypical anorexia nervosa. In *Anorexia Nervosa* (ed. R. A. Vigersky), pp. 11–19. Raven Press: New York.

Beck, J. C. & Brøchner-Mortensen, K. (1954). Observations on the prognosis in anorexia nervosa. *Acta Medica Scandinavica*, 149:409–430.

Beumont, P. J. V., George, G. C. W. & Smart, D. E. (1976). "Dieters" and "vomiters and purgers" in anorexia nervosa. *Psychological Medicine*, 6:617–622.

Bhanji, S. & Thompson, J. (1974). Operant conditioning in the treatment of anorexia nervosa. *British Journal of Psychiatry*, 124:166–172.

Blitzer, J. R., Rollins, N. & Blackwell, A. (1961). Children who starve themselves: anorexia nervosa. *Psychosomatic Medicine*, 23:369–383.

Brady, J. P. & Rieger, W. (1975). Behavioral treatment of anorexia nervosa. In *Applications of Behavior Modification* (ed. T. Thompson and W. S. Dockens III), pp. 45–63. Academic Press: New York.

Browning, C. H. & Miller, S. I. (1968). Anorexia nervosa: a study in prognosis and management. *American Journal of Psychiatry*, 124:1128–1132.

Bruch, H. (1973). Outcome and outlook. In *Eating Disorders* (ed. H. Bruch), pp. 377–387. Basic Books: New York.

Cantwell, D. P., Sturzenberger, S., Burroughs, J., Salkin, B. & Green, J. (1977). Anorexia nervosa—an affective disorder? *Archives of General Psychiatry*, 34:1087–1093.

Cremerius, J. (1978). Zur Prognose der Anorexia nervosa. *Zeitschrift für psychosomatische Medizin und Psychoanalyse*, 24:56–69.

Crisp, A. H. (1965). Some aspects of the evolution, presentation and follow-up of anorexia nervosa. *Proceedings of the Royal Society of Medicine*, 58:814–820.

Crisp, A. H. (1966). A treatment regime for anorexia nervosa. *British Journal of Psychiatry*, 112:505–512.

Crisp, A. H., Harding, G. & McGuiness, B. (1974). Anorexia nervosa. Psychoneurotic characteristics of parents: relationship to prognosis. *Journal of Psychosomatic Research*, 18:167–173.

Dally, P. J. (1969). *Anorexia Nervosa*. Heinemann Medical Books: London.

Dally, P. J. & Sargant, W. (1966). Treatment and outcome of anorexia nervosa. *British Medical Journal* ii, 793–795.

Farquharson, R. F. & Hyland, H. H. (1966). Anorexia nervosa: the course of 15 patients treated from 20 to 30 years previously. *Canadian Medical Association Journal*, 96:411–419.

Feighner, J., Robins, E., Guze, S., Woodruff, R., Winokur, G. & Munoz, R. (1972). Diagnostic criteria for use in psychiatric research. *Archives of General Psychiatry*, 26:57–63.

Frahm, H. (1965). Ergebnisse einer systematisch durchgeführten somatisch orientierten Behandlungsform bei Kranken mit Anorexia nervosa. In *Anorexia Nervosa* (ed. J. E. Meyer and H. Feldman), pp. 64–70. Thieme: Stuttgart.

Frazier, S. H. (1965). Anorexia nervosa. *Diseases of the Nervous System*, 26:155–159.

Fries, H. (1977). Studies on secondary amenorrhea, anorectic behavior and body-image perception: importance for the early recognition of anorexia nervosa. In *Anorexia Nervosa* (ed. R. A. Vigersky), pp. 163–176. Raven Press: New York.

Garfinkel, P. E., Moldofsky, H. & Garner, D. M. (1977). The outcome of anorexia nervosa: significance of clinical features, body image and behavior modification. In *Anorexia Nervosa* (ed. R. A. Vigersky), pp. 315–329. Raven Press: New York.

Goetz, P. L., Succop, R. A., Reinhart, J. B. & Miller, A. (1977). Anorexia nervosa in children: a follow-up study. *American Journal of Orthopsychiatry*, 47:597–603.

Halmi, K. A., Brodland, G. & Loney, J. (1973). Prognosis in anorexia nervosa. *Annals of Internal Medicine,* **78**:907–909.

Halmi, K. A., Brodland, G. & Rigas, C. (1976). A follow-up study of seventy nine patients with anorexia nervosa: an evaluation of prognostic factors and diagnostic criteria. *Life History Research in Psychopathology,* Vol. 4 (ed. R. Writ, G. Winokur and M. Roff), pp. 290–300. University of Minnesota Press: Minneapolis.

Hsu, L. K. G., Crisp, A. H. & Harding, B. (1979). Outcome of anorexia nervosa. *Lancet* i, 61–65.

Kalucy, R. S., Crisp, A. H., Chard, T., McNeilly, A., Chen, C. N. & Lacey, J. H. (1976). Nocturnal hormonal profiles in massive obesity, anorexia nervosa and normal females. *Journal of Psychosomatic Research,* **20**:595–604.

Kalucy, R. S., Crisp, A. H. & Harding, B. (1977). A study of 56 families with anorexia nervosa. *British Journal of Medical Psychology,* **50**:381–395.

Kay, D. W. (1953). Anorexia nervosa: a study in prognosis. *Proceedings of the Royal Society of Medicine,* **46**:669–674.

Kay, D. W. & Schapira, K. (1965). The prognosis in anorexia nervosa. In *Anorexia Nervosa* (ed. J. E. Meyer and H. Feldman), pp. 113–117. Thieme: Stuttgart.

Lesser, L. I., Ashenden, B. J., Debushey, M. & Eisenberg, L. (1960). Anorexia nervosa in children. *American Journal of Orthopsychiatry,* **30**:572–580.

Meyer, J. E. (1961). Das Syndrom der Anorexia nervosa. Katamnestische Untersuchungen. *Archiv für Psychiatrie und Nervenkrankheiten,* **202**:31–59.

Morgan, H. G. & Russell, G. F. M. (1975). Value of family background and clinical features as predictors of long-term outcome in anorexia nervosa: four-year follow-up study of 41 patients. *Psychological Medicine,* **5**:355–371.

Niederhoff, H., Wiesler, B. & Kuenzer, W. (1975). Somatisch orientierte Behandlung der Anorexia nervosa. *Monatsschrift für Kinderheilkunde,* **123**:343–344.

Niskanen, P., Jääskeläinen, J. & Achté, K. (1974). Anorexia nervosa, treatment results and prognosis. *Psychiatria Fennica,* 57–263.

Pertschuk, M. J. (1977). Behavior therapy: extended follow-up. In *Anorexia Nervosa* (ed. R. A. Vigersky), pp. 305–314. Raven Press: New York.

Petzold, E. (1979). *Familienkonfrontationstherapie bei Anorexia nervosa.* Verlag für medizinische Psychologie Dr C. J. Hogrefe: Göttingen.

Pierloot, R. A., Wellens, W. & Houben, M. E. (1975). Elements of resistance to a combined medical and psychotherapeutic program in anorexia nervosa. *Psychotherapie-Psychosomatik,* **26**:101–117.

Rollins, N. & Blackwell, A. (1968). The treatment of anorexia nervosa in children and adolescents. Stage I. *Journal of Child Psychology and Psychiatry,* **9**:81–91.

Rollins, N. & Piazza, E. (1978). Diagnosis of anorexia nervosa. *Journal of the American Academy of Child Psychiatry,* **17**:126–137.

Rollins, N. & Piazza, E. (1981). Anorexia nervosa. A qualitative approach to follow-up. *Journal of the American Academy of Child Psychiatry,* **20**: 167–183.

Rosman, B. L., Minuchin, S., Liebman, R. & Baker, L. (1976). Input and outcome of family therapy in anorexia nervosa. In *Successful Psychotherapy* (ed. J. L. Claghorn), pp. 128–139. Brunner/Mazel: New York.

Schütze, G. (1980). *Anorexia Nervosa,* pp. 121–131. Huber: Bern.

Seidensticker, J. & Tzagournis, M. (1968). Anorexia nervosa—clinical features and long-term follow-up. *Journal of Chronic Diseases,* **21**:366–367.

Silverman, J. A. (1974). Anorexia nervosa: clinical observations in a successful treatment plan. *Journal of Pediatrics,* **84**:68–73.

Slade, P. D. & Russell, G. F. M. (1973). Awareness of body dimensions in anorexia nervosa: cross-sectional and longitudinal studies. *Psychological Medicine*, **3**:188–199.

Sours, J. A. (1969). Anorexia nervosa: nosology, diagnosis, developmental patterns, and power-control dynamics. In *Adolescence: Psychosocial Perspectives* (ed. G. Caplan and S. Lebovici), pp. 185–212. Basic Books: New York.

Stonehill, E. & Crisp, A. H. (1977). Psychoneurotic characteristics of patients with anorexia nervosa before and after treatment and at follow-up 4–7 years later. *Journal of Psychosomatic Research*, **21**:187–193.

Sturzenberger, S., Cantwell, P. D., Burroughs, J., Salkin, B. & Green, J. K. (1977). A follow-up study of adolescent psychiatric inpatients with anorexia nervosa. *Journal of the American Academy of Child Psychiatry*, **16**:703–715.

Theander, S. (1970). Anorexia nervosa a psychiatric investigation of 94 female patients. *Acta psychiatrica scandinavica* Supp. 214.

Thomä, H. (1961). *Anorexia Nervosa*. Huber: Bern.

Tolstrup, K. (1965). Die Charakteristika der jüngeren Fälle von Anorexia nervosa. In *Anorexia Nervosa* (ed. J. E. Meyer and H. Feldman), pp. 51–59. Thieme: Stuttgart.

Valanne, E. H., Taipale, V., Larkio-Miettinen, A.-K., Morén, R. & Aukee, M. (1972). Anorexia nervosa. A follow-up study. *Psychiatria Fennica*, 65–269.

Warren, W. (1968). A study of anorexia nervosa in young girls. *Journal of Child Psychology and Psychiatry*, **9**:27–40.

Willi, J. & Hagemann, R. (1976). Langzeitverläufe von Anorexia nervosa. *Schweizerische Medizinische Wochenschrift*, **106**:1459–1465.

Williams, E. (1958). Anorexia nervosa: a somatic disorder. *British Medical Journal* ii, 190–195.

Ziegler, R. & Sours, J. (1968). A naturalistic study of patients with anorectic nervosa admitted to an university medical center. *Comprehensive Psychiatry*, **9**:644–651.

Ziolko, H. U. (1978). Zur Katamnese der Pubertätsmagersucht. *Archiv für Psychiatrie und Nervenkrankheitten*, **225**:117–125.

28

An Overview of Anorexia Nervosa, Bulimia, and Obesity in Children and Adolescents

Michael J. Maloney, and William M. Klykylo

University of Cincinnati College of Medicine

The authors present a critical reivew of recent clinical literature on eating disorders in children and adolescents. Anorexia nervosa, bulimia, and obesity appear to be reaching such epidemic proportions that up to 25% of teenagers will demonstrate one of these eating disorders. Long-term follow-up studies of these eating disorders document a fall of mortality rates but no improvement in morbidity rates. The authors critically review techniques of weight stabilization during short-term and long-term treatment, including individual psychodynamic, behavioral, somatic, and family therapies.

ANOREXIA NERVOSA

Epidemiology

The prevalence of anorexia nervosa appears to be increasing. According to Hill (1977), 4% of female teenagers will at some time show enough weight loss to cause amenorrhea. Using strict diagnostic criteria,

---

Reprinted with permission from the *Journal of the American Academy of Child Psychiatry*, 1983, Vol. 22, No. 2, 99–107. Copyright 1983 by the American Academy of Child Psychiatry.

This work was supported in part by Public Health Service Grant MH–13882–06 from the National Institute of Mental Health, Psychiatry Education Branch.

The authors would like to thank Linda Lewis Lemming and Ann Byrd Maloney.

Crisp et al. (1976) found severe anorexia nervosa in 1% of female British students aged 16–18 years; Nylander (1971) in 1 of every 150 Scandinavian adolescent females. Heightened diagnostic awareness of anorexia nervosa may play a role in the absolute increase of this disorder. The diagnostic criteria used in this article include (a) the elective restriction of food causing weight loss of at least 20% of premorbid weight; (b) overwhelming fears of becoming fat; (c) distorted body image; (d) amenorrhea; (e) fine lanugo hair, bradycardia, hypotension, hypothermia with cold intolerance, constipation; (f) unusual hoarding of food or vomiting with bulimia; and (g) absence of other psychiatric and medical illness. This list integrates the criteria of Feighner et al. (1972), Rollins and Piazza (1978), Kirstein (1981), and the American Psychiatric Association (1980).

Approximately 90% of the cases of primary anorexia appear in females (Halmi, 1974; Hay and Leonard, 1979). The boys who develop anorexia tend to be more schizoid and paranoid. They are not uniformly good students and often are more resistant to treatment (Sours, 1980).

Recent studies suggest genetic factors may play a role in anorexia nervosa. Theander (1970) and Garfinkel et al. (1980) found an increased prevalence (6%) of anorexia nervosa in sisters of patients, but this may be due to environmental rather than genetic factors (Winokur et al., 1980). Garfinkel and Garner (1982) reviewed the literature on anorexia in twins and found 36 twin pairs. The total monozygous concordance rate was 52%. Of the 9 dizygous twin pairs in the literature, there has been only one concordant dizygous twin pair (11%) reported by Morgan and Russell (1975). These authors correctly warn that the numbers are too few, and the zygosity and concordance too uncertain, to permit any scientific conclusion about genetic predisposition.

Primary anorexia nervosa (King, 1963; Sours, 1979) is a devastating illness for the patient and family. Long-term studies (Hsu, 1980; Swift, 1982) indicate that after 5 years only 35% are eating normally and free of neurotic fixations on body weight. Most patients (75% eventually find full time employment and improve in terms of weight and menses (75%) and are well-adjusted socially (40-75%). Mortality rates vary from 3.6 to 6.6%, although some report up to 22% deaths (Lucas et al., 1976).

Treatment during the Acute Phase

Patients with anorexia nervosa may not come for medical attention until they have lost considerable weight. It is often necessary for a child psychiatrist who is working up an emaciated patient to refer the child to a pediatric gastroenterologist or other experienced specialist for a thorough medical evaluation. A physical examination and laboratory studies are necessary in order to monitor starvation effects including: hypotension, syncope, hypothermia, dry skin, lanugo hair, diminished triceps skin-fold thickness, hypoglycemia, hair loss, sensitivity to noise, leukopenia, and fatigue (Halmi et al., 1981); arrhythmia (Mitchell and Gillum, 1980); electrolyte and hypothalamic dysfunction (Vigersky and Lorioux, 1977); gastric ulcer (Kline, 1979); hyperactivity (Kron et al., 1978); sucrose sensitivity (Lacey et al., 1977); superior mensenteric artery syndrome (Sours and Vorhaus, 1981); and amenorrhea (Jeuniewic et al., 1978). Starvation can cause psychological and cognitive disturbances including food preoccupation, poor concentration, social isolation, depression, and labile moods (Casper and Davis, 1977; Garfinkel and Garner, 1982; Keys et al., 1950; Maloney and Farrell, 1980). These signs and symptoms of starvation usually require medical management in a hospital when weight loss reaches more than 25% of premorbid weight. The medical management in the hospital involves returning the patient's weight to a safe level. This treatment may include behavioral modification (Agras and Werne, 1977; Halmi et al., 1975; Stunkard, 1972); hyperalimentation (Maloney and Farrell, 1980; Pertschuk et al., 1981); forced nasogastric tube feeding (Crisp, 1965); and/or psychopharmacotherapy including antidepressants (Kendler, 1978; Needleman and Waber, 1977); chlorpromazine (Maxmen et al., 1974), and experimental use of cyproheptadine (Vigersky and Lorioux, 1977), metocloparamide (Moldofsky et al., 1977) and diphenylhydantoin (Green and Rou, 1977). However, most anorexics will not take medications (Sours, 1981). The goal of medical management during hospitalization is weight gain. A typical patient is admitted at 70% of ideal body weight and discharged at 80–85%. Recently, some institutions are attempting to feed patients in the hospital until they achieve 90% of ideal weight (Sours, 1980).

Whichever treatment regimen is planned, the patient is usually hospitalized on a unit with nurses, physicians, and support staff who are experienced with anorexic patients. The nurses learn to understand and deal patiently with the covert food-related behavior of the anorexic. The treatment plan is usually based on a strong diagnostic and dynamic-structural formulation of the patient's disturbance, along with a careful assessment of the patient's medical and metabolic status (Silverman, 1974; Sours, 1980). Without this psychotherapeutic support, many patients will not tolerate weight gain (Maloney et al., 1982).

Although hospitalization is required for many starved anorexics, most clinicians stress the need for post-hospital treatment (Reinhart et al.,

1972). It is generally agreed that psychotherapy is the cornerstone of long-term management (Bruch, 1978b; Garner et al., 1982; Goodsitt, 1977). As with other psychological disorders, the "uniformity myth" (Keisler, 1966) has been applied to anorexia nervosa. The dramatic weight loss and the effects of starvation superimpose superficial similarities between patients. However, with weight gain and progress in psychotherapy, differences between patients emerge and require diversity in psychotherapeutic approaches (Garner et al., 1982). We shall review psychodynamic, behavioral, and family therapy approaches.

Psychodynamic Approaches

For a period of time, classical psychoanalytic psychotherapy was judged to be ineffective in altering anorexic behavior (Bruch, 1973; Palazzoli, 1978; Ross, 1977). Most of these criticisms were directed toward the outmoded "id analyses" of the 1930s and 1940s. Bruch (1978b) claimed that psychoanalytic therapy was ineffective in anorexia because it interpretively "force feeds" the patient and provides no opportunity for self-exploration and development of an effective sense of self. Sours (1980) and Bruch (1982) herself rebuts her earlier statements by describing advances in analytic theory over the last 2 decades. Recent advances in object relations theory have emphasized ego-structural and narcissistic defects which interfere with separation, individuation, and autonomous functioning (Kohut, 1977; Mahler et al., 1975). These advances in psychodynamic theory can be utilized to elaborate negative transference and to interpret pathological defenses during long-term outpatient psychotherapy with anorexics (Goodsitt, 1977; Kernberg, 1976; Masterson, 1977).

During long-term individual psychotherapy, the anorexic may demonstrate regressions to any level of psychosexual development. The syndrome of anorexia nervosa can be embedded in a variety of defenses and personality organizations. Freud (1918) pointed out the anorexic's aversion to sexuality. Others have studied ego boundary problems (Strober and Goldenberg, 1981); oral drive regression (Friedman, 1972); pathological sense of self, related to disturbance at the level of mirroring phase (Casper et al., 1981; Edgecumbe and Burgner, 1975; Rizzuto et al., 1981); body image distortion (Garner et al., 1981); asceticism (Galdston, 1974; Mogul, 1980); intrapersonal paranoia (Palazzoli, 1978); fantasies associated with an internal abdominal mass in the context of a close mother-child relationship (Rollins and Blackwell, 1968); incapacitating sense of ineffectiveness (Bruch, 1978a); weight phobias (Crisp, 1970);

and depression (Cantwell et al., 1977; Sours, 1981). The advances in psychodynamic theory as related to anorexia nervosa are providing a scientific base for long-term, outpatient psychotherapy in this eating disorder.

Behavioral and Cognitive Approaches

Behavioral modification is commonly used on inpatient settings. Techniques include operant reinforcement methods with contracts, negative contingencies, practicing avoided behavior, role playing, relaxation techniques, and systematic desensitization. Because of its potential for rapid weight gain, behavioral modification is frequently utilized (Agras and Werne, 1977). There have been some criticisms of behavioral approaches in anorexia nervosa for being too coercive (Bruch, 1974); for the inappropriate emphasis on extremely rapid weight gain which may lead to bulimia; and for the ethical dilemma posed by enforced treatment with prolonged isolation and deprivation of normal rights (Bemis, 1978). A significant criticism of many behavioral studies is the failure to conduct adequate follow-up assessments. In fact, one of the most comprehensive follow-up studies of a behavioral program (Bhanji and Thompson, 1974) is also the most pessimistic: "Operant conditioning techniques are often inadequate for long-term maintenance of normal eating habits and weight, and they are probably best used simply as a means of rapid weight restoration at times of nutritional crisis."

Some clinicians are attempting to integrate behavioral therapy and psychotherapy (Geller, 1975). Garner et al. (1982) integrate both approaches in a "multimodal cognitive psychotherapy" using reality-oriented feedback to help the patient learn to identify, evaluate, and change faulty thinking patterns and erroneous beliefs. There are no follow up studies of this cognitive approach.

Family Therapy

Family therapy has been increasingly recognized as an important clinical approach for some patients with anorexia nervosa. Minuchin et al. (1978) and Palazolli (1978) use it as the principal mode of treatment. Minuchin states that anorexic eating behavior should be viewed as an interpersonal rather than an individual problem and maintains that successful treatment must be directed toward a restructuring of the dysfunctional family system as a whole. Minuchin (1974) and Liebman et al. (1974) proposed a technique called "the family therapy lunch session," in which the family therapist may take advantage of the emotionally charged mealtime situation to carry out on-the-spot interventions to change patterns of enmeshment, rigidity, and poor conflict resolution in the family. Minuchin et al. (1978) asserts that his treatment is effective in 86% of the cases, regardless of age, symptomatology, and character structure. With family treatment, Minuchin claims that anorexic symptomatology ceases in 2–8 weeks; hospitalization is seldom necessary; individual treatment is unnecessary; and rarely does treatment last more than 10 months. Sours (1980), Swift (1982), Tseng and McDermott (1979), and Malone (1979) criticize Minuchin on several levels: (1) Minuchin views anorexia nervosa as a unitary concept and diagnostically ignores the heterogeneity of the syndrome, (2) some anorexics request individual psychotherapy after the family system is stabilized, (3) Minuchin's follow-up evaluations lack face to face interviews with a majority of the patients, (4) his mean duration of follow-up is not adequate (2⅔ years rather than 4–5 years), (5) no reports of menses are included, and (6) no systematic assessment of eating difficulties, psychosexual adjustment, or psychiatric symptoms are carried out. Furthermore Bemis (1978) doubts the conclusions of most family studies about dysfunctional anorexic family systems because of the virtual absence of controlled studies. Despite these weaknesses in family studies, family therapy can be useful for some patients as long as the heterogeneity of the syndrome is kept in focus.

Conclusions About Anorexia Nervosa

Anorexia nervosa appears to be reaching epidemic proportions in upper socioeconomic level girls. These girls may have a psychophysiological vulnerability which remains latent until the onset of pubertal changes. Clinicians treating these patients need to utilize a biopsychosocial approach in order to manage the medical complications of starvation, the intrapsychic character problems, and the interpersonal stresses which trouble these patients. Whether individual, behavioral, and/or family therapy is utilized, the therapist usually faces a long-term, and often frustrating, treatment process. Countertransference problems may arise related to the patients silences, food refusal, and the therapist's tendency to act like a parent rather than a doctor (Schowalter, 1981). Also frustrating is the eventual discovery by therapists that "relapses and final outcome are similar, whatever initial treatment is given" (Dally,

1969). Perhaps recent improvements in the methodology of follow up studies (Hsu, 1980; Rollins and Piazza, 1981; Swift, 1982) will lead to precision in treatment planning.

BULIMIA

Bulimia literally means "ox hunger" or voracious appetite but in recent years has come to mean binge-eating. The syndrome of bulimia is exhibited mostly by women who alternatively binge on food and then purge by forced vomiting, fasting, laxative or amphetamine abuse. Alternative names for this syndrome are "bulimarexia" (White and Boskind-White, 1981); "purger-vomiters" (Beumont et al., 1976); "bulimia nervosa" (Russell, 1979); "dysorexia" (Guiora, 1967); and "the abnormal normal weight control syndrome" (Crisp, 1982). What distinguishes the bulimic from the anorexic patient is that the bulimic patient has no history of excessive weight loss or amenorrhea, although she may demonstrate food preoccupation and mild weight fluctuations. Schwartz et al. (1982) found that 10% of women at a private, coeducational college practice weight control by regular self-induced vomiting and 3% attempt to control weight with periodic laxative abuse.

Bulimia in Anorexia Nervosa

Some patients with anorexia nervosa demonstrate rapid consumption of large amounts of food in a short period of time. In two large clinical studies, the percentage of anorexics who admitted binge-vomiting was 48% (Garfinkel et al., 1980) and 47% (Casper et al., 1980). The other anorexics in these studies achieved weight loss by consistently fasting (restricters). According to Garfinkel et al. (1980), the anorexic patients with bulimia display a wide variety of impulsive behaviors including the use of alcohol and street drugs, stealing, suicide attempts, and self-mutilation. Comparing the bulimic patients with the fasting patients, Casper et al. (1980) found the builimia patients were more extroverted, admitted more frequently to a strong appetite, tended to be older, to admit kleptomania, to have greater anxiety, depression, guilt, interpersonal sensitivity, more somatic complaints, and a significantly higher prevalence of maternal obesity than the fasting patients. Strober (1980) found bulimic anorexics to have less self-control than abstainers. It is noteworthy that Casper et al. (1980) found that, once they were diagnosed, the bulimic patients were more willing to enter into psychotherapy.

Bulimia with No History of Anorexia Nervosa

The diagnosis of normal weight bulimia is often difficult because the bulimic patient, ashamed of her behavior, will frequently withhold information about her symptoms. Herzog (1982) warns that health professionals in psychiatry, medicine, pediatrics, and dentistry should be aware that the bulimia syndrome exists, and that it should be considered in the differential diagnosis of any patient presenting with a depressive picture or with otherwise unexplained hypokalemia or parotid enlargement (Levin et al., 1980), rectal bleeding, alopecia, or dental enamel loss (Brady, 1980; House et al., 1981; Hurst et al., 1977).

Bulimia patients often demonstrate borderline features (Gunderson and Singer, 1975; Masterson, 1977) including labile affect, loss of control and a sense of emptiness. Garfinkel and Garner (1982) found that bulimics' interpersonal relationships fluctuate between transient, superficial ones and intense dependent ones that lead to further personal devaluation and anger.

Treatment of Bulimia

Once the patient with bulimia has been accurately diagnosed and agrees to treatment, she may be subjected to a wide variety of interventions including hospitalization (Russell, 1979), group therapy with an existential-behavioral format (White and Boskind-White, 1981), multidimensional psychotherapy (Garner et al., 1982), individual psychoanalytic psychotherapy (Sours, 1980), diphenylhydantoin or antidepressants (Mitchell and Pyle, 1982). The data is equivocal on these interventions with bulimia patients. Whichever approach is utilized, the therapist should keep in mind that binge-vomiters can become particularly depressed, and that suicide is the most common cause of death in this disorder (Crisp, 1982).

OBESITY

Obesity is defined as a condition in which body weight exceeds ideal weight for height by 20% or more. For children, ideal weights are usually taken from National Center for Health Statistics growth charts (Merritt, 1979). In recent years, obesity has also been defined in terms of triceps skin fold thickness (Frisancho, 1974). Disparate criteria have complicated estimates of the prevalence of this disorder, but it is commonly reckoned to be present in 5–10% of preschool age children, 10% of school age children, and 15% of adolescents. By comparison, 30% of American adults are obese. Like its adult counterpart, juvenile obesity seems related to socioeconomic status (Goldblatt et al., 1965), occurring much more frequently in lower socioeconomic groups.

Perhaps the most common observation made about juvenile obesity is its persistence. Although a majority of obese infants do not become obese children, most obese children were obese infants. At least 60–80% of obese teenagers become and remain obese adults. Merritt (1979) notes that "It is unusual for an obese child who becomes an obese teenager ever to attain normal weight status."

Many syndromes and medical diseases may cause or contribute to obesity, although they afflict only a very small portion of obese children. These include CNS disease or brain damage secondary to tumor, trauma, or infection; endocrine disorders such as diabetes, Cushing's syndrome, and hypothyroidism; syndromes including Lawrence-Moon-Biedl, Alstrom's, and Praeder-Willi; many chromosomal abnormalities; and obviously any condition causing physical inactivity.

A multitude of clinical studies, case reports, and clinical formulations abound concerning the psychodynamic and psychopathologic bases and correlates of juvenile obesity. In her seminal book *Eating Disorders: Obesity, Anorexia Nervosa and the Person Within*, Bruch (1973) describes a considerable lack of uniformity in the dynamics of the many obese children she studied. No particular psychiatric diagnosis nor set of individual or family dynamics seems to be especially related to juvenile obesity. Some of Bruch's obese subjects became well-adjusted adults, while many others developed serious psychopathology. Wilkinson et al. (1977) have implicated vicissitudes of the separation process in the young child, beginning perhaps with early separation. We have observed the use of food by some parents to protract the period of an infant's absolute dependence. However, it is difficult to generalize such notions into a universal theory. Even the common belief of clinicians that obese children are more disturbed than their normal weight counterparts is difficult to prove statistically. The elaboration of strict DSM-III diagnostic criteria has afforded researchers [notably Halmi et al. (1980)] the opportunity to demonstrate no increased prevalence of psychiatric disorders in obese adults. To our knowledge, no such work involving obese children has been published. Although Bruch (1973) has noted that childhood obesity carries with it psychological sequellae, these seem in some cases to be mitigated by caring, sensitive parents.

What, then, does cause obesity in children? The answer seems to include a complicated assemblage of biopsychosocial factors. Stunkard in his authoritative reviews (1975a, 1980) delineated six major determinant areas. Two of these, the emotional and socioeconomic factors in obesity, have already been noted here. The other areas are genetics, development, physical activity, and brain damage.

Genetics. Davenport (1923) documented that obesity "runs in families." Other work has suggested that somatotypes which are familially transmitted can predispose or protect against obesity (Seltzer and Mayer, 1964).

Development. Coddington and Bruch (1970) have proposed that obesity involves a faulty learning of "gastric perceptivity," developing from a series of miscommunications between infant and caretaker. Similarly, Stunkard (1975b) and Booth (1976) proposed the existence of a special form of "alimentary learning" in which obese children at a very early age "learn" to perceive satiety at a different level of gastric distention or to respond to this perception in a different fashion from nonobese children. Another developmental area of investigation involves adiposity. Observers have recognized two different histologic types of obesity: hyperplastic, wherein the body has an abnormally high number of adipose cells, and hypertrophic, where the adipose cells are of normal number, but of increased fat volume. Adults whose obesity began in childhood tend to suffer from the hyperplastic or a mixed hyperplastic-hypertrophic variety. It has been suggested that weight reduction for these adult hyperplastic individuals would be more difficult than for their hypertrophic obese colleagues. Much of this work has been done in laboratory rats (Knittle, 1972). A review by Stern and Johnson (1978) suggests that there are at least two periods of cellular proliferation in human children, ages 0–2 and 10–14 years. These periods could be protracted in overfed children with ensuing hyperplastic development of adipose cells, although it is possible that a genetic predisposition may be requires.

Activity. The relative contribution of overeating versus inactivity in the development of obesity has long been a matter of controversy. Obese adults have been observed to be less active than normal weight colleagues, and recent work suggests that activity may actually reduce appetite. With children, the picture is much less clear. Bruch (1978a) noted inactivity among her patients. Recent work by Drabman et al. (1979), Stunkard (1980), and Waxman and Stunkard (1980) reaffirms that obese children, even those as young as 1½–2 years of age, eat faster than normal weight controls. In general, however, this area remains confusing.

Brain Damage. The neuroendocrinological foundations of appetite and satiety have been investigated in great detail, and a comprehensive review of this area is beyond the scope of this article. Multiple theories of appetite have been proposed, based upon the use of metabolic signals to the hypothalamus, such as metabolites of protein (aminostatic theory), fat (lipostatic), carbohydrate (glucostatic), or postprandial hypothalamic temperature increase (thermostatic). Work with stereotactic lesions has indicated that the venteromedial nucleus is associated with satiety, while hunger is related to the lateral area of the hypothalamus. The psychopharmacologic research of Wurtman et al. (1981) implicates serotoninergic transmission in the mediation of carbohydrate craving, and suggests the possibility of alteraction by administration of tryptophan (to enhance serotonin synthesis) or fenfluramine (to enhance release). One may speculate that such work will reveal subtypes of obesity related to various biochemical lesions of the hypothalamus.

In surveying this array of data and hypotheses one must conclude that the pathogenesis of obesity, including its juvenile form, may be considered as a multifactorial process. Not surprisingly a plethora of treatment approaches continue to be employed in an attempt to keep obese children from consuming as many calories as they expend. These treatments may be grouped into somatic, educational (including diet and exercise education), and psychotherapeutic (including behavioral) therapies.

Somatic Treatment. We note no recent controlled studies of surgery for the treatment of juvenile obesity, although Blackburn and Bistrian (1975) and Halmi et al. (1981) reported its use in adolescents. In their uncontrolled study, Halmi et al. (1981) found that a group of 80 patients including some adolescents claimed a mean weight loss 2 years post surgery of 44 kg ($\pm$ 20.7 kg S.D.), along with a selective reduction in calorie-dense high carbohydrate foods. This represented a mean weight loss of 55% of excess weight. This report suggests that gastrointestinal surgery may alter mechanisms of appetite feedback, particularly of the glucostatic variety. Despite its promise, such surgery poses significant risks and should be reserved only for the most morbidly obese. The use of pharmacotherapy, particularly of stimulants, for weight reduction in children and adolescents is uncommon. Furthermore, the safety and efficacy of stimulants in obesity are unsupported at this time (Grollman, 1975). By contrast the abuse potential of these drugs is well known.

Educational Treatments. A multitude of strategies to educate parents and children about the value of a proper diet to ameliorate obesity have been attempted. In general, these have been unrewarding. Only 5 of 142 of Hilda Bruch's subjects reported in 1940 lost more than 9 kg (20 lb) after 6 months of active follow-up in a clinic, including psychotherapy as well as education. Subsequent studies have yielded little better results, if sufficiently long-term follow up is pursued. The work of Kirscht et al. (1978) who attempted to study belief and behavior in regard to obesity, typifies the difficulties in this area. They attempted to measure the effects of learned parental communications varying in degrees of threat upon weight change in obese children. They found that high-threat messages from mothers to children could be efficacious in yielding weight loss, more so than low-threat messages. However, their patients were only followed for an average of 61 days and the weight losses during this period were relatively modest.

Concern continues over the possibility of psychic harm befalling children as a result of undue parental and societal pressure for weight loss (Stunkard and Mendelson, 1967; Wooley et al., 1979). Such concern, when juxtaposed with the relative lack of long-term success of exhortational and educational programs for weight loss, warrants that these programs be truly educational rather than primarily coercive.

Psychotherapeutic. In reviewing a large number of behavioral studies, Stunkard (1978) tempered the early enthusiasm which behavioral treatment engendered. Behavioral therapy in adults can lower the number of dropouts and the incidence of emotional complications of treatment compared to alternate regimen. However, mean weight losses in most of these programs have tended to be modest and impermanent. Parental obesity may play a dynamic role in the development of childhood obesity according to Epstein et al. (1980), who recently reported a study of behavior modification and nutrition education programs for overweight children (ages 6–12) and their mothers. Again, however, the weight losses in this study were modest and the follow-up period was short (3 months).

There is still no evidence that psychodynamically oriented psychotherapy is of statistically significant value in the treatment of juvenile obesity. Rand and Stunkard (1978) noted the subjective report of lasting weight loss in patients undergoing psychoanalysis. Similar findings might obtain among children undergoing long-term intensive psychodynamic psychotherapy. Dynamic therapy can assist patients around issues of self-esteem and body image disparagement, and its value in these areas should not be minimized. The value of cognitive therapeutic approaches in these areas may also warrant investigation.

Conclusion in Obesity

The current state of knowledge in childhood obesity suggests a number of areas of promise for investigation including the early development of feeding patterns between infants and mothers, the influence of family dynamics upon overeating, and the elaboration of more specific pharmacologic agents working directly upon centers of hunger and satiety.

OVERALL CONCLUSION

The frequency with which eating disorders appear in the general population may equal 25% if the reported prevalence of anorexia nervosa, bulimia, and obesity are added together. These three conditions, despite their disparate presentations, are similar in that they result from the conjunction of multiple causative factors characterized by intense, although heterogeneous, emotional issues combined with equally intense social and somatic concerns. Their treatment is always arduous and often inadequate and requires a truly biopsychosocial approach.

REFERENCES

Agras, S., & Werne, J. A. (1977). Behavior modification of anorexia nervosa: research foundations. In *Anorexia Nervosa*, ed. R. Vigersky. New York: Raven Press.

American Psychiatric Association (1980). *Diagnostic and Statistical Manual of Mental Disorders DSM-III*), Ed. 3, APA, Washington, DC.

Bemis, M. (1978). Current approaches to the etiology and treatment of anorexia nervosa. *Psychol. Bull., 35:593–617.*

Beumont, P. J. V., George, G. C. W. & Smart, D. E. (1976). Dieters and vomiters and purgers in anorexia nervosa. *Psychol. Med.*, 6:617–622.

Bhanji, S. & Thompson, J. (1974). Operant conditioning in the treatment of anorexia nervosa: a review and retrospective study of 11 cases. *Brit. J. Psychiat.*, 124:166–172.

Blackburn, G. L. & Bistrian, B. R. (1975). Surgical techniques in the treatment of adolescent obesity. In *Childhood Obesity*, ed. P. J. Collipp. Acton, Mass.: Publishing Sciences Group.

Booth, D. A. (1976). Satiety and appetite are conditioned reactions. *Psychosom. Med.*, 39:76.

Brady, W. F. (1980). The anorexia nervosa syndrome. *Oral Surg.*, 50:509–516.

Bruch, H. (1973). *Eating Disorders: Obesity, Anorexia Nervosa and the Person Within.* New York: Basic Books.

———— (1974). Perils of behavioral modification in the treatment of anorexia nervosa. *This Journal*, 230:1419–1422.

———— (1978a). Obesity and anorexia nervosa. *Psychosomatics*, 19:208–212.

———— (1978b). *The Golden Cage: The Enigma of Anorexia Nervosa.* Cambridge, Mass. Harvard University Press.

———— (1982). Psychotherapy in anorexia nervosa. *Int. J. Eating Disord.*, 1:3–14.

Cantwell, D. P., Sturzenberger, S., Burroughs, J. Salkin, B. & Green, J. K. (1977). Anorexia nervosa: an affective disorder? *Arch. Gen. Psychiat.*, 34:1087–1093.

Casper, R. C. & Davis, J. M. (1977). On the course of anorexia nervosa. *Amer. J. Psychiat.*, 134:974–978.

———— Eckert, E. D., Halmi, K. A., Goldberg, S. C. & Davis, J. M. (1980). Bulimia: its incidence and clinical importance in patients with anorexia nervosa. *Arch. Gen. Psychiat.*, 37:1030–1035.

—— Offer, D. & Ostrov, E. (1981). The self-image of adolescents with acute anorexia nervosa. *J. Pediat.*, 98:656–661.

Coddington, R. D. & Bruch, H. (1970). Gastric perception in normal, obese, and schizophrenic subjects. *Psychosomatics*, 11:571–579.

Crisp, A. H. (1965). A treatment regimen for anorexia nervosa. *Brit. J. Psychiat.*, 112:505–512.

—— (1970). Premorbid factors in adult disorders of weight, with particular reference to primary anorexia nervosa (weight phobia): a literature review. *J. Psychosom. Res.*, 14:1–22.

—— Palmer, R. L. & Kalucy, R. S. (1976). How common is anorexia nervosa? A prevalence study. *Brit. J. Psychiat.*, 128:549–554.

—— (1982). Anorexia nervosa at normal body weight: the abnormal normal weight control syndrome. *Int. J. Psychiat. Med.*, 11:203–233.

Dally, P. J. (1969). *Anorexia Nervosa*. New York: Grune & Stratton.

Davenport, C. B. (1923). *Body Build and Its Inheritance*, Publication No. 329. Washington, DC: Carnegie Institute.

Drabman, R. S., Cordua, G. D., Hammer, D., Jarvie, G. J. & Horton, W. (1979). Developmental trends in eating rates of normal and overweight preschool children. *Child Developm.*, 50:211–216.

Edgecumbe, R. & Burgner, M. (1975). The phallic-narcissistic phase. *The Psychoanalytic Study of the Child*, 30:161–181.

Epstein, L. H., Wing, R. R., Steranchak, L., Dickson, B. & Michelson, J. (1980). Comparison of family-based behavior modification and nutrition education for childhood obesity. *J. Pediat. Psychol.*, 5:25–36.

Feighner, J. P., Rubin, E., Guze, S. B. & Munoz, R. (1972). Diagnostic criteria for use in psychiatric research. *Arch. Gen. Psychiat.*, 26:57–63.

Freud, S. (1918). *Standard Edition*, 17:106. London: Hogarth Press, 1978.

Friedman, S. (1972). On the presence of a variant form of instinctual regression: oral drive cycles in obesity-bulimia. *Psychoanal. Quart.*, 41:364–383.

Frisancho, A. R. (1974). Triceps skin fold and upper arm muscle size norms for assessment of nutritional status. *Amer. J. Clin. Nutr.*, 27:1052–1058.

Galdston, R. (1974). Mind over matter: observations on 50 patients hospitalized with anorexia nervosa. *This Journal*, 13:246–263.

Garfinkel, P., Moldofsky, H. & Garner, D. M. (1980). The heterogeneity of anorexia nervosa: bulimia as a distinct subgroup. *Arch. Gen. Psychiat.*, 37:1036–1040.

Garfinkel, P. E. & Garner, D. M. (1982). *Anorexia Nervosa: A Multidimensional Perspective*. New York: Brunner/Mazel.

Garner, D. M. & Garfinkel, P. E. (1981). Body image in anorexia nervosa: measurement, theory and clinical implications. *Int. J. Psychiat. Med.*, 11(3):263–284.

—— —— & Bemis, K. M. (1982). A multidimensional psychotherapy for anorexia nervosa. *Int. J. Eating Disord.*, 1:3–47.

Geller, J. L. (1975). Treatment of anorexia nervosa by the integration of behavior therapy and psychotherapy. *Psychother. Psychosom.*, 26:167–177.

Goldblatt, P. B., Moore, M. E. & Stunkard, A. J. (1965). Social factors in obesity. *J. Amer. Med. Assn.*, 192:97–102.

Goodsitt, A. (1977). Narcissistic disturbances in anorexia nervosa. In: *Adolescent Psychiatry*, ed. S. C. Feinstein & P. L. Giovacchini. New York: Jason Aronson.

Green, R. S. & Rou, J. (1977). The use of diphenylhydantoin in compulsive eating disorders: further studies. In: *Anorexia Nervosa*, ed. R. Vigersky. New York: Raven Press.

Grollman, A. (1975). Drug therapy of obesity in children. In: *Childhood Obesity*, ed. P. J. Collipp. Acton, Mass.: Publishing Sciences Group.

Guiora, A. S. (1967). Dysorexia: a psychopathological study of anorexia nervosa and bulimia. *Amer. J. Psychiat.*, 124:391–393.

Gunderson, J. G. & Singer, M. T. (1975). Defining borderline patients: an overview. *Amer. J. Psychiat.*, 132:1–10.

Halmi, K. A. (1974). Anorexia nervosa: demographic and clinical features in 94 cases. *Psychosom. Med.*, 36:18–26.

—— Powers, P. & Cunningham, S. (1975). Treatment of anorexia nervosa with behavior modification. *Arch. Gen. Psychiat.*, 32:93–96.

—— Long, M., Stunkard, A. J. & Mason, E. (1980). Psychiatric diagnosis of morbidly obese gastric bypass patients. *Amer. J. Psychiat.*, 127:470–472.

—— Mason, E., Falk, J. R. & Stunkard, A. J. (1981). Appetitive behavior after gastric bypass for obesity. *Int. J. Obesity*, 5:457–465.

Hay, G. G. & Leonard, J. C. (1979). Anorexia nervosa in males. *Lancet*, :574–575.

Herzog, D. B. (1982). Bulimia: the secretive syndrome. *Psychosomatics*, 23:481–487.

Hill, O. W. (1977). Epidemiologic aspects of anorexia nervosa. *Advan. Psychosom. Med.*, 9:48–62.

House, R. C., Crisius, R. & Bliziotes, M. M. (1981). Perimolysis: unveiling the surreptitious vomiter. *Oral Surg.*, 51:152–155.

Hsu, L. K. G. (1980). Outcome in anorexia nervosa. *Arch. Gen. Psychiat.*, 37:1041–1048.

Hurst, P. S., Lacey, J. A. & Crisp, A. H. (1977). Teeth, vomiting, and diet: a study of dental characteristics of seventeen anorexia nervosa patients. *Postgrad. Med. J.*, 53:298–305.

Jeuniewic, N., Brown, G. M., Garfinkel, P. E. & Moldofsky, H. (1978). Hypothalamic functions as related to body weight and body fat in anorexia nervosa. *Psychosom. Med.*, 40:187–187.

Keisler, D. J. (1966). Some myths of psychotherapy research and the search for a paradigm. *Psychol. Bull.*, 65:110–136.

Kendler, K. S. (1978). Amitriptyline-induced obesity in anorexia nervosa: a case report. *Amer. J. Psychiat.*, 135:1107–1108.

Kernberg, O. (1976). *Object Relations Theory and Clinical Psychoanalysis*. New York: Jason Aronson.

Keys, S., Brozek, J., Henschel, A., et al. (1950). *The Biology of Human Starvation*. Minneapolis, Minn.: University of Minnesota Press.

King, A. (1963). Primary and secondary anorexia nervosa syndrome. *Brit. J. Psychiat.*, 109:470–479.

Kirscht, J. P., Becker, M. H., Haefner, D. P. & Maiman, L. A. (1978). Effects of threatening communications and mothers' health beliefs on weight change in obese children. *J. Behav. Med.*, 1:147–157.

Kirstein, L. (1981). Diagnostic issues in primary anorexia nervosa. *Int. J. Psychiat. Med.*, 11(3):235–244.

Kline, C. L. (1979). Anorexia nervosa: death from complications of ruptured gastric ulcer. *Canad. J. Psychiat.*, 24:153–156.

Knittle, J. L. (1972). Obesity in childhood: a problem in adipose tissue cellular development. *J. Pediat.*, 81:1048–1059.

Kohut, H. (1977). *The Restoration of the Self*. New York: International Universities Press.

Kron, L., Katz, J. L., Corzynski, G. & Weiner, H. (1978). Hyperactivity in anorexia nervosa: a fundamental clinical feature. *Comp. Psychiat.*, 19(5):433–440.

Lacey, J. A., Stanley, P. A., Crutchfield, M. & Crisp, A. H. (1977). Sucrose sensitivity in anorexia nervosa. *J. Psychosom. Res.*, 21:17–21.

Levin, P. A., Falko, J. M., Dixon, K., Gallup, E. M. & Saunders, W. (1980). Benign parotid enlargement in bulimia. *Ann. Intern. Med.*, 93:827–829.

Liebman, R., Minuchin, S. & Baker, L. (1974). The role of the family in the treatment of anorexia nervosa. *This Journal*, 13:264–274.

Lucas, A. R., Duncan, J. W., Piens, V. (1976). The treatment of anorexia nervosa. *Amer. J. Psychiat.*, 133:1034–1038.

Mahler, M. S., Pine, F. & Bergman, A. (1974). *The Psychological Birth of the Human Infant Symbiosis and Individuation.* New York: Basic Books.

Malone, C. A. (1979). Child psychiatry and family therapy. *This Journal*, 18:4–21.

Maloney, M. J. & Farrell, M. K. (1980). Treatment of severe weight loss in anorexia nervosa with hyperalimentation and psychotherapy. *Amer. J. Psychiat.*, 137(3):310–314.

——— Pettigrew, H. & Farrell, M. (1982). Treatment sequence for severe weight loss in anorexia nervosa. *Int. J. Eating Disord.* (in press).

Masterson, J. F. (1977). Primary anorexia nervosa in the borderline adolescent—an object relations view. In: *Borderline Personality Disorders*, ed. P. Hartocollis. New York: Intern. U. Press.

Maxmen, J. S., Siberfarb, P. M., & Ferrell, R. B. (1974). Anorexia nervosa: practical initial management in a general hospital. *J. Amer. Med. Assn.*, 29:801–808.

Merritt, R. J. (1979). Obesity in pediatric patients. *Comprehen. Ther.*, 5:26–34.

Minuchin, S. (1974). *Families and Family Therapy.* Cambridge, Mass.: Harvard University Press.

——— Rosman, B. L. & Baker, L. (1978). *Psychosomatic Families.* Cambridge, Mass.: Harvard University Press.

Mitchell, J. E. & Gillum, R. (1980). Weight-dependent arrhythmia in a patient with anorexia nervosa. *Amer. J. Psychiat.*, 137:377–378.

——— & Pyle, R. L. (1982). The bulimic syndrome in normal weight individuals: a review. *Int. J. Eating Disord.*, 1:61–73.

Mogul, L. S. (1980). Asceticism in adolescence and anorexia nervosa. *The Psychoanalytic Study of the Child*, 35:155–175.

Moldofsky, H., Jeuniewic, N. & Garfinkel, P. E. (1977). Preliminary report on metoclopramide in anorexia nervosa. In *Anorexia Nervosa*, ed. R. A. Vigersky. New York: Raven Press.

Morgan, H. G. & Russell, G. F. M. (1975). Value of family background and clinical features as predictors of long-term outcome in anorexia nervosa: four-year follow-up study of 41 patients. *Psychol. Med.*, 5:355–372.

Needleman, H. & Waber, D. (1977). The use of amitriptyline in anorexia nervosa. In *Anorexia Nervosa*, ed. R. A. Vigersky. New York: Raven Press.

Nylander, T. (1971). The feeling of being fat and dieting in a school population. *Acta Sociomed. Scand.*, 3:17–26.

Palozzoli, M. S. (1978). *Self-Starvation.* New York: Jason Aronson.

Pertschuk, M. J., Forster, J., Buzby, G. & Mullen, J. L. (1981). The treatment of anorexia nervosa with total parenteral nutrition. *Biol. Psychiat.*, 16:539–550.

Rand, C. S. W. & Stunkard, A. J. (1978). Obesity and psychoanalysis. *Amer. J. Psychiat.*, 135:547–551.

Reinhart, J. B., Kenna, M. D. & Succop, R. A. (1972). Anorexia nervosa in children outpatient management. *This Journal*, 12:114–131.

Rizzuto, A., Peterson, R. K. & Reed, M. (1981). The pathological sense of self in anorexia nervosa. *Psychiat. Clin. N. Amer.* 4:471–487.

Rollins, N. & Blackwell, A. (1968). The treatment of anorexia nervosa in children and adolescents. *J. Child Psychol. Psychiat.*, 9:81–91.

—— & Piazza, E. (1978). Diagnosis of anorexia nervosa: a critical reappraisal. *This Journal.* 17(1):126–137.

—— —— (1981). Anorexia nervosa: a quantitative approach to follow-up. *This Journal,* 20:167–183.

Ross, I. L. (1977). Anorexia nervosa—an overview. *Bull. Menninger Clin.*, 41:418–436.

Russell, G. (1979). Bulimia nervosa: an ominous variant of anorexia nervosa. *Psychol. Med.,* 9:429–448.

Schowalter, J. (1981). Psychoanalytic psychotherapy in anorexia nervosa. Presented at the Annual Meeting of the American Academy of Child Psychiatry, Dallas, Tex.

Schwartz, D. M., Thompson, M. G. & Johnson, C. L. (1982). Anorexia nervosa and bulimia: the socio-cultural context. *Int. J. Eating Disor.*, 1:20–36.

Seltzer, C. C. & Mayer, J. (1964). Body build and obesity—who are the obese? *J. Amer. Med. Assn.*, 189:677–684.

Silverman, J. A. (1974). Anorexia nervosa: clinical observations in a successful treatment plan. *J. Pediat.*, 84:68–73.

Sours, J. A. (1979). Primary anorexia nervosa syndrome. In: *Basic Handbook of Child Psychiatry*, ed. J. Noshpitz, New York: Basic Books.

—— (1980). *Starving to Death in a Sea of Objects: The Anorexia Nervosa Syndrome*, New York: Jason Aronson.

—— (1981). Depression and the anorexia nervosa syndrome. *Psychiat. Clin. N. Amer.*, 4:145–158.

—— & Vorhaus, L. J. (1981). Superior mesenteric artery syndrome in anorexia nervosa: a case report. *Amer. J. Psychiat.*, 138:519–520.

Stern, J. S. & Johnson, P. R. (1978). Size and number of adipocytes and their implications. In: *Advances in Modern Nutrition*, ed. H. Katzer & R. Mahler. New York: John Wiley & Sons.

Strober, M. (1980). Personality and symptomatological features in young, nonchronic anorexia nervosa patients. *J. Psychosom. Res.*, 24:353–359.

—— & Goldenberg, I. (1981). Ego boundary disturbance in juvenile anorexia nervosa. *J. Clin. Psychol.*, 37:433–438.

Stunkard, A. (1972). New therapies for eating disorders: behavioral modification of obesity and anorexia nervosa. *Arch. Gen. Psychiat.*, 26:391–398.

—— (1975a). Obesity. In: *Amer. Handbook of Psychiat.*, ed. M. F. Reiser. New York: Basic Books.

—— (1975b). Satiety is a conditioned reflex. *Psychosom. Med.*, 37:383.

—— (1978). Behavioral treatment of obesity: the current status. *Int. J. Obesity*, 2:237.

—— (1980). Obesity. In: *Comprehensive Textbook of Psychiatry/III*, ed. H. I. Kaplan, A. M. Freedman & B. J. Sadock. Baltimore: Williams & Wilkins.

—— & Mendelson, M. (1967). Obesity and body image: I. Characteristics of disturbances in the body image of some obese persons. *Amer. J. Psychiat.*, 123:10.

Swift, W. J. (1982). The long-term outcome of early onset anorexia nervosa: critical review. *This Journal*, 21:38–46.

Theander, S. (1970). Anorexia nervosa: a psychiatric investigation of 94 female cases. *Acta Psychiat. Scand. (Suppl.), 214:1–194.*

Tseng, W. & McDermott, J. E. (1979). Triaxial family classification: a proposal. *This Journal*, 18:22–43.

Vigersky, R. A. & Lorioux, D. L. (1977). Anorexia nervosa as a model of hypothalamic dysfunction. In: *Anorexia Nervosa*, ed. R. A. Vigersky. New York: Raven Press.

Waxman, M. & Stunkard, A. J. (1980). Caloric intake and expenditure of obese boys. *J. Pediat.* 96:187–193.

White, W. C. & Boskind–White, M. (1981). An experiential-behavioral approach to the treatment of bulimarexia. *Psychother. Theory Res. Pract.*, 18:501–507.

Wilkinson, P. W., Parkin, J. M., Pearlson, J., Philips, P. R. & Sykes, P. (1977). Obesity in childhood: a community study in Newcastle upon Tyne. *Lancet*, 1:350.

Winokur, A., March, V. & Mendels, J. (1980). Primary affective disorder in relatives of patients with anorexia nervosa. *Amer. J. Psychiat.*, 137:695–698.

Wooley, S. C., Wooley, O. W. & Dyrenforth, S. R. (1979). Theoretical, practical and social issues in behavioral treatments of obesity. *J. Appl. Behav. Anal.*, 12:3–25.

Wurtman, J. J., Wurtman, R. J., Growdon, J. H., Henry, P., Lipscomb, A. & Zeisel, S. H. (1981). Carbohydrate craving in obese people: suppression by treatment affecting serotoninergic transmission. *Int. J. Eating Disord.*, 1:2–15.

Part VIII

PUBLIC POLICY ISSUES

This section discusses a number of issues of public policy which are of concern to mental health professionals as advocates for children and as advisers to parents.

Maccoby and her coauthors point out that research findings can have a major impact in influencing the thinking of many people who shape the political climate. To do so, however, requires not only that good research be done, but that the findings be disseminated at the right time to the right people in the right language. The authors point up the considerations researchers must keep in mind in communication with policymakers if they are to act as a constituency on behalf of children.

Now that an increasing number of mothers of young children work outside the home—the fastest growing segment of the work force is among mothers of children under age three—substitute quality day care for their children becomes an imperative for public policy. Yet, as Zigler and Muenchow point out in their trenchant criticism, federal subsidies for low-income families have been reduced and federal commitments to setting minimum standards for such centers have been abandoned. Beyond this, the United States stands alone among advanced industrial nations in not having statutory maternity leave provisions which would give mothers the alternative opportunity to stay home and take care of their young children themselves. Zigler and Muenchow spell out these issues and their implications, and challenge mental health professionals to lend their influence to this profoundly important question. Ironically, the United States has sometimes been called a "child-centered" nation, but the facts clearly justify an opposite label.

In his article on child custody and divorce, Henry Foster, an attorney with a wealth of experience and wisdom in family law, reviews the many issues that can become sources of contention in child custody cases. He welcomes the shift from the former emphasis on family fitness to a concern with the child's welfare, and discusses the implications of this shift. He underlines the importance of the recommendations of child psychiatrists in custody cases, discusses specific aspects of the psychiatrist's role, and makes thoughtful recommendations. We should take to heart his final statement: "Psychiatric generalizations should not decide concrete cases. It should be the dynamics of the individual case that controls the particular result".

The use and abuse of commercial television by children continues to be a hotly debated issue. The Singers review the psychological literature and summarize their own findings in their article "Psychologists Look at Television". They point out that the current heavy viewing of television by children is likely, if anything, to increase as the use of cable television, videodiscs, and home-video recording expands. The authors are concerned about the psychological consequences for children of heavy television viewing and the fact that the potential benefits of the medium for education and constructive development have not generally been translated into regular age-specific programming for children by the television industry. Avenues for intervention by parents and professionals and directions for future research are reviewed.

29

The Role of Psychological Research in the Formation of Policies Affecting Children

Eleanor E. Maccoby

Stanford University

Alfred J. Kahn

Columbia University

Barbara A. Everett

Society for Research in Child Development, Washington Liaison Office

This article considers some of the factors that determine whether, and how, psychological research will have an impact on public policies regarding children. Factors discussed include the following: (a) consistencies and inconsistencies in research findings, especially cases in which early results are greatly modified, or even reversed, by later ones; (b) cases in which documentation of a problem is not accompanied by information on the costs and benefits of possible remedial measures; (c) in evaluation research, failure to monitor the implementation as well as the expected outcomes of interventions; (d) disjunctions in timing between the appearance of a research finding and congressional schedules, executive decision processes, and the agendas of interest groups. The importance of the political climate is stressed, as well as the need for researchers to know the right times and places for introducing their information to the policymaking process.

Reprinted with permission from *American Psychologist*, 1983, Vol. 38, No. 1, 80–84. Copyright 1983 by the American Psychological Association, Inc.

The relationship between researchers and policymakers is essentially an uneasy one. Policymakers sometimes see researchers as impractical, and may be skeptical about policy recommendations coming from researchers who seem not to understand the complexities of achieving a consensus among rival constituencies or administering programs once they have been legislated. Researchers, on the other hand, often see policymakers as disingenuous and too willing to compromise on matters where compromise does not seem justified on the basis of research evidence. Frustrations can go so deep that informed people throw up their hands and conclude that rational decision making on a societal level is impossible, at least on certain issues (see Steiner, 1981). Yet when a variety of political and social forces converge with empirical findings at a crucial moment in time, research has a clear impact on policy. This article considers the relationship of research to the other elements involved in formulating policy affecting children.

At the outset we should note that "policy research" is not a distinct category. Much of the research drawn upon in public policy formation was not intended for that purpose. Research can be utilized for identifying needs, for setting new objectives, for clarifying what works and what does not, or for understanding the nature of the phenomena that give rise to a problem or set limits on its solution. In pursuing these questions, policymakers draw on a wide variety of data sources, including statistical series; descriptive studies of institutions or life circumstances of different segments of the population; evaluation studies which compare the alternative consequences of different interventions; and basic research such as studies that clarify cognitive development or analyze family interaction and socialization. All these kinds of research become "policy research" when utilized during one of the steps in the policy-formation process.

Public policies affecting children are formed and implemented in an intensely political atmosphere. Overarching political and economic ideologies are involved, as are pressures from interest groups. Policy formation occurs in legislative committees, in offices of the executive branches of national, state, and local governments, and in public, private, and semiprivate service agencies, boards, and commissions. Outcomes inevitably reflect compromises between conflicting values of various constituencies, and the role played by research depends on what groups are involved and how they are aligned. Consider, for example, the following policy questions, all of which are currently under active debate:

1. When parents abuse or neglect their children, should their legal rights be terminated quickly, so that their children can be placed in

permanent adoptive homes? Or should the rights of natural parents be protected against arbitrary bureaucratic action by providing a variety of judicial restraints on removal and a slower decision process that calls for efforts to reconcile the child with the natural parents?

2. Should the public welfare structure be geared toward providing support at home for impoverished mothers of young children, or should it be designed to enable these mothers to work (e.g., by providing day care)?

3. Should federal funds to support day care be made contingent on providers' meeting certain quality standards? If so, who should formulate the standards, what should they require, and how should compliance be monitored?

4. What standard should the law apply in awarding custody of children in contested cases when both parents are judged fit? Is a general "best interest of the child" standard workable? Should there be a presumption for joint custody? Or for maternal custody when the child is "of tender years"?

5. What are the costs and benefits of preschool education programs, particularly for children at risk for subsequent school failure? Is it more efficient to invest in remedial education at later ages, or does the impact of later interventions depend on earlier ones?

6. Should handicapped children, or children who are slow learners, be put into special education classes or kept in mainstream classrooms? If minority children are overrepresented among slow learners, does this have any implications for which solution should be chosen? (See Heller, Holzman, & Messick, 1982.)

7. In programs designed to detect health problems as early as possible, should children be "screened" for emotional and behavioral problems as well as physical ones? Should screening be done even if no mechanism exists for treating disorders once they are detected?

8. Should physicians be required to inform parents when teenagers are treated for venereal disease or provided with contraceptive information?

9. What should be the responsibility of police, courts, social agencies, and schools for children who are truant or run away from home? Under what circumstances, if any, should such children be put in secure detention? (See Handler & Zatz, 1982.)

All of these questions involve value choices. In considering any of them, information is needed from a variety of knowledge areas, so psychological research is only one source of relevant data. There are psychological studies that bear on all these issues and many more, and their findings have played a part in the debates. Whether a particular piece of research is drawn upon, however, depends greatly on its timing in relation to various aspects of the sociopolitical climate. A finding that will fall on deaf ears at one time may become salient at another. For example, an early report on the sexist bias in school textbooks (Child, Potter, & Levine, 1946) was virtually ignored, whereas similar reports appearing in the 1970s, when feminist concerns had become focal, received widespread attention and were used in efforts to reform the content of textbooks in the interests of greater gender equity.

Although available knowledge is frequently not utilized because the political climate is not receptive to it, the reverse situation may also occur. That is, a piece of information may be badly needed to allow policy formation to proceed, so that when this information becomes available it is quickly taken up and acted upon. An instance of this kind is reported in detail in the National Research Council (NRC) report, *Making Policies for Children* (Hayes, 1982). One of the case studies in this report deals with federal standards for day care (Issue 3 above). The NRC analysis shows that although legislation passed in the late 1960s called for the establishment of such standards, the process of formulating them was stalemated for many years. Many experts in early childhood education wanted to require that the ratio of adult caregivers to the number of children being cared for should be high, but it soon became clear that if federal funds to support day care were made contingent on care centers' having high ratios, many existing facilities would have to go out of business and the overall child care system would be weakened. A national study of the factors contributing to favorable outcomes of day care was commissioned. When the results of this study showed that the staff-child ratio was relatively unimportant compared to other factors, a leading element in the policy dilemma was resolved, and it became possible to proceed with the development of federal standards. Although this process has recently become moot (because of channeling federal funds for the support of day care into block grants to states, thus foreclosing the federal role in standard setting), at one point in the process there was a high state of readiness to receive and utilize the findings that the National Day Care Study happened to provide.

There is an issue in the area of divorce and custody where policy formation is perhaps too ready to receive a specific research finding. Legal scholars studying custody cases have recognized that judges are in a poor position to make good decisions in most cases of contested custody. They are looking for an easy formula which will short-circuit the painful and time-consuming adjudication process that now exists, and have moved quickly toward a presumption for joint custody. The studies of divorce and its impact on children (Hetherington, Cox, & Cox, 1982; Wallerstein & Kelley, 1980) have shown that children in maternal custody fare better if they are able to maintain contact with their fathers after the divorce. In their eagerness to find a way to simplify the decision process for judges, legal scholars have interpreted these findings as though they constituted evidence for joint custody in contested cases, which (in our opinion and that of the researchers being cited) they do not. We may presume that if negative findings on the feasibility of joint custody in contested cases emerge as time goes on, it will be much more difficult for them to get a hearing. Thus when research is "needed" by a powerful interest group, as it was in the day-care standards case, it may contribute greatly to the policy-fomation process by breaking a deadlock. But this state of readiness may result in research being used prematurely or inappropriately.

The results of the National Day Care Study may have been particularly salient because they ran counter to conventional wisdom about the importance of child-staff ratios. A similar recent instance comes from testimony by Greenberger (1983) on legislation designed to foster adolescent employment. Greenberger reported studies showing that contrary to common belief, teenage employment may *not* foster the long-range occupational achievements of youth. This testimony coincided with the interests of an important interest group (organized labor) that opposed the revision of child labor laws, with a resulting strong impact.

Research is a continuous process, whereas legislation tends to be episodic. New results may call for modifications in programs that drew upon earlier research when they were established. The recent reforms in legislation having to do with adoption and foster care (P.L. 96–272, 198) provide a case in point. This legislation rests on a considerable research base. Surveys and descriptive studies, as well as testimony and some data concerning the experiences of children in institutions and foster homes, suggested that too many children were remaining in long-term foster care without positive results or with detriment. Clearly, not enough was being done to free them for adoption, to strenghthen their natural homes, to seek to return them to their parents, or to avoid taking them away in the first place. Reform thus combated well-defined and documented evils. But the reform embodied remedies (strongly backed by financial sanctions) that were not yet documented by research. We do not know whether the subsidized adoptions supported by the new law will be better for children than long-term foster care. And we do not know whether the required efforts to return children to their natural homes will be a successful alternative. Research is now beginning to cast doubt on how successfully children can be reunited with some abusing or neglecting parents, and to show comparatively good outcomes from foster care. These new studies do not detract from the need for reform in our adoption and foster-care procedures, but they do illustrate the problem faced by legislators when research documents the existence of problems but has only begun to explore possible solutions.

The case of the Head Start and Follow Through programs illustrates some of the difficulties of integrating the slow cumulation of research knowledge with the differently timed policy-formation process. Head Start was one of the first social programs to have a requirement for evaluation built in to its founding legislation. At the outset, Head Start instructional programs for preschoolers were put in place with extraordinary haste, and evaluation began before a shakedown period could occur. An early study (Westinghouse, 1969) very nearly killed the program. This study reported that although there had been some health gains for children served by the program, intellectual gains (assessed primarily through IQ scores) were small and temporary. The report came in just before President Nixon's first message to Congress in 1969. He had planned to give an unqualified endorsement to Head Start, but changed the message toward a more neutral position on the basis of the Westinghouse study. The momentum of the program faltered, and Head Start was rescued by pressure from parents and other child advocates in spite of, rather than because of, research. Gradually, replicable positive findings from evaluation studies of early educational intervention programs began to come in. Two reports published in 1975, one generally positive (Stallings) and one showing few sustained effects (Miller & Dyer), illustrated some of the complexities of conducting such evaluations. It was not until 1982 that a monograph became available summarizing some positive long-term outcomes from 12 different early-intervention studies (Lazar & Darlington, 1982). The reports by this consortium are not without their critics: the high attrition rates raise questions; one cannot be sure to what extent teachers in the later grades were aware of the children's early educational histories; and the achievments of "model" programs may not generalize to widely disseminated programs. For our present purposes, however, we will set these questions aside, and consider some of the lessons that have emerged from the history of this and other evaluation research. In this summary, we draw on a National Research Council report on the evaluation of early-childhood programs (Travers & Light, 1982). Some of the major lessons are:

1. Immediate effects and delayed effects of a program may be quite different, and early effects may not be good predictors of later effects. These facts pose problems for the utilization of research results in the policy-formation process, since policy formation often has its own time-table, geared to the politics of election cycles and to the cycles for reauthorization of specific legislation.

2. Different instructional programs have been shown to have different outcomes. Thus there is no way in which an omnibus set of interventions of the sort involved in Head Start and Follow Through can be pronounced successful or unsuccessful. It is necessary to ask which program element is successful with respect to which outcome.

3. Assessment of intervention programs must include evaluation of the degree to which planned programs have actually been implemented. Implementation varies by site and program, and quite often failures to achieve gains via an intervention program have not meant that the program was ineffective; rather, failures have stemmed from the fact that a program was never actually put into place.

4. The verdict with regard to the effectiveness of a program depends heavily on the outcome measures selected for study. (a) Long-term positive effects of early intervention programs have been shown in terms of lower rates of absence from school, lower rates of repeating grades or being assigned to remedial classes, and greater incorporation of academic values into self-concepts. If research attention had been confined to gains in IQ or improvements in achievement scores on specific academic tests, the impact of the programs would have been greatly underestimated. (b) It has been repeatedly noted that the impact of early interventions on social-emotional development has not been adequately assessed. The problem here is not merely a psychometric one having to do with a lag in test development. Rather, it reflects a lack of basic knowledge concerning the cross-age stability and predictive validity of various aspects of social-emotional functioning—knowledge that would guide both the selection of measures and the design of programs (Travers & Light, 1982). (c) The choice of outcomes depends on values. Legislators are understandably interested in getting demonstrations of short-term effects within their terms of office, but researchers can sometimes get them to attend to the values entailed in longer-term outcomes. The reverse also applies: Advocates are often concerned with establishing programs that involve intervening in childhood so as to lower the subsequent rates of juvenile delinquency, mental illness, or economic dependency. It has been argued that we have been overly preoccupied with

such outcomes and that we ought to be concerned as well with the impact of programs on children's concurrent "quality of life" (assuming that this can be defined and measured).

The impact of a piece of research depends greatly on its timing, its scope in relation to the policy issue at hand, and its concordance or discordance with political forces. It is also true that the degree of agreement among researchers makes a difference. When studies come up with divergent findings, protagonists for various points of view comb through the research literature and select items that best support their own position. They also take as much advantage as possible of any critique of the opposition's research base. In a sense, researchers limit their own effectiveness by reporting nonreplications of other people's findings or mounting heavy methodological critiques of studies that might otherwise play a useful role. It has been suggested that they should attempt to come to some sort of agreement among themselves in advance of public discussion, rather than being caught in the embarrassing position of testifying on both sides of a debate. It seems to us that complexities, critiques, and even contradictions are an inevitable part of the scientific process. Researchers cannot suppress findings, nor can they refrain from criticizing flawed studies. There will always be solid evidence to support more than one side of a debate. We see no way in which researchers can speak with a single voice. It may be hoped, however, that they will be responsibly aware of the ways in which their findings may be interpreted, and try to restrain distortions in the application of their work whenever possible.

Even when there is a reasonably high degree of consensus among researchers and other experts, their knowledge does not always have an impact on policy implementation. If researchers want their work to be utilized on behalf of children, they need to be aware of the timetables governing the decision-making process in legislative and administrative bodies, and they must take the initiative in making their information available at appropriate times. In addition, they will sometimes have to consider how adequate the organizational structure of legislatures and executive offices is for the utilization of information. Is there an appropriate committee in Congress, or an office or agency in the executive branch, that is clearly required and empowered to carry out the policy-formation process with respect to children's issues? Continuous vigilance on the part of informed citizens is necessary if such agencies are to be created, maintained, and given the support necessary to carry out their tasks.

In the long run, we believe, the continuing accumulation of findings from both basic and applied research may have its major impact by influencing the thinking of many people who form the political climate. We have a representative form of government, and both legislators and administrators are responsive to inputs from informed members of their constituencies. With this fact in mind, it becomes important that researchers not only continue to do good work but also translate their findings into readable English and disseminate them not only to legislators and adminstrators but to influential members of the lay public. These persons can then act in an informed way as a constituency on behalf of children.

REFERENCES

Child, I., Potter, E. G., & Levine, E. M. (1946). Children's textbooks and personality development: An exploration in the social psychology of education. *Psychological Monographs, 60*(3, Whole No. 279).

Greenberger, E. (1983). A researcher in the policy arena: The case of child labor. *American Psychologist, 38,* 104–111.

Handler, J. F., & Zatz, J. (1982). *Neither angels nor thieves: Studies in deinstitutionalization of status offenders.* Washington, D.C.: National Academy Press.

Hayes, C. D. (Ed.) (1982). *Making policies for children: A study of the federal process* (National Research Council report). Washington, D.C.: National Academy Press.

Heller, K. A., Holzman, W. G., & Messick, S. (Eds.) (1982). *Placing children in special education: A strategy for equity* (National Research Council report). Washington, D.C.: National Academy Press.

Hetherington, E. M., Cox, M., & Cox, R. (1982). Effects of divorce on parents and children. In M. Lamb (Ed.), *Non-traditional families.* Hillsdale, N.J.: Erlbaum.

Lazar, I., & Darlington, R. (1982). Lasting effects of early education: A report from the Consortium for Longitudinal Studies. *Monographs of the Society for Research in Child Development, 47,* 1–139.

Miller, L. B., & Dyer, J. L. (1975). Four preschool programs: Their dimensions and effects. *Monographs of the Society for Research in Child Development, 40*(5 & 6, Serial No. 162).

Stallings, J. (1975). Implementation and child effects of teaching practices in Follow-Through classrooms. *Monographs of the Society for Research in Child Development, 40*(7 & 8, Serial No. 163).

Steiner, A. Y. (1981). *The futility of family policy.* Washington, D.C.: Brookings Institution.

Travers, J. R., & Light, R. J. (Eds.) (1982). *Learning from experience: Evaluating early childhood demonstration programs* (National Research Council report). Washington, D.C.: National Academy Press.

Wallerstein, J. S., & Kelley, J. B. (1980). *Surviving the breakup: How children and parents cope with divorce.* New York: Basic Books.

Westinghouse Learning Corporation & Ohio University (1969). *The impact of Head Start: An evaluation of the effects of Head Start on children's cognitive and affective development* (Executive Summary). Report to the Office of Economic Opportunity [EDO 36321]. Washington, D.C.: Clearinghouse for Federal Scientific and Technical Information.

30

Infant Day Care and Infant-Care Leaves: A Policy Vacuum

Edward Zigler and Susan Muenchow

Yale University

Current U.S. policy supports neither high-quality infant day care nor alternatives, such as paid leaves for infant care. Psychologists, on the basis of research showing the importance of quality care for infants, should support measures to protect day care quality and to help families afford decent care. At the same time, there are compelling child and family health reasons for psychologists to support voluntary, part-paid, six-month leaves for infant care. For four weeks preceding and six weeks following childbirth, working mothers would be eligible for a fully paid maternity leave. The remainder of the leave would be made available on a part-paid basis to either parent in any combination they chose.

There is a Catch-22 in current public policies affecting day care in the United States. High-quality infant day care is expensive (if it is available at all), with fees ranging between $3,000 to $4,000 a year in many communities (*Child Care and Equal Opportunity for Women*, 1981). While good-quality infant day care thus remains beyond the reach of many working families, taking time out from the work force to care for a newborn is increasingly a luxury parents cannot afford.

Current public policy toward infant day care in the United States can best be summed up as "let the buyer beware." Not only have direct federal subsidies for day care for low-income families been reduced by

*Reprinted with permission from *American Psychologist*, Vol. 38, No. 1, 91–94. Copyright 1983 by the American Psychological Association, Inc.

20%, but also, under block grants, the federal standards designed to provide a minimum standard for the quality of care have been abandoned. As a result, some states, like Mississippi, have no statutory requirements regulating infant day care. Others, like Arizona, have extremely loose state licensing requirements, allowing one adult to care for as many as 10 children under two years of age even in federally funded centers (Administration for Children, Youth & Families, 1981).

Indirect subsidies for day care, in the form of a child-care tax credit, have expanded slightly to help offset the cost of care for some families. Working parents now qualify for a credit that ranges, depending on family income, from 20% to 30% of child-care expenses up to $2,400 a year for one child. But this credit benefits least the very lower-middle-income families who most need assistance with child care expenses, because the credit is nonrefundable and their tax liability may not be great enough to reap the full value of the credit. Furthermore, given the high cost of infant day care, the maximum $720 tax credit does not begin to make high-quality infant day care affordable.

At the same time, despite the reluctance to help make infant day care affordable, or even to minitor its quality, the United States does little to make the use of out-of-home care for infants less necessary. This nation has one of the highest rates of female participation in the labor force in the world, and the fastest growing segment of the work force is among mothers of children under age three. Yet the United States stands alone among advanced industrialized nations in having no statutory maternity leave policy. Unlike 75 other countries, including Canada, France, and West Germany, the United States has no provision guaranteeing a woman the right to leave work for a specified period to care for a baby, and no job protection or cash benefit to help compensate for not working because of pregnancy or childbirth (Kamerman, 1980; Kamerman & Kahn, 1981).

Nor do the majority of employed women in the United States have access to maternity leaves under private insurance or company benefits. Despite passage of the Pregnancy Discrimination Act in 1978, which requires that companies provide the same disability benefits to women who must take time off because of childbirth as they do to employees temporarily disabled for other reasons, only 40% of employed women have access to any maternity benefits (Kamerman & Kahn, 1981). These private disability benefits rarely involve full wage replacement and tend to cover no more than six weeks of time. Moreover, the disability benefits, by definition, amount to a medical leave, not a newborn child-care leave. There is no recognition that a healthy parent may have a psychological need for some time off to be with a new baby, or that a baby, in turn, may need some time to establish a relationship with at least one parent.

How have we come to such an impasse, where mothers and fathers of infants must be in the work force, psychologically safe day care is prohibitively expensive, and yet there is no funding to help either parent stay home for even a few months to take care of a baby? Unlike many European countries that have adopted day-care and maternity-leave policies as a pronatalist tool, the United States has at least until recently not been concerned about counteracting a declining birth rate. Nor has this nation, except in times of national crisis such as World War II or to combat rising welfare rolls, been motivated to advance day care as a device for encouraging women to join the work force. Furthermore, unlike many European countries, where there is a sense that society should help share the costs of childbearing, the United States has tended to believe that parents alone should finance the costs of bearing and raising children.

But there is also another important reason for the current policy impasse on infant day care in the United States, and that is the genuine difference of opinion among psychologists as to whether early group care is harmful to young children. Perhaps the late Selma Fraiberg (1977) best sums up one side of this debate when she, reflecting on her clinical experience, worries about "babies . . . who are delivered like packages to neighbors, to strangers, to storage houses like Merry Mites" and about what she sees as a resulting increase in the "diseases of non-attachment." On the other side, Jerome Kagan argues, on the basis of a study of children who entered day care as early as age three-and-half months, that day-care children are no more or less attached to their mothers than are young children raised exclusively at home (Kagan, Kearsley, & Zelazo, 1978).

Although empirical studies have produced little evidence that infant day care disrupts parent-child attachment or impedes the infant's cognitive development (Rutter, 1982), most of these studies have been conducted in high-quality, university-based centers with plenty of trained caregivers, not the kind of care most infants are in. Only 17% of children in out-of-home care are in licensed day-care facilities; the rest are in unlicensed family day-care homes (Ruopp & Travers, 1982). Few of the licensed facilities meet the conditions for safe infant day care laid down by Rutter (1982), who recommends that one adult caregiver be responsible for no more than three infants (the same staff-child ratio proposed by a coalition of child advocacy groups for revisions in the Federal Interagency Day Care Requirements in 1978). As for unlicensed family day care, this type of infant care varies the most in quality, with care ranging from the excellent to the horrible (Keyserling, 1972). Finally, few of the existing studies include children who entered day care as early as a few weeks after birth, a relatively recent phenomenon. To sum up, the amount of research on infant day care is not commensurate with the seriousness of the issue, and few of the existing longitudinal studies focus on the type of day care most infants actually experience.

While disturbingly little is known about the quality of infant day care in the United States, there is increasing evidence that the quality of care matters. And this is where psychologists should be able to agree and to join together to support measures to protect day care quality and to help families afford decent care. Small group size and a sufficient number of adult child-care workers are crucial to the quality of care, according to the National Day Care Study (Ruopp, Travers, Glantz, & Coelen, 1979). The study found that when infants were placed in too large groups with too few adults, the babies cried more or became withdrawn and apathetic. Lack of sufficient attention even led to exposure of infants to potential physical danger. Furthermore, as a study by Farber and Egeland (1982) indicates, infants who experience frequent changes in caregivers do exhibit the kinds of anxiety and insecure attachments to their mothers that critics of infant day care have long predicted.

There are also indications that caregiver training influences the outcome of infant day care. According to the National Day Care Study, child care workers with some training in early childhood education, child development, or day care spend more time playing and talking with children and praising, comforting, and instructing them. The children, in turn, do better on standardized tests (Ruopp et al., 1979). Sufficient verbal interaction between caregiver and child seems to be one of the keys to day care quality, with positive effects not only on children's language development, but also on their emotional adjustment (McCartney, Scarr, Phillips, Grajek, & Schwarz, 1982). Although more research is needed to identify other special features of day care quality, these preliminary findings should be brought home to Congress to show why federal standards for day care, particularly infant day care, are so vital.

Attention to infant day care standards alone is not enough, however. Given the expense of providing good-quality infant day-care (Ruopp & Travers, 1982) and the risks of settling for anything less, psychologists should also support alternatives to infant day care, such as a voluntary, six-month infant-care leave. Part of what we are advocating is a fully paid maternity leave to be taken up to four weeks prior to the birth and six weeks after. This option would help many working mothers through the fatigue that frequently accompanies the last weeks of pregnancy, and the initial recovery from childbirth up to the standard postpartum checkup following delivery. The six-week paid maternity leave would also contribute to the baby's physical well-being. There is a growing body of medical evidence concerning the protective benefits of breast-feeding (Udall et al., 1981). Given adequate job and income protection, many mothers would choose to stay at home for at least the first six weeks, when feedings take place at close, frequently irregular intervals.

The remainder of the six-month leave, on a part-paid basis, could be taken by either parent in any combination they chose, and its purpose would be to help ensure that the parent-infant relationship gets off to a smooth start. Recognizing the nonmedical reasons for the infant-care leave, it should be made available to adoptive as well as biological parents.

Although the six-month time limit on the proposed leave may seem arbitrary, and certainly deserves further study and consideration, we offer several reasons for proposing it. First, the process by which parents and infants communicate with each other is a subtle one in which each partner has to learn to pick up the other's cues. It takes time for this process to develop, and both parent and infant could benefit from a six-month get-acquainted period. By the age of six months, the infant's sleeping patterns are better established, and many breast-fed infants are weaned. Until a baby reaches six months of age, both parents are apt to suffer from frequent interruptions in their own sleep, and there is the added stress of just making room for a new human being. Although family coping strategies vary greatly, and although no parent should be forced to take an infant-care leave, there are compelling family as well as child-health reasons to make this leave available for a period of up to six months.

Support for offering a six-month infant-care leave also comes from the second thoughts many countries seem to be having about early entry into day care. Partly, the Europeans seem to have adopted maternity leaves as a way of making childbearing more attractive to working parents; partly, there has been a continuing concern about relatively high rates of infection in day-care centers (Kamerman & Kahn, 1981). In short, there seems to be a general consensus in many countries that it is better for the physical and emotional well-being of the mother and child if women stay home for at least a few months before returning to work.

Finally, we propose an optional six-month leave for infant care because this seems to be a feasible length of leave from work. In a study of child-care policies in 75 countries, Kamerman (1980) found that the average length of paid leave is between four and five months—the longest being nine months and the shortest being three months. Benefits average between 60% and 90% of a woman's wage, and the vast majority of women take advantage of the option. In Sweden, where child-care leave is available to fathers as well as to mothers, only 5% of fathers take at least one month of paid leave (Lamb, 1982). However, male eligibility for the benefit is said nonetheless to have mitigated against possible employment discrimination against young women (Kamerman & Kahn, 1981). None of the countries seem to think in terms of paid child-care leaves of more than a year, both because few working parents, even with their seniority and job protected, could afford any more interruption in their work.

Precisely what methods should be used to expand access to decent-quality infant day care and infant-care leaves will require further debate. But it is a debate psychologists have a responsibility to inform. With respect to infant day care, one possible method would be to alter the current child-care tax credits so that larger credits are granted for infant care, which is more expensive than preschool or after-school care because it is even more labor-intensive. This recommendation would be in keeping with a developmental approach to day care. Representative Barber Conable (R-New York), one of the original sponsors of the child-care tax credit legislation, has also proposed making the credit refundable and raising the maximum credit to 50% for those with incomes under $10,000 per year.

As for paid maternity and infant-care leaves, thinkers like Secretary of Health, Education and Welfare Wilbur Cohen, as well as Kamerman and Kahn, strongly urge making such benefits available through some form of social insurance. If efforts to extend maternity or infant-care leaves are confined to the private sector alone, they argue, large numbers of working parents will continue to go without coverage. One possible method would be to extend maternity leaves through state disability insurance. Five states (California, New Jersey, Rhode Island, Hawaii, and New York) already extend some maternity benefits to women under their statutory provisions for short-term and temporary disability leave (Catalyst, 1981). Although benefits are low, and although they would, by definition, cover only the first few weeks of *maternal* disability after childbirth, this may well be the place to begin (Kamerman, Kingston, & Kah, Note 1).

Another possible method for extending maternity and infant-care benefits, which has won favor with some conservatives, is to increase the personal tax exemption for the year in which a child is either born or adopted. As a small step in this direction, the Economic Recovery Tax Act of 1981 contained a provision allowing a $1,500 exemption for the adoption of certain children with special needs (Muenchow & Mc-Farland, 1982).

Any recommendation to extend social insurance or tax benefits to cover maternity and infant-care leaves may seem hopelessly out of touch with current fiscal realities. Although research is needed to determine the precise costs of extending such benefits (along with the cost of *not* doing so), there are some indications that part-paid six-month leaves for infant care would not be too costly. First, women's participation in the work force increasingly resembles that of men. When women are given maternity leaves, they do not stay out of the labor force permanently, but rather return soon after, perhaps with increased company loyalty. Furthermore, the new demographics show that an increasing number of married women are delaying childbirth until their careers are more established and that they are having fewer children—closer to two children than to three. Thus, when we recommend offering infant-care leaves, what we are really talking about is subsidizing two six-month leaves per family—not a very large amount of time when we consider that women, like men, have approximately a 45-year work span.

Women are in the work force to stay, and it is long past time for the United States to make some accommodations in policy to recognize this fact. Childless families may ask what stake they have in subsidizing infant-care leaves or day care for other people's children. But as families have fewer children, both present and future generations will have to rely on a proportionately smaller adult labor force to support both the very young and the very old. As Nicholas Hobbs often states, now that Americans are having fewer children, it behooves us to invest as much as we can in the children we have.

REFERENCE NOTE

1. Kamerman, S. B., Kingston, P., & Kahn, A. J. (1983). *Maternity policies and working women.* Book in preparation.

REFERENCES

Administration for Children, Youth and Families, Day Care Division (1981). *Report to Congress: Summary report of current state practices in Title XX-funded day care programs* (OHDS-81-30331). Washington, D.C.: U.S. Department of Health and Human Services, Office of Human Development.

Catalyst (May 1981). Parental leaves for child care. *Career and Family Bulletin*, No. 2, pp. 1–4.

Child care and equal opportunity for women (Clearinghouse Publication No. 67) (1981). Washington, D.C.: U.S. Commission on Civil Rights.

Farber, E. A., & Egeland, B. (1982). Developmental consequences of out-of-home care for infants in a low-income population. In E. F. Zigler & E. W. Gordon (Eds.), *Day Care: Scientific and social policy issues*. Boston: Auburn House.

Fraiberg, S. (1977). *Every child's birthright: In defense of mothering*. New York: Basic Books.

Kagan, J., Kearsley, R., & Zelazo, P. (1978). The effects of infant day care on psychological development. In J. Kagan (Ed.), *The growth of the child*. New York: W. W. Norton.

Kamerman, S. B. (Fall 1980). Maternity and parental benefits and leaves: An international review. *Impact on Policy Series*, Columbia University Center for the Social Sciences. (1).

Kamerman, S. B., & Kahn, A. J. (1981). *Child care, family benefits, and working parents. A study in comparative policy*. New York: Columbia University Press.

Keyserling, M. (1972). *Windows on day care*. New York: National Council of Jewish Women.

Lamb, M. (October 1982). Why Swedish fathers aren't liberated. *Psychology Today*, pp. 74–77.

McCartney, K., Scarr, S., Phillips, D., Grajek, S., & Schwarz, J. C. (1982). Environmental differences among day care centers and their effects on children's development. In E. F. Zigler & E. W. Gordon (Eds.), *Day care: Scientific and social policy issues*. Boston: Auburn House.

Muenchow, S., & McFarland, M. L. (Eds.) (1982). *What is pro-family policy? Proceedings of the Bush interest group/symposium*. New Haven, Conn.: Bush Center in Child Development and Social Policy, Yale University. (ERIC Document Reproduction Service No. PS 012 783).

Ruopp, R., & Travers, J. (1982). Janus faces day care: Perspectives on quality and cost. In E. F. Zigler & E. W. Gordon (Eds.), *Day care: Scientific and social policy issues*. Boston: Auburn House.

Ruopp, R., Travers, J., Glantz, F., & Coelen, C. (1979). *Children at the center* (Final rep. of the National Day Care Study). Cambridge, Mass.: Abt Books.

Rutter, M. (1982). Social-emotional consequences of day care for pre-school children. In E. F. Zigler & E. W. Gordon (Eds.), *Day care: Scientific and social policy issues*. Boston: Auburn House.

Udall, J. N., Colony, P., Fritze, L., Pang, K., Trier, J. S., & Walker, W. A. (1981). Development of gastrointestinal permeability to macro-molecules. *Pediatrics Research*, 15:245–249.

31

Child Custody and Divorce: A Lawyer's View

Henry H. Foster

New York University

The recommendations of child psychiatrists provide the substance and much of the content for the legal conclusion regarding the best interests of the child which must be reached by the court in cases where the contending parties cannot reach an agreement. In addition to his or her role as forensic expert, the child psychiatrist may be needed for treatment or therapy before, during, and after the divorce. Counseling may promote settlement of previously disputed issues. The applicable legal principles in child custody cases are amorphous but reflect current socioeconomic values. The former emphasis on parental fitness fortunately has given way to an emphasis of the child's welfare, which requires a prediction of the child's developmental needs and an assessment of interfamily relationships. The history of custodial law is summarized, the usual criteria that courts apply is examined, and the role of the expert witness is discussed.

The sociological function of law is to resolve disputes in accordance with the dominant values of the given time and place. Family law in general, and custodial law in particular, demonstrates the impact of social change upon legal principles. Alternative or new legal principles (mutations) appear once a new and strongly held consensus develops. This is possible due to the eclecticism and remarkable flexibility of the com-

Reprinted with permission from the *Journal of the American Academy of Child Psychiatry*, 1983, Vol. 22, No. 4, 392–398. Copyright 1983 by the American Academy of Child Psychiatry.

mon law, which, as Professor Paul Freund (1961) observed, has legal principles that march in battalions. It is this phenomenon which enables the common law to both change and to remain stable.

We are not here concerned with divorce or dissolution as such, since custodial disputes may arise within or outside of matrimonial actions. But it should be noted at the outset that the parties themselves determine custodial and visitation arrangements in over 90% of the cases and that such issues are litigated in but a small fraction of separations and divorces.

PREFERENCES AND PRESUMPTIONS

Due to principles derived from feudalism and religion, the father was the favored custodian of his children at common law. His claim, however, was conditioned upon his moral fitness, and able judges also referred to the best interests of children. Of course, only a few cases reached court and it is likely that the mother often retained custody where her circumstances permitted. It is also probable that, due to family, social and religious pressures, many fathers relinquished their prerogatives.

If we look behind the common law's preference for the father in child custody disputes, we find socioeconomic explanations. It was not pure whimsy or tradition. Religion and feudalism combined to make the father "lord and master" of his own household. Under the feudal system he was protector and guardian of his family. Under the common law property system, he controlled the family's purse strings. Upon marriage he acquired most of his wife's personal property, managed her real estate, and pocketed the profits. The wife (*feme covert*) was not a legal person; she could not make contracts, nor sue or be sued in her own name. Moreover, children became "young adults" at age 12, and could be put to work. Divorce, except for peers and the very wealthy theoretically was unobtainable, although there were other escape routes from "holy deadlock" such as annulment or desertion.

By mid-19th century, the industrial revolution, the change in wealth from land to property (tangible and intangible), and the migration to urban centers changed the structure of the family. Married Women's Property Acts were passed in most states which emancipated (at least in part) wives from their identity crisis. They achieved legal status, could own and dispose of property, make contracts, and sue and be sued in their own name. Compulsory school attendance laws were enacted, and a few states experimented with child labor laws.

The typical household consisted of a breadwinner husband and a homemaker wife and mother, and middle class children were expected to complete high school. The law's reaction to such significant social and economic change was to adopt as a model the typical household and division of labor. It logically followed that the mother was the preferred custodian for the children and the father, if he wanted to, could get visitation rights. This was the effect of the "tender years doctrine."

As had been true in the case of the paternal preference, the mother's entitlement to custody was not absolute. In both cases the claimant had to be a "fit" parent, and especially during the Victorian age that meant moral and sexual orthodoxy. Percy Bysshe Shelley, in 1817, lost custody of his and Harriet's daughters because of his professed atheism and notorious profligacy, and some 62 years later Mary Besant was deprived of custody because she had publicly espoused birth control. Moral activism was rampant during the 19th century, and only a few persons had heard of Sigmund Freud.

Commencing in the 1920s, American custodial law became more concerned about "best interests" and less worried about meting out rewards and punishments. In most states, the mere fact that the husband established a fault ground for divorce no longer qualified him for custody, even though the divorce ground was adultery. The "tender years doctrine" was applied except where the mother's immorality was believed to jeopardize the future well-being of the children.

As long as most husbands worked outside the home and most wives worked within, the preference for the mother in child custody decisions was functional, and it was backed up by a consensus. The emergence of the new Women's Movement after World War II and the phenomenal increase in the number of women in the work force changed the 19th century image into an obsolete stereotype. The sexual revolution, the switching of parental roles and division of labor, necessitated some changes in custodial law. And the law, somewhat reluctantly, gave in to the emerging consensus.

Legitimate demands for racial and sexual equality gained a fixed basis in the Equal Protection Clause of the Federal Constitution and E.R.A. amendments to some state constitutions. Egalitarian principles achieved popular acceptance despite difficulties of implementation. Laws that discriminated *for* as well as *against* women fell under constitutional challenges. This meant that the "tender years doctrine" was no longer viable as a preference or a presumption.

The current situation in the United States is that, theoretically, fathers and mothers have equal claims to child custody, and the best interests of the child determine the choice. In perhaps 90% of the cases, however, custody is still awarded to the mother and visitation to the father. In part this is because most fathers do not want custody. In some cases, however, judges are prejudiced in favor of mothers or against fathers and the "best interests" test is so amorphous that the result may be rationalized. A few judges may privately agree with the Utah court even though they keep their bias off the record. The Utah court said that it would agree that fathers had an equal claim to child custody once it was established that men could lactate (*Arends* v. *Arends*, 1974).

Even though the father defeats the mother and prevails only in rare instances, courts are becoming accustomed to paternal claims for sole custody and for joint custody. Such claims no longer are quixotic. A Dr. Salk may obtain sole custody (especially where the children prefer the father), and under proper circumstances most courts will consider joint custody as a possibility.

Thus, in response to social change and functional considerations the pendulum has swung from father to mother to either or to both. We have reached, or are reaching, the point where the facts of the individual case, rather than a presumption or preference, determine the result.

We have been discussing the law of child custody thus far in terms of "preferences" rather than "presumptions" because the latter seems to be too strong a term where the conflict is between parents and the claim of either is conditioned on parental fitness. Where the contest is between a parent and a "stranger" (meaning any nonparent), however, it is appropriate to say that there is a *presumption* favoring the parent. The stranger must, even today, introduce strong and convincing proof of paternal unfitness in order to win a custody dispute against a natural parent. He must rebut the presumption that a child belongs with his parent. The mere fact that the child might be better off with the stranger is insufficient; there must be proof of abandonment, neglect, or abuse for the stranger to win.

To phrase it differently, for a stranger to prevail, it is not enough to show that the child's best interests would be served by an award of custody to the stranger. The legal concept of abandonment, however, permits some flexibility. If the natural parent is deemed to have relinquished parental rights voluntarily it may be tantamount to an abandonment. For example, in the leading New York case of *Bennett* v. *Jeffreys* (1975), a 15-year-old natural mother had placed her baby with a family friend for 8 years before she demanded her return. The New York Court of Appeals held: "[the] State may not deprive a parent of the custody of a child absent surrender [for adoption], abandonment, persistent neglect, unfitness or *other like extraordinary circumstances*. If any such extraordinary circumstances are present, the disposition of custody is influenced or controlled by what is in the best interests of the child" [emphasis supplied]. The case was remanded to the Family Court for further hearing while the child stayed with the natural mother. The testimony of some 26 witnesses over a 4-week trial resulted in the finding that the child [Gina Marie] should be returned to the foster mother, but with liberal visitation privileges for the natural mother. The record in the extensive hearing established that while the natural mother met the physical needs she could not supply the emotional needs of Gina Marie, who still referred to the foster parent as "mother" and insisted that she wanted to return "home" after spending some 15 months with the natural mother until, at last, there was a final disposition.

In addition to the outmoded maternal preference and presumption favoring a natural parent over a stranger, there are additional considerations in child custody disputes that may be called "factors" which enter into the court's determination. Formerly, the one who prevailed in a divorce case ordinarily got custody of the children if he or she wanted it. This no longer is the case, especially where there are no-fault grounds for divorce.

The wishes of the child regarding custody and visitation is called the child's "preference." At most, the child's preference will be considered in the exercise of the court's discretion in determining custody and visitation, and the weight it receives will depend upon the maturity of the particular child and the circumstances of the case.

Still another factor is that, where possible, courts avoid splitting siblings and prefer that they remain in the same household. Of course, in some cases for practical reasons this cannot be done. Still another factor is the court's inclination to award custody to the parent who intends to remain in the community and to deny custody to a parent who plans to move to another jurisdiction.

Closely related to the factor of geographical location is the consideration of which parent or contestant is most cooperative in providing access to the other in order to maintain an on-going relationship with the child, including telephonic communication. This factor is gaining increasing recognition and sometimes is couched in terms of the child's right to know and associate with both parents after the parents separate or divorce.

Finally, although the proprietary rights of parents in children are somewhat muted, they still exist. At its 1982 term, the Supreme Court held that before a parent could be *permanently* deprived of his or her parental rights, abandonment, neglect or unfitness must be established by *clear and convincing evidence* and that a mere preponderance of evidence was not enough. Exactly what impact this decision may have in contests between a natural parent and a psychological parent remains to be seen.

BASIC CRITERIA FOR DECISION

Courts depend upon counsel, in large measure, to develop the facts in a custody dispute. Unfortunately perhaps, skill and advocacy are influential as to outcome. Not all lawyers are equal. Not all expert witnesses are equally articulate and effective. The glib lawyer or expert witness may be most convincing even though greater merit is on the other side. Form (of presentation) as well as substance is important in a courtroom, in politics, and in most activities of life.

Judges, like academics or psychiatrists, have their own scales of value and accord different weight to different factors or criteria. Today, at least in metropolitan areas, medical or psychiatric evidence is crucial in the trial of most noncommercial cases. In custody disputes, as often as not, it is the testimony of the psychiatrist or psychologist that determines the result. Where impressive experts appear for each side, they may cancel each other out. Moreover, the testimony of a court-appointed psychiatrist or psychologist may be regarded as more "impartial" and hence entitled to receive greater credibility than the testimony of a party's expert.

The ultimate question in most custody cases is what decision regarding custody and visitation serves the best interests of the children. All other considerations are subordinate to that ultimate issue where the contest is between parents. The difficulty with the "best interests" rule is that it is so broad and amorphous that it may encompass any result. It has not been shown, however, that "the least detrimental alternative" test would be an improvement, and it too is largely a matter of subjective judgment. In any event, the courts still adhere to the "best interests" formulation.

The practical problem is to break up the abstract "best interests" concept into smaller components. A court or lawyer having access to expert psychiatric opinion will be inclined to emphasize the psychological best interest of the child in question. Heed will be taken as to which contestant has the closer bond with the child and the child's needs as to care, nurture, and training. To whom does the child turn in case of need? Which one does the real parenting? The quality as well as the quantity of time spent with the child may be significant. The willingness of each to cooperate in maintaining an on-going meaningful relationship with the other parent is significant.

Currently, courts are constrained not to get involved in comparing material advantages or disadvantages unless it has a bearing on the health of a child. Today, most courts are tolerant of alternative lifestyles, although prejudice has not been completely eliminated. Lesbian mothers have been deprived of custody but perhaps the weight of authority requires some proof of actual detriment to the child. For example, a New York court understandably was upset by proof that the live-in lover of the lesbian mother was constantly running down the father and was attempting to undermine his relationship with his children. Illinois, however, in *Jarrett* v. *Jarret* (1979), took a long step backward when it took three protesting daughters from their mother's home merely because after divorce she had a live-in male lover. Where there is a judicial overreaction to what a particular court may regard as gross immorality (usually meaning sex life), the gravest harm and injustice may be occasioned by self-righteous moral activists.

Another situation which invites error is where chauvinism (in its original sense) is operative. The California court, after the death of the father, awarded children to the custody of relatives rather than to their Czechoslovakian mother who had remained behind the "iron curtain" when the father fled to America with the children. The highly publicized Chicago case of Walter Polovchal in 1980 also had chauvinistic overtones when the Department of State intervened to block the minor son's return to the USSR. Recent press reports related that a Georgia court took the children away from two Harvard graduates who had turned "hippy." Of course, it may have been their educational background rather than their lifestyle that the Georgia court found most offensive.

In sum, the most relevant criteria in child custody cases are those that have a direct bearing on the child's development and maturation in a warm and loving environment. Matters that have no direct bearing, such as the private sex life of the custodian, should be ignored. The focus should be placed upon the child's emotional and psychological well being, not upon the alleged moral unfitness of the particular custodian. Of course, parental unfitness sometimes may be one side of the coin and detriment to the child may be the other side of the same coin. The court, however, may best promote justice to the child by concentrating on the *child's* welfare and detriment.

One of the most comforting things to a judge who handles custody disputes is the knowledge that if he makes a mistake it is subject to later correction. Custody and visitation awards in most states are not final; they may be, and frequently are, modified. There have been criticisms regarding the lack of finality in custody decisions and it has been recommended that, once an award is made, it should not be subject to modification. Texas, by statute, forbids modification for 6 months after the initial order. From a lawyer's point of view, this is throwing the baby out with the bathwater. The margin for error in the initial disposition is too great, and to protect the child there must be power to modify. This does not mean, however, that there should not be strict requirements of proof in order to obtain modification, nor that the security and continuity of the parent-child relationship is not an important and often decisive factor in modification proceedings.

TYPES OF CUSTODIAL ARRANGEMENTS

In divorce cases the favored placement is an award of the child (or children) to one parent for custodial purposes with visitation rights granted to the other. The legal custodian usually is granted autonomy and does not have to share decision making with the other parent, although by agreement or decree some issues such as schooling or religious training, may be subjects for mutual decision. The terms of visitation depend upon numerous factors, including geographic proximity, school and work schedules, the desires and needs of the parents and children, and how visitation previously worked out in practice.

Courts generally seek to accord "reasonable visitation" to the noncustodial parent and to perpetuate meaningful on-going parent-child relationships. What is deemed to be "reasonable" depends upon all of the facts and circumstances of the individual case. However, it is quite common to award weekend visitation every other weekend in the case of school-age children, plus alternating holidays and a period of some weeks during the summer vacation. Sometimes a weekday dinner is added for the parent having visitation. Preschool-age children are accorded more selective treatment and in the case of many teenage adolescents, they visit when and if they feel like it, no matter what the court decree provides.

Within the past decade there had been a tremendous increase in the number of cases where the father seeks either sole custody or joint custody with the mother. Occasionally, courts have awarded joint custody in contested proceedings but ordinarily joint custody occurs where the parties consent to that arrangement. The term "joint custody" comprehends (a) joint decision making on major child rearing issues, and (b) a sharing of physical possession. Of course, minor issues may have to be decided on an *ad hoc* basis by the one in immediate control, and the sharing of physical possession need not be on an equal time basis. Some "joint custody" arrangements are difficult to distinguish on an operational level from sole custody plus "reasonable visitation." Moreover, some separate families have tried a "nesting" arrangement where the parents take turns moving into and out of the family home while the children stay put.

There is little disagreement over joint custody as an ideal. As often stated, it most closely resembles the situation which existed when there was an intact family, and a child should have the right to an on-going and meaningful relationship with both parents. The problem, however, is workability. The experience of most judges and lawyers has been that, to be workable, joint custody requires optimal conditions. There must be geographical proximity, a favorable school and work schedule, suitable physical arrangements, and a spirit of parental cooperation that places the child's welfare foremost. Unfortunately, these favorable conditions usually do not exist. Moreover, samplings of public opinion suggest that most fathers do not want sole or joint custody.

Notwithstanding the practical problems inherent in joint custody arrangements, since the publication of Roman and Haddod's (1978) book, *The Disposable Parent*, concerted efforts have been made throughout the country to make joint custody the preferred arrangement. A few states, including California, New Hampshire, Nevada, and New Mexico, have statutes that seek to make joint custody the norm and mandate that, where both parents agree, a presumption arises in its favor. If the court fails to award joint custody, it must set forth its reasons. If sole custody is awarded, the court is directed to favor the parent most likely to give frequent access to the other parent. Other states have passed statutes that in effect merely authorize the court to consider and award joint custody.

Joint custody should be reserved for exceptional circumstances, such as where civilized parents generally agree as to what is for the best interests of the children and feel free to communicate regarding their welfare. Moreover, court ordered joint custody may be a "cop out" for a particular court that wishes to avoid a meticulous assessment of the facts of the individual case. A father's demand for sole or joint custody also may be part of an overall strategy in divorce litigation.

Although I question the practicality and wisdom of California-type statutes, I do agree that lawyers and therapists as well as courts should be alert to the fact that joint custody may be a viable alternative when conditions are favorable. Far too often in the past the alternative was overlooked. Finally, the emphasis upon maintaing access to both parents generally is in the child's best interests, and usually it would be highly detrimental to give the custodial parent a veto over visitation as recommended in Goldstein et al. (1973, p. 38).

JUDICIAL ATTITUDE TOWARD EXPERT TESTIMONY

Courts react to expert testimony in various ways depending in part on the training, background, and experience of the individual judge. A few judges are psychiatrically oriented; perhaps more are cynical about expert testimony in general and psychiatric testimony in particular. One reason for cynicism is the so-called "battle of the experts" which is often staged in court. The court's own staff or witness may be more convincing than forensic stars.

The model judge keeps an open mind, hears both sides, is skeptical regarding expert testimony, and conscientiously weighs the evidence. The judge is no amateur when it comes to fact finding. Moreover, the court, under our form of government, is the agency responsible for the community's conscience and that is answerable to a consensus. Whether an accused should be convicted or acquitted upon his defense of insanity ordinarily is a social and moral decision, and the same often is true on the issue of who gets custody.

Thus, the role or function of the expert in child development, when he testifies as a witness, is to provide grist for the judicial mill. Often the expert testimony will be crucial or decisive, but at other times it will be offset by competing expert testimony or significant facts and circumstances. In Europe, the prevalent model is to hear the testimony of the senior professor at the forensic science institute and rarely is the senior contradicted. In this country, however, cross examination and rebuttal testimony are at the heart of our due process.

There are frequent proposals that we abandon the adversary process for a panel of experts, especially in child custody disputes. Even if constitutional, the wisdom of such a move is highly questionable. Far better and more acceptable under our system is the adaptation of the adversary process in the handling of child placement issues. Such may be done by helping to ensure that the court has access to all relevant facts and opinions in custody cases. Two techniques may accomplish that end:

first, for such cases the court needs a competent professional staff to investigate and report; and, second, in contested cases ordinarily the child or children need and deserve their own counsel.

ROLE OF THE CHILD PSYCHIATRIST

From the lawyer's point of view, the child psychiatrist or other expert on child development may have two functions in connection with custody litigation. The two roles are distinct but interrelated. One involves evaluation, treatment, counseling, or therapy. The other is forensic: the specialist is a potential witness.

With regard to evaluation, the individual child psychiatrist must determine whether or not he must see the family and its members or merely the child or children. For purposes of testimony, ordinarily, where possible, it is better for the expert to see the entire family constellation since then his or her findings and opinions will carry greater weight and conviction. He will have seen the whole picture, including the interrelationships among family members.

Due to the trauma occasioned by the divorce and postdivorce process to children as well as parents, a program of treatment may be in order for the children. The potential legal difficulty in such situations is that there may be a conflict of interests. The psychiatrist should make it clear, preferably in writing, what his or her ground rules are when he accepts such a child as a patient, and what, if any, disclosures he or she intends to make to a particular parent. If properly handled, confidentiality will be owed to the child patient, not to his parent, even though the latter pays the bills. A parent's waiver of confidentiality (such as by bringing a custody action) may not be held to be a waiver by the patient-child.

In some states, moreover, a rule has developed that the psychiatrist may come under the larger umbrella of lawyer-client privilege where the lawyer engages the psychiatrist to assist him by interviewing the lawyer's client or the child before trial. If the psychiatrist takes the witness stand, however, there may be a waiver of confidentiality.

The child psychiatrist or other expert also serves an important function in trial preparation. Lawyers differ as to their levels of sophistication (if any) with reference to psychiatric knowledge and insights. The experienced forensic expert may be valuable for determining trial strategy and tactics in general as well as the form and content of his own testimony. Similarly, the experienced trial lawyer may help the expert to articulate his facts and opinions in most convincing fashion. The fact that the expert is subjected to cross-examination by the other side should not be viewed as an insult, because if no questions are forthcoming, it could mean that the expert's testimony was ineffectual.

PRACTICAL TIPS FOR THE EXPERT WITNESS

The child psychiatrist who is called upon to testify in a custody dispute should be aware that as an "expert" he is a privileged character. Most of us are not free to voice opinions from the witness stand. The "expert" is an exception, whether his testimony is in response to hypothetical questions or in normal fashion. Moreover, the individual psychiatrist may testify as a treating physician at one point, and as an expert at another, in which event he or she is entitled to ordinary witness fees for the former and the fees of an expert for the latter.

It is an old ruse for the cross-examining attorney to ask the expert if he is being paid for his opinion, and if so, how much? Although it is tempting to respond that he is being paid for his time not his opinion, be wary of fencing with lawyers. They are on their own turf, and the odds are against you. It is best to state accurately the financial facts and not to give hostile counsel an opening. Badgering a witness often is counter-productive. Do not play into the cross-examiner's hands by showing anger, justified or not.

If you have overgeneralized or failed to note exceptions or qualifications in your testimony, freely admit such to be the case. Remember, the lawyer who called you will have a chance to "rehabilitate" your testimony if need be on re-direct examination. The favorite tactic of the cross-examiner is to get you out on a limb and have *you* saw it off. The fall may be precipitous. That may be avoided by sticking to facts and opinions you can back up and document. If there is room for a difference in opinion, graciously acknowledge such to be the case.

Insist upon a careful briefing and preparation before trial so that you will know in general and in advance what the questions will be on direct examination and what the probable questions will be on cross-examination. Do not get up tight about challenges to your professional status or reputation. Attacking the credibility of a witness is standard practice and should not be taken personally.

With regard to custody and visitation issues, show flexibility, because you may be dealing with a *prediction* as to future behavior. Where possible, speak in terms of the child's needs and desires, apart from those of a parent. For example, a child's need to know and associate with both parents may carry more weight than a parent's need to see the child. There are some things you may say with more assurance than others. As for the latter, be prepared to qualify or explain.

The expertise of the child psychiatrist that may be decisive is his other awareness of the dynamics of particular relationships. If the expert is able to describe fairly what is going on within the family and its inter-relationships, it will be a positive aid to the court's decision. Reasons and examples supporting any recommendation or evaluation and, in some cases, psychological testing, may give weight to expert testimony. Courts are more interested in family dynamics than in psychiatric labels.

Finally, remember the compromising character of law. In most custody cases neither contestant wins a clear-cut victory. One (usually the mother) gets custody and the other (usually the father) gets reasonable visitation rights. Unless there are exceptional facts or circumstances, that result is predictable.

CONCLUSION

The law of child custody is not written in stone. In a given case a particular judge weighs and balances all of the facts and evidence presented before him. The opinion or recommendation of a child psychiatrist regarding custody is only one of the elements considered. Increasingly, however, such testimony is crucial and decisive.

The recommendations of the Group for the Advancement of Psychiatry, Committee on the Family (1981), set forth criteria to be used in decision making in custody cases:

The court's determination should aim at providing the child with an ongoing relationship with as many members of his or her family of origin as possible. . . .

The court should not confirm the moral condemnation of one parent by the other since the child's welfare is badly served by the loss of trust such condemnations engender. . . .

In determining parental competence, the court should seriously consider the comparative willingness of the two contestants to provide the child access to the other parent, to siblings, grandparents, and other relatives.

The child should not be considered merely a passive recipient of parental care but also a concerned and willing source of support for both parents . . . the child has a need to express and channel concern about all family members, including the noncustodial parent (146–147).

The above criteria were respectfully recommended to courts that adjudicate custody matters. Of course, they are not the only factors for decision making and due to the eclectic nature of law they are not the only guidelines courts will consider. Moreover, it may be somewhat naive to suggest that courts should not "confirm the moral condemnations of one parent," especially if the claimed immorality has a direct bearing on the child's welfare. At best we may hope that courts will focus on detriment to the child rather than upon parental "unfitness" as such.

Both law and psychiatry get into the business of predicting future human behavior. That is dangerous territory. There are so many variables. And humility is in short supply. A custody decision is a prediction as to what is best for the child. Fortunately, if there be egregious error, the prediction is subject to modification upon review. Although from the psychiatric point of view continuity, stability, and the security of child placement may be paramount, from the legal point of view it is a blessing that where need be child custody may be changed.

Goldstein et al. (1973) in *Beyond the Best Interests of the Child* pose the case of the Dutch Jews who left their children with gentile surrogates during World War II and what was to be done with the children when surviving Jewish parents returned. The Dutch authorities handed the children over to their natural parents. The eminent authors suggest that the children remain with the surrogates. From this lawyer's point of view, there should be no rule of thumb; each case should be decided on the basis of its individual facts. Psychiatric generalizations should not decide concrete cases. It should be the dynamics of the individual case that controls the particular result. And the psychiatric recommendation or prediction is but grist for the mill.

REFERENCES

Arends v. *Arends*, 517 P.2d 1019, 1020 (Utah, 1974).

Bennett v. *Jeffreys*, 40 N.Y. 2d 543, 387 N.Y.S. 2d 821, 356 N.E. 2d 277 (1975).

Freund, P. (1961). *The Supreme Court of the United States: Its Businesses, Purposes and Enforcement.* Cleveland: World Publishing.

Goldstein, J., Freud, A. & Solnit, A. J. (1973). *Beyond the Best Interests of the Child.* New York: The Free Press.

Group for the Advancement of Psychiatry, Committee on Family Law (1981). *Divorce, Child Custody and the Family.* San Francisco: Jossey-Bass. Reprinted as: *New Trends in Child Custody Determinations.* New York: Law & Business Inc./Harcourt Brace Jovanovich, 1981.

Jarrett v. *Jarret*, 78 Ill.2d 337, 36 Ill. Dec 1, 400 N.E.2d 421 (1979).

Roman, M. & Haddod, W. (1978). *The Disposable Parent.* New York: Penguin Books.

32

Psychologists Look at Television: Cognitive, Developmental, Personality, and Social Policy Implications

Jerome L. Singer

Yale University

Dorothy G. Singer

Yale University and University of Bridgeport

The omnipresence of the television set in American homes and its extensive use suggest that it may now be considered a basic source of input for the growing child. This article points to some issues concerning the continuing exposure of the child to this special medium that require examination by cognitive, developmental, and personality psychologists. A series of studies are reviewed dealing with the structural format and content of commercial television and the problems that they pose for the developing child—the possible influences on cognitive skills, imagination, beliefs, motor controls, and aggression. The relationships between family lifestyle and television viewing by the child are also considered. Evidence accumulates suggesting that heavy viewing of currently available television fare by children may

Reprinted with permission from *American Psychologist*, 1983, Vol. 38, No. 7, 826–834. Copyright 1983 by the American Psychological Association, Inc.

A portion of this article was presented by the first author as the Leonard S. Kogan Memorial Lecture at the City University of New York, October 21, 1980.

Some of the research described herein was supported by grants from the National Science Foundation, the Spencer Foundation, the American Broadcasting Company, and the Teleprompter Corporation.

be harmful. Research suggesting potential benefits of the medium for education and constructive development has not generally been translated into regular age-specific programming for children by the television industry. Avenues for intervention by psychologists with parents, educators, and industry are reviewed and possible further exploration of social policy involvements by resarchers are considered.

Our collaboration on investigations of television and child development emerged from interests in tracing the origins of adult consciousness and imagination back to early manifestations of children's make-believe play and to the cognitive developmental stages and social influences on the emergence of fantasy (D. Singer & Revenson, 1978; J. Singer, 1973). In direct observations of children at play and in talks with parents and nursery school teachers, it became increasingly apparent that the content and structure of children's fantasy activities were reflecting consistent and extensive exposure to television. As we began to explore through direct research some of the possible influences of television on young children, we found ourselves drawn further and further into confrontation with problems and possibilities bearing on the cognitive, developmental, personality, and social policy implications of the medium.

We found ourselves trying to understand basic issues of the cognitive processing sequence in relation to the structural format of television; for example, how much sense do children at different ages make of the rapidly paced, much interrupted, nonrepetitive quality of most commercial television and also of programs designed presumably especially for children (J. Singer, 1980; J. Singer & D. Singer, 1976, 1983; Tower, Singer, Singer, & Biggs, 1979)?

In attempting to understand television's impact on overt behavior as well as on imagination, we felt it necessary to conduct longitudinal field studies correlating children's naturalistic behavior with the frequency and type of home television viewing that characterized them in preschool and early elementary school ages (D. Singer & J. Singer, 1980; J. Singer & D. Singer, 1981).

Recognizing that television viewing might itself reflect patterns of a broader family life-style, we were led further into considering parental values and household routines that might separately or in association with television viewing influence children's cognitive, affective, and behavioral patterns (J. Singer & D. Singer, 1981).

We also found it necessary to look at elementary school performances such as reading, academic adjustment, and so forth, as correlates of parent and child home-viewing patterns (Zuckerman, Singer, & Singer, 1980).

Inevitably we were drawn to considering whether particular kinds of programming might have constructive possibilities in stimulating imaginativeness, positive emotionality, and greater social or ethical awareness (Tower, Singer, Singer, & Biggs, 1979; D. Singer, J. Singer, & Dodsworth-Rugani, Note 1).

When our data as well as related research by others increasingly pointed to potential hazards of heavy viewing (especially of aggressive content) for young children and also to some constructive possibilities of selective viewing with parental guidance, we were drawn into applied research designed to evaluate methods of influencing parents and educators toward a more effective use of the medium (D. Singer & J. Singer, 1982; D. Singer, J. Singer, & Zuckerman, 1980; J. Singer & D. Singer, 1981). This led to actual preparation of a series of school lesson plans with associated videotape demonstrations designed to orient children about the television medium, its structure, hazards, and potentials, and how to approach it more critically (D. Singer, J. Singer, & Zuckerman, 1981).

Our increasing sense of the importance of the medium and of the gap between developmental psychology research evidence and the lore of the industry led us to consultation with writers, producers, and industry executives, and eventually to social policy conferences with communication lawyers, federal commissioners, and industry self-regulatory agencies.

As social scientists our stance has been that opinions are cheap but that systematic data collection and careful evaluation of evidence is the special contribution we can bring to these fields. We have tried wherever possible to propose and to carry out research relevant to questions that arise.

In what follows we should like to examine some specific areas that are being increasingly studied not only in our own work but by a slowly growing number of investigators. In highlighting our own research, we do not mean in any way to minimize others' work but to exemplify that once one gets to carefully looking at the television medium, one cannot avoid issues that touch on basic theoretical and applied psychology.

COGNITIVE AND AFFECTIVE ISSUES IN THE STRUCTURE OF TELEVISION

A special property of American television certainly, and perhaps increasingly of television production in other nations, is the rapid pace of presentation of material with constant intercutting, interruption, and shifts in sound levels. Our commercial television is primarily designed to keep the viewers' attention on the screen. This is accomplished quite skillfully by producers who know to shift sequences rapidly, zoom in and zoom out, and suddenly introduce new settings, loud music, new characters, and a variety of special effects. Foreigners not used to American television, watching the brief segments, the constant interruptions by brief rapid-fire commercials, and the quick changes of pace even within plot sequences, as well as the heavy emphasis on physical action, report that it is disorganizing and often arouses anger or almost physical distress. But American children have grown up with this pattern of quick-paced stimulus presentation, and this must indeed be a new kind of experience never before a part of the perceptual environment of the child in civilization.

Here, then, we confront the major question about this medium. A cognitive analysis suggests that because cognitive processing takes place over time, effective learning and storage of material presented requires some mental replaying and rehearsal with an occasional opportunity to shift one's attention away from the set and reflect on what was seen. If new material is piled on top of other material, particularly irrelevant contents, can one really intelligently sit and reexamine information? (See Wright & Huston, 1983, in this issue and Collins, 1982.)

Our own studies with deliberately slow-paced, repetitively structured preschool children's programs such as *Mr. Rogers' Neighborhood* or the Australian *Here's Humphrey* suggest that carefully designed, age-specific formats are not only well-received by children but yield gains in cognitive and affective areas (J. Singer & D. Singer, 1976; Tower, Singer, Singer, & Biggs, 1979; D. Singer, J. Singer, & Dodsworth-Rugani, Note 1). Researchers are increasingly defining an area of study examining how children's attention and comprehension are influenced by the formal features of the television medium. A related question of increasing interest in the area of developmental cognition bears on how children come to identify and to make sense of the special codes of television; for example, when and how do children learn to discriminate a pictorial flashback or reminiscence scene from a mere change of location (Bryant & Anderson, 1983; Collins, 1982; see also Wright & Huston, 1983, in this issue)? There has been concern that the powerful visual components of television may create an atmosphere conducive to a passive, nondiscriminating viewing set or that the story-telling of television may lead to an easy escape for persons whose own inner lives are troubled or dysphoric (Csikszentmihalyi & Kubey, 1981; McIlwraith & Schallow, 1983, in press; J. Singer, 1980). Salomon (1981) has proposed that television does not demand as strong an amount of invested mental effort

(AIME) as does reading and that often it does not therefore contribute as well to learning or to the experience of personal self-efficacy. Changes in television format or the encouragement of children to watch more actively may enhance their capacity to gain useful knowledge from the medium. Examining the special properties of television can teach us about children's processing capacities but can also point the way toward more effective use of the medium to promote learning and prosocial skills.

BEHAVIORAL CORRELATES OF HOME TELEVISION VIEWING IN YOUNG CHILDREN: RESULTS OF FIELD STUDIES

A major conclusion of the recent update of the 1972 Surgeon General's report on television was that evidence supports a general learning effect of exposure to television. Heavy viewing especially of violent programming is consistently associated with aggressive behavior in children and adults, but there is also considerable evidence of prosocial learning, for example, cooperativeness, sharing, and imaginativeness under specific conditions (Pearl, Bouthilet, & Lazar, 1982; see also Rubinstein, 1983, in this issue). A recent analysis of a large number of studies by Hearold (1979) does suggest, however, that imitation of aggressive material seems to generalize more extensively, whereas prosocial behavior is more specifically and narrowly enhanced by television exposure. Increasing efforts have been made to control for a range of alternative explanations of the correlations linking heavy viewing to aggression (Eron, 1982; Huesmann, 1982; Milavsky, Kessler, Stipp, & Rubens, 1982). Such alternative possibilities include the likelihood that aggressive children may simply prefer more violent programming or that aggressive children imitate parents who are themselves overtly violent and may also prefer violent television. Statistical analyses involving cross-lag correlational procedures and multiple regression analyses in which sociocultural and familial variables are partialed out are therefore increasingly employed.

In our own earlier studies, two groups of preschool children were each followed over a year's time. Home television logs were sampled for a 2-week period several times during the year while direct observations of the spontaneous play and aggression of the children were recorded by observers (blind to the home-viewing scores) during these periods. We consistently found that heavy viewing especially of aggressive action adventure or cartoon shows was linked to overt aggression and that neither the preferential-viewing hypothesis nor the family aggression pattern could explain away such results (D. Singer & J. Singer, 1980; J. Singer & D. Singer, 1981).

Family Patterns and the Television Environment: Toward a Broader Model

More recently, in collaboration with Wanda Rapaczynski, we have attempted a longer term look at how parental patterns, household routines, and the child's television environment may interact to yield predictions across time of later cognitive and behavioral patterns in children studied over a period from ages 4 through 9. From a sample of somewhat more than 100 children whom we could study through home TV-logs, direct observation, and parent interviews at home and at the TV Center at various times, we will briefly describe results for the 84 children for whom we have complete data on the dependent and independent variables. These children's television-viewing patterns as preschoolers in 1976–1977 were available, and they were again observed and interviewed in 1980, 1981, and 1982. TV-logs were also available for those years, and parents were interviewed about family life-style patterns and filled out questionnaires about childrearing patterns, personal values, and so forth, during each of those years.

Table 1 presents the structural format of our approach. The left-hand column reflects the various kinds of home factors that could conceivably influence or predict a series of dependent variables—the children's cognitive, imaginative, motoric, aggressive, and attitudinal orientations, which are represented in the right-hand column. The growing child experiences parents who emphasize or value certain characteristics in their own personalities, for example, reliability (e.g., stability or conventionality), social relationships, resourcefulness (e.g., independence, curiosity, creativity, imagination [Tower, 1980]). The parents also show specific belief systems, for example, a sense of a mean and scary world (Gerbner, Gross, Morgan, & Signorielli, 1980a). Parents also adopt particular disciplinary and childrearing attitudes, for example, emphasis on physical punishment or related power-assertive methods. The family may be under continuing stress, for example, bereavement, divorce, illness, unemployment of breadwinner. Finally, daily household routines and life-styles may vary and children may experience more or less regular sleep patterns and so forth. Factor analyses reduced the measures assessing these characteristics to a manageable number of independent variables.

A second category of potential influence or prediction of later behavior

TABLE 1

Home Influences and Cognitive or Behavioral Measures in a Longitudinal Study

Home influences (Independent variables)	Cognitive and behavioral patterns (Dependent variables) 1980, 1981, 1982
Family characteristics Parents' self-described values, e.g., resourcefulness (imagination, curiosity, adventurousness, creativity). Parents' attitudes toward discipline and child-rearing, e.g., power-assertive versus inductive methods. Parents' belief-systems: mean and scary world test. Family structure and stress level: single-parent family, etc.	Cognition Reading scores (recognition and comprehension) Language use Academic adjustment Beliefs
Daily life-style sleep patterns organized daily routines diverse cultural activities emphasis on outdoor sports, etc.	Imagination Inkblots, interview, block play, birthday party script Comprehension of television content (1982) *Swiss Family Robinson* plot Commercial understanding
Television environment Average weekly viewing (1977, 1980, 1981, 1982) Type of programming, e.g., action-adventure (realistic or fantasy), cartoons, etc. Home emphasis on television, e.g., parent-viewing, cable or HBO, number of sets, attempts to control child's viewing	Waiting ability Astronaut; delaying ability Motor restlessness during spontaneous waiting period Aggression School behavioral adjustment

represents the television environment. How much and what kind of television was watched as preschoolers and then annually in the early school years? How much emphasis did parents place on television? Was it important enough in the home to necessitate multiple sets or even a set in or near the child's room? Was it worth the investment of extra money for cable television and Home Box Office or a related service? Were efforts made to control and monitor what was watched and how often, or were the children in control of their own viewing? These variables formed a single factor labeled the *television environment*, but we looked at frequency and type of programming viewed by the child separately as well.

The right-hand column in Table 1 identifies the major dependent variables. Measures of reading comprehension, language usage and understanding, academic school adjustment, and beliefsystems made up the cognitive category. The child's ability to answer questions about the plot of an episode from a television series (not previously seen) or to identify and explain the purpose of a television commercial reflected knowledge about the medium. A group of measures of imagination forming a single factor included seeing human movement (Rorschach's *M* response) on inkblots, self-described imaginativeness, providing divergent, low-probability details beyond the usual features of the birthday party script employed in artificial intelligence research, and fantasy block play in a semi-standardized procedure. To estimate the restlessness or poor delaying capacity often attributed by critics of television to the pace of the medium, measures of ability to sit quietly as an astronaut might have to in a capsule or the amount of random and lively motor activity shown during a period of waiting were employed. Aggression was measured annually by parents' reports on the children's patterns of daily response in a variety of situations, and school behavior was also based on parents' accounts of school reports on their children.

Space does not permit a detailed account here of findings or procedures. For present purposes our results can be summarized as follows:

Reading comprehension. Our data suggested that the best prediction of good reading comprehension by the 2nd or 3rd grades emerges from a combination of (a) familial factors such as parental reliance on inductive rather than power-assertive discipline, the mother's own self-description as resourceful (e.g., curious, creative, imaginative), and a more orderly household routine with more hours of sleep and (b) television variables, specifically, fewer hours of television watching during the preschool years. This result is particularly clear for the brighter or more middle-class cohorts in our study; for lower socioeconomic status (SES) children better reading comprehension in the early school years is predicted by a combination of heavier preschool television watching and a mother who represents herself as curious and imaginative. These findings seem to conform to those reported by Morgan and Gross (1982) suggesting that television viewing may have a leveling effect or what Gerbner, Gross, Morgan, and Signorielli (1980b) term *cultivation*.

Comprehension of television plots and commercials. Here our data suggest that children whose families strongly emphasize television, whose mothers are less imaginative, and who have less regular bedtime routines and more power-assertive parental discipline perform more poorly in grasping plot details and understanding commercials. Thus sheer exposure to television may not benefit one in making sense of the medium.

Effectiveness of language usage. We found that more facile use of language was best predicted by less television viewing and less family emphasis on television, a father who self-describes as resourceful, and a more flexible daily household routine.

Beliefs. In support of earlier findings mainly with adults (Hawkins & Pingree, 1982), our data suggest that children who report a belief in an unfriendly or dangerous world are more likely to be in families emphasizing heavy television viewing, to have viewed more of the realistic action-adventure programming (e.g., police shows), and to have a father who does not emphasize resourcefulness. Exposure to more television and to a world depicted therein that emphasizes violence does appear linked to the child's beliefs about neighborhood dangers.

Imagination. The combined measures of imaginativeness in the 8-year-old are best predicted by less preschool television viewing, less recent viewing of realistic action-adventure programming, greater self-description as imaginative and creative by both parents, and less parental emphasis on power-assertive disciplinary methods. These data provide even clearer evidence than earlier research reviewed by D. Singer (1982a), which suggested an inverse relationship between heavy television viewing and self-generated imaginative capacities.

Waiting ability and motoric restlessness. In keeping with the anecdotal reports by teachers, our data suggest that heavy preschool television viewing, more recent viewing of violent programming, a father who does not value imagination, and minimal family involvement in varied cultural activities are the best predictors of an inability to sit quietly in the astronaut test or of greater spontaneous motor restlessness during a natural waiting situation.

Aggressive behavior. Our data continue to implicate early heavy television viewing as a preschooler or heavy viewing of action-adventure programming in that period as relevant to measures of aggressive behavior in the 2nd and 3rd grades. Parental emphasis on force in discipline and fewer hours of sleep for the child also contribute independently to the prediction that the child will be characterized as hitting other children with or without provocation.

Poor school adjustment. Essentially the same variables, heavy television viewing and parental power-assertive discipline, predicted more behavioral problems at school.

Summary. Our longitudinal data continue to suggest that the following combination of television and family variables puts a child at risk for problematic behavior by early elementary school age: (a) a home in which television viewing of an uncontrolled type is emphasized; (b) heavy viewing of television in the preschool years; (c) more recent heavy viewing of violent programming; (d) parents who themselves emphasize physical force as a means of discipline; and (e) parents whose self-descriptions or values do not stress imagination, curiosity, or creativity, traits that might offer alternatives to the direct imitation of the television content or to reliance on television as a major source of entertainment. The children in our study who were reared in such a combined family and television environment seem to be making less progress cognitively, to be more frightened or suspicious of the outside world, and to show less imagination and more restlessness and aggression as well as poor behavioral adjustment at school.

INTERVENTION EFFORTS: REACHING THE PARENTS

With at least circumstantial evidence of potentially noxious influences of television, as well as with indications from some of our *Mr. Rogers' Neighborhood* studies that useful programming for children is available, we have attempted studies designed to more directly influence parents to (a) monitor and significantly limit the heavy viewing patterns of their children and (b) provide alternative sources of educational entertainment that might moderate the effects of children's television viewing. In a rather carefully controlled study with various training groups of parents, we found that consciousness-raising sessions geared to having parents drastically reduce television viewing by their preschool children were relatively unsuccessful. In contrast, by providing parents with training skills for the children in imaginative play or in cognitive skills of various kinds, we were more successful and found that there was some decrease in television-viewing patterns, some increase in spontaneous language ability expressed by the children over a year, and other positive benefits for the children's social behavior (J. Singer & D. Singer, 1981). On the whole, however, we have found that direct interventions with parents built primarily around cutting down the viewing patterns of their children are largely unavailing. Instead we have been forced to recognize that the babysitting function of television is so attractive and pervasive for parents, both in middle and lower socioeconomic groups, that we have had to turn our attention in other directions to intervene. Our major current research efforts are focused on a more intensive look at how parents mediate the external world, filtering material for the cognitive capacities of children. To what extent do they include television in the process?

Brief mention can also be made of a type of intervention with parents whose impact, if potentially widespread, cannot be properly evaluated. We have attempted to present some of our experience on consciousness raising about the medium and about constructive uses of television to parents for developing imaginative and cognitive skills through a book (D. Singer, J. Singer, & Zuckerman, 1980) and through popular articles written in a variety of magazines. We have also produced monthly columns on how parents can relate to problems of violence or the prosocial uses of the medium in magazines like *Highlights* or *TV Guide*. In writing these materials we have tried within the constraints imposed by limited space and vocabulary range to refer regularly to research evidence. We believe that although this is a difficult task for the self-critical investigator, it is necessary for behavioral scientists because the field is otherwise open to self-styled experts or journalists who largely are presenting anecdotal experiences or essentially undocumented opinions.

DIRECT INTERVENTION WITH CHILDREN IN SCHOOL

In the study with preschoolers from lower SES backgrounds, we trained teachers at day-care centers to provide lessons designed to encourage imaginative, cognitive, and prosocial behavior, such as sharing, taking turns, or empathy, by the use of special game playing and also of brief segments taken from children's programming that highlighted these behaviors. Other control conditions were included to assess whether the inclusion of the television segments made a difference in the training of the children. We also hoped that including television segments would ultimately sensitize children to watch for such behaviors more extensively in their home television viewing. In general, our lessons were well-received by teachers and worked well within the school setting.

We do not, however, have adequate evidence that our efforts generalized to consistent home-viewing patterns of the children.

In a second study we developed special programming for cognitive skills using programming imported from Australia under circumstances in which children in the school watched for several weeks and in one condition had additional teacher follow-up on the viewing patterns. Particularly those children with the teacher follow-up showed gains in concept knowledge upon posttesting compared to control groups.

In still another study with 78 3rd graders and 93 5th graders, we employed special programming designed to see whether regular viewing in the schools of episodes from *Fables of the Green Forest* and *Swiss Family Robinson* would modify some of the moral reasoning and friendship and family attitudes displayed by the children (Singer, Singer, & Dodsworth-Rugani, Note 1). Our evidence suggested that although children did not exhibit a change in global stages of moral reasoning, those children who had exposure to appropriate material on television as well as teacher follow-up in these areas made significant gains in reducing selfish attitudes and in modifying some sex-stereotyped orientations. They showed gains in more positive concepts about family interaction patterns. Appropriate television materials may have a useful place when the teacher uses the material to exemplify certain constructive social attitudes.

It has become increasingly clear to us that children are growing up in a world of television that covers a whole array of attitudes and orientations without any explanation from parents or school about what that box is doing in the home. That is to say, we need more attention paid to the very medium of television as part of the learning process. In the study to be described next, we were concerned with teaching 3rd, 4th, and 5th grade children about television as part of their regular school curriculum (D. Singer, D. Zuckerman, & J. Singer, 1980). Approximately 230 middle-class children were involved in a study representing 82% of children enrolled in those grades in two Connecticut schools.

Lessons were designed to teach the children the different types of programs, to understand the difference between reality and fantasy on television, to understand special effects (e.g., how a superhero could jump to a building top), to learn about commercials, to learn how television works and how programs are produced, to understand how television influences our ideas and feelings, to understand how television presents violence, and to encourage children to control their viewing habits. Teachers were given training in use of lesson plans of approximately 40 minutes. There were, in addition, associated homework assignments involving writing and reading for the children. Special 10-minute videotapes were produced highlighting points made in each lesson. Lessons were designed to provide practice in language arts skills such as reading, punctuation, analogies, critical thinking, and summary skills.

Pretest and posttest measures focused on evaluating such types of learning as defining lesson-related vocabulary words such as audio, fiction, and props; identifying videotape examples of effects such as slow motion and close-up; understanding advertising in terms of special effects; interpreting messages; differentiating among real people, realistic characters, and fantasy characters; developing opinions regarding television programs and characters; developing attitudes toward reading; and assessing sex and race prejudices. Following eight lessons over a 2-month period we then compared scores on the series of tests and looked for generalizations from the material for experimental and control groups.

Results indicated that children in the experimental group showed a greater increase in knowledge than children in the control group on special effects, commercials, and advertising. The experimental group found out how television characters could disappear, how advertising was used to enhance products, who pays for television programs, and where to write letters regarding programs or commercials. They also learned vocabulary words relative to television and could identify camera techniques and effects such as dissolve, edit, zoom, and cut. Children also learned how to distinguish among real people, realistic people, and fantasy figures. Lessons were successful too in helping children understand that violence on fictional television programs is not real and that alternative methods for coping with conflicts were available in the real world. Homework assignments and classroom activities demonstrated the children's significant gains in learning about television. They wrote scripts, stories, and letters to celebrities; illustrated special effects; and used critical thinking in such exercises as categorizing and analogy usage. When the curriculum was then instituted for the control group, they showed comparable gains, and retesting also indicated maintenance of gains by the experimental group after several months.

By and large the students and teachers were enthusiastic about the curriculum and appeared to enjoy the television tie-in to the language arts curriculum. Of course, we cannot answer the longer-range question of whether these children will go on to be more discriminating viewers, but at least a beginning has been made by demonstrating that classroom lessons about television can be intriguing to students and also effective in producing a better understanding of the medium.

We have subsequently developed lesson plans suitable for kindergarten through 2nd grade, have recently completed evaluation of experiments in groups with this curriculum, and have completed further testing of the 3rd, 4th, and 5th grade curricula (Rapaczynski, Singer, & Singer, 1982). Our special curricula were then further tested in 10 school districts around the United States employing newly developed and more professional videotapes. Newspaper reports indicate that our television curriculum has been adopted in about 100 schools since then.

MEDDLING IN THE MEDIA: IMPLICATIONS FOR SOCIAL POLICY

As we have tried to suggest so far, the basic research on the nature of the television medium leads inevitably to some kinds of attempts at intervention with children, parents, and teachers. There is, however, a broader kind of intervention possible for psychologists. Major forces in the society have created antagonistic positions on the nature of the television medium. Keep in mind that in the United States television functions by a kind of giveaway of the air waves through licensing by the Federal Communications Commission to private companies. With the exception of public television, which has statistically only a slight influence on national viewing, the networks and other local stations are commercially run enterprises that are on the whole extremely profitable and among the most successful businesses in the united States. They exist primarily to communicate commercial advertising to the public. Programming must be geared wherever possible to attracting the broadest number of viewers, since pricing of advertising is chiefly determined by Nielsen ratings.

Although the Federal Communications Commission has required some degree of public service and news presentation from local stations, withdrawal of a license for noncompliance with some of these rather general rules is rare indeed over the almost 50 years of broadcasting history. So powerful is the network influence that when the Federal Trade Commission some years ago proposed a ban on advertising during children's programming, Congress responded to network pressure by withholding the Commission's funds and almost putting the entire FTC out of action. During the Carter administration the Federal Communications Commission, responding to consumer group pressure, raised the question as to whether local stations should be required to provide better quality programming for children as part of the licensing requirement. A special concern has been that programming should be geared to be age-specific, that is, that different programs are needed for children at preschool or elementary school ages and at the junior high school level and early adolescence.

At the Yale TV Center we have been involved at the social policy level on a number of fronts. One of us (JLS) has served as an advisor along with other psychologists in the drawing up of industry self-regulations concerning advertising for the Council of Better Business Bureau's Children's Review Unit, which oversees advertising in broadcast and print media. Our committee sought to apply the best available knowledge of child development research to helping advertisers make decisions about whether certain types of advertising would be fair or unfair to children. Although some of us might have reservations about any advertising at all to children, it is obvious that it is hopeless to attempt at this time to change that policy, and it is better to enforce adequate industry self-regulation.

Another of the authors (DGS) has served for several years on the National Council for Children and Television, a group that brings together representatives from government, the communications industry, foundations, major television advertising industry, education associations such as the PTA, and various consumer advocate groups as well as some researchers on television. This group has held numerous forums and attempts in various ways to reach public figures. Our role in connection with groups like this has been again to emphasize the importance of adequate data collection and research to resolve questionable issues. Especially valuable opportunities afforded by the National Council involve regular 2- or 3-day conferences with writers, producers, and industry executives. At these meetings it has been possible to point to specific ways in which developmental or television research findings can lead to modifications in format or plot content to enhance the constructive value of the medium for children of different ages as well as adults (D. Singer, 1982b).

Other examples of such policy-related consultations include serving on the National Institute of Mental Health's committee to update the research on television and behavior, which has recently produced a two-volume report (Pearl, Bouthilet, & Lazar, 1982); testifying before the Federal Communications Commission on cognitive development and the importance of age-specific programming for children; and meeting directly with specific industry executives, producers, and writers to discuss programming possibilities for children. In general, one of our concerns has been the necessity for prior evaluation of programming through more careful research directly with children. Producers often make judgments about what will entertain children or what will be educationally valuable for children based on adult reactions. Occassionally they may pull together a panel of children, but from what we can ascertain they often lack sophistication in asking appropriate questions or in observing spontaneous behavior of children in sufficiently objective fashion to permit adequate judgment. With such groups we have been advocating more extensive, careful, and controlled research as part of the overall process of program development.

A recent issue of great import for public policy has been the recognition highlighted in the Surgeon-General's report *Healthy People* that maladaptive health behavior may be partially fostered by television representations. Although advertising hard liquor is banned from television, it is not necessary for liquor companies to foster interest in drinking when all of the good guys or heroines in fictional stories spend so much time modeling that indulgence. Psychology has a significant role to play in educating television producers and writers about the possibilities for reducing gratuitous representations of unsafe behaviors or maladaptive health practices and for finding opportunities to model constructive health behavior (Rubinstein, 1982). Often gestures such as taking a drink or lighting a cigarette are employed by writers simply to give actors something to do with their hands or to manage scene transitions. We have met personally with individual producers such as Garry Marshall (*Happy Days; Laverne and Shirley*) and have also addressed groups of writers and producers under the aegis of the National Council for Children and Television to review possibilities for changing story content in a positive health-oriented direction without interfering with plot creativity. Why not have a character refuse an alcoholic drink and order plain soda or juice instead, as many people now do in the real world? It has been gratifying that following a meeting on health issues and the media at the National Academy of Medicine, the appearance of the NIMH report, and a series of individual efforts of researchers in contacts with industry representatives, some change is evident. Some commercials are now appearing urging viewers to buckle up; fictional heroes are refusing drinks on occasion; and in a recent episode of Hill Street Blues, Captain Furillo took severe offense at the cigar smoking of an adjoining diner in a restaurant scene.

In conclusion, we can see that taking a hard look at the television medium leads inevitably to a full range of psychological challenges. We confront the possibility of basic studies on how the omnipresence of television has influenced the nature of our cognitive functioning. We need more understanding of its effects on our fears and worries, our perception of the outside world and, especially for children, the direct effect on their spontaneous behavior of the particular heavy load of certain kinds of antisocial content in the programming. We must recognize constructive possibilities of the medium and accept the reality that there is unlikely to be a mass movement toward turning off the set by parents. Instead, if anything, with increased use of cable television and videodisc or home video recording, we are likely to see more emphasis on this type of medium as a part of daily life. Given this reality, psychologists are going to have to make even more serious attempts to study various effects of the types of programming, to participate actively in commissions and groups examining such influences, and perhaps even to take somewhat stronger advocacy stands once research evidence points in fairly conclusive directions.

REFERENCE NOTE

1. Singer, D., Singer, J., & Dodsworth-Rugani, K. (1979). Fables of the Green Forest *and* Swiss Family Robinson: *An experimental evaluation of their educational and prosocial potential.* (Report to the Teleprompter Corporation.) Unpublished manuscript, Yale University. (Available from the authors.)

REFERENCES

Bryant, J., & Anderson, D. R. (1983). *Children's understanding of television: Research on attention and comprehension.* New York: Academic Press.

Collins, W. A. (1982). Cognitive processing in television viewing. In D. Pearl, L. Bouthilet, & J. Lazar (Eds.), *Television and behavior: Ten years of scientific progress and implications for the eighties.* Washington, D.C.: U.S. Government Printing Office.

Csikszentmihalyi, M., & Kubey, R. (1981). Television and the rest of life: A systematic comparison of subjective experience. *Public Opinion Quarterly,* 45:317–328.

Eron, L. D. (1982). Parent-child interaction, television violence, and aggression of children. *American Psychologist,* 37:197–511.

Gerbner, G., Gross, L., Morgan, M., & Signorielli, N. (1980). The "mainstreaming" of America: Violence profile. No. 11. *Journal of Communications,* 30:10–29.(a)

Gerbner, G., Gross, L., Morgan, M., & Signorielli, N. (1980). Some additional comments on cultivation analysis. *Public Opinion Quarterly,* 44:408–411.(b)

Hawkins, R. P., & Pingree, S. (1982). Television's influence on social reality. In D. Pearl, L. Bouthilet, & J. Lazar (Eds.). *Television and behavior: Ten years of scientific progress and implications for the eighties* (Vol. 2). Washington, D.C.: U.S. Government Printing Office.

Hearold, S. L. (1979). *Meta-analysis of the effects of television on social behavior.* Unpublished doctoral dissertation, University of Colorado.

Huesmann, L. R. (1982). Television violence and aggressive behavior. In D. Pearl, L. Bouthilet, & J. Lazar (Eds.), *Television and behavior: Ten years of scientific progress and implications for the eighties* (Vol. 2). Washington, D.C.: U.S. Government Printing Office.

McIlwraith, R., & Schallow, J. (1983). Adult fantasy life and patterns of media use. *Journal of Communications*, 33:78–91.

McIlwraith, R., & Schallow, J. (in press). Television viewing and styles of children's fantasy. *Imagination, Cognition and Personality*.

Milavsky, J. R., Kessler, R., Stipp, H., & Rubens, W. S. (1982). Television and aggression: Results of a panel study. In D. Pearl, L. Bouthilet, & J. Lazar (Eds.), *Television and behavior: Ten years of scientific progress and implications for the eighties* (Vol. 2), Washington, D.C.: U.S. Government Printing Office.

Morgan, M., & Gross, L. (1982). Television and educational achievement. In D. Pearl, L. Bouthilet, & J. Lazar (Eds.), *Television and behavior: Ten years of scientific progress and implications for the eighties* (Vol. 2). Washington, D.C.: U.S. Government Printing Office.

Pearl, D. Bouthilet, L., & Lazar, J. (Eds.). (1982). *Television and behavior: Ten years of scientific progress and implications for the eighties* (Vols. 1 & 2). Washington, D.C.: U.S. Government Printing Office.

Rapaczynski, W., Singer, D. G., & Singer, J. L. (1982). Teaching television: A curriculum for young children. *Journal of Communications*, 32:46–55.

Rubinstein, E. A. (1983). Television and behavior: Conclusions of the 1982 NIMH report and their policy implications. *American Psychologist*, 38:820–825.

Salomon, G. (1981). Introducing AIME: The assessment of children's mental involvement with television. In H. Gardner & H. Kelly (Eds.), *Children and the worlds of television*. San Francisco: Jossey-Bass.

Singer, D. G. (1982). Television and the developing imagination of the child. In D. Pearl, L. Bouthilet, & J. Lazar (Eds.), *Television and behavior: Ten years of scientific progress and implications for the eighties* (Vol. 2). Washington, D.C.: U.S. Government Publishing Office. (a)

Singer, D. G. (1982). The research connection. *Television and Children*, 5:25–35. (b)

Singer, D. G., & Revenson, T. (1978). *A Piaget primer: How a child thinks*. New York: International Universities Press and New American Library.

Singer, D. G., & Singer, J. L. (1980). Television viewing and aggressive behavior in preschool children: A field study. *Annals of the New York Academy of Science*, 347:289–303.

Singer, D. G., & Singer, J. L. (1981). Television and the developing imagination of the child. *Journal of Broadcasting*, 41:373–387.

Singer, D. G., & Singer, J. L. (1982). *Getting involved: Your child and TV. A Head Start initiative in collaboration with elementary schools*. Belmont, Mass.: Contract Research Corporation.

Singer, D. G., Singer, J. L., & Zuckerman, D. (1980). *Teaching television: How to use television to your child's advantage*. New York: Dial.

Singer, D. G., Singer, J. L., & Zuckerman, D. (1981). *Getting the most out of television*. Chicago, Ill.: Good Year Books, Scott, Foresman.

Singer, D. G., Zuckerman, D., & Singer, J. L. (1980). Helping elementary school children learn about TV. *Journal of Communications*, 30:84–93.

Singer, J. L. (1973). *The child's world of make-believe: Experimental studies of imaginative play*. New York: Academic Press.

Singer, J. L. (1980). The powers and limitations of television: A cognitive-affective analysis. In P. Tannenbaum (Ed.), *The entertainment function of television*. Hillsdale, N.J.: Erlbaum.

Singer, J. L., & Singer, D. G. (1976). Fostering creativity in children: Can TV stimulate imaginative play? *Journal of Communications*, 26:74–80.

Singer, J. L., & Singer, D. G. (1981). *Television, imagination and aggression: A study of pres-*

choolers. Hillsdale, N.J.: Erlbaum.

Singer, J. L., & Singer, D. G. (1983). Implications of childhood televsion viewing for cognition, imagination and emotion. In J. Bryant & D. R. Anderson (Eds.), *Children's understanding of television: Research on attention and comprehension*. New York: Academic Press.

Tower, R. B. (1980). Parents self-concepts and preschool children's behaviors. *Journal of Personality and Social Psychology*, 39:710–718.

Tower, R. B., Singer, D. G., Singer, J. L., & Biggs, A. (1979). Differential effects of television programming on preschoolers' cognition, imagination and social play. *American Journal of Orthopsychiatry*, 49:265–281.

Wright, J., & Huston, A. (1983). A matter of form: Potentials of television for young viewers. *American Psychologist*, 38:835–843.

Zuckerman, D., Singer, D. G., & Singer, J. L. (1980). Television viewing, children's reading and related school behavior. *Journal of Communications*, 30:166–174.